REEFER WELLNESS

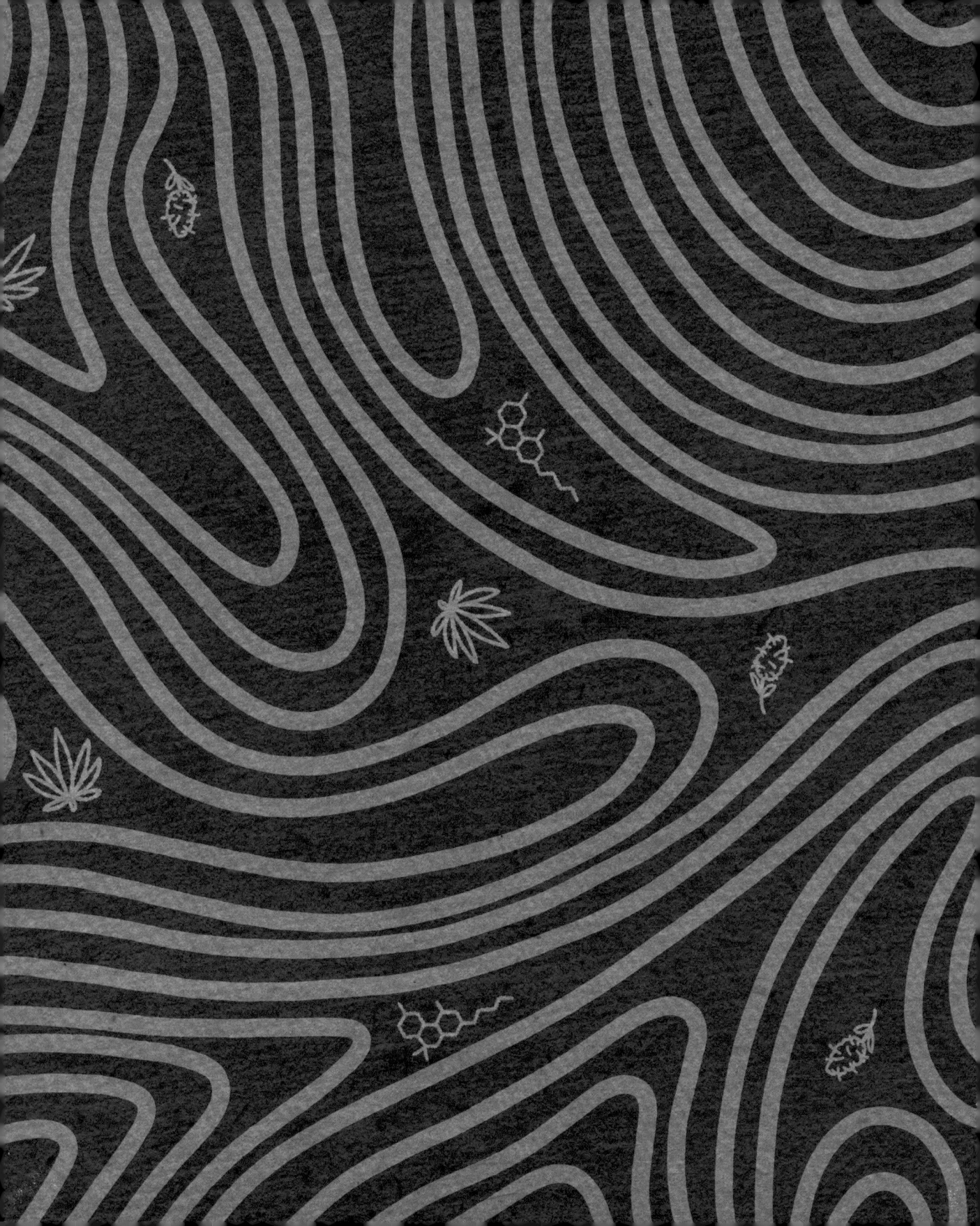

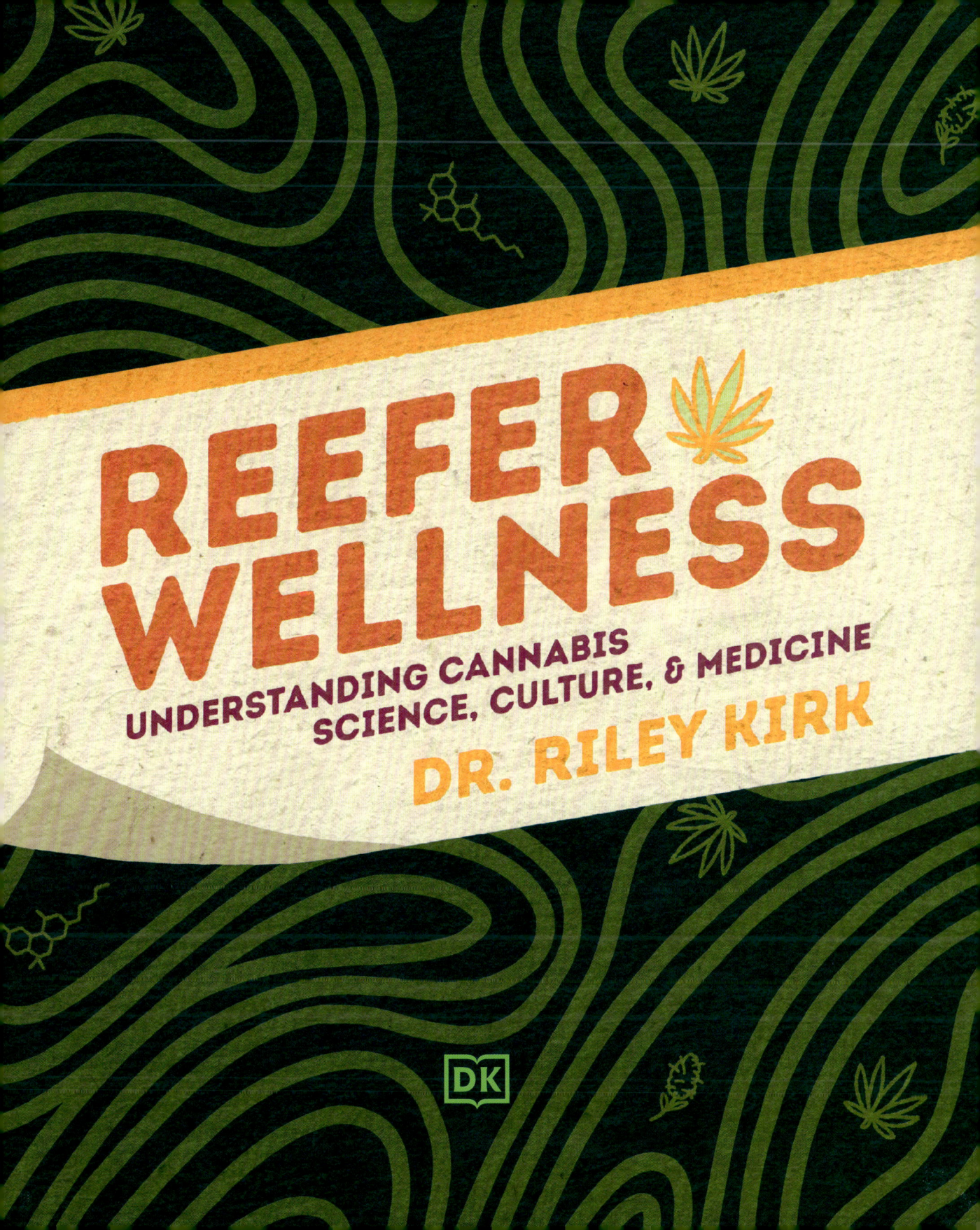

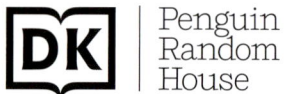

Publisher Mike Sanders
Art & Design Director William Thomas
Editorial Director Ann Barton
Senior Editor Molly Ahuja
Designer Lindsay Dobbs
Illustrator Mallory Heyer
Copy Editor Claire Safran
Proofreaders Megan Douglass and Christina Guthrie
Indexer Beverlee Day

First American Edition, 2025
Published in the United States by DK Publishing
1745 Broadway, 20th Floor, New York, NY 10019

The authorized representative in the EEA is Dorling Kindersley
Verlag GmbH. Arnulfstr. 124, 80636 Munich, Germany

A catalog record for this book
is available from the Library of Congress.
ISBN 978-0-5938-4715-2

DK books are available at special discounts when purchased
in bulk for sales promotions, premiums, fund-raising, or
educational use. For details, contact SpecialSales@dk.com

Printed and bound in China

www.dk.com

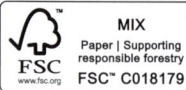

THIS BOOK IS DEDICATED TO THOSE WHO HAVE EMBRACED THIS MEDICINE LONG BEFORE SCIENCE CONFIRMED ITS VALUE—TO THOSE WHO LISTENED TO THEIR BODIES AND PLACED THEIR TRUST IN NATURE, EVEN WHEN DOING SO WAS DEEMED UNLAWFUL.

TO THE MILLIONS OF PEOPLE WHO HAVE SERVED TIME AND WHO ARE STILL INCARCERATED FOR GROWING, SMUGGLING, SELLING, OR CONSUMING THIS PLANT. TO THOSE WHO ARE TARGETED AND DISCRIMINATED AGAINST EVERY SINGLE DAY FOR LOOKING, SMELLING, OR ACTING LIKE A STONER.

THIS BOOK IS DEDICATED TO THE AMAZING ADVOCATES IN OUR COMMUNITY WHO HAVE SPENT THEIR ENTIRE LIVES PUSHING TO INCREASE ACCESS TO THIS PLANT, AND CONTINUE TO SHOW UP EVERY SINGLE DAY.

I HOPE THE WORDS IN THIS BOOK CAN HELP US ALL COMMUNICATE OUR PASSION AND LOVE FOR THE PLANT, AND HELP REPRESENT AND PROTECT OUR COMMUNITY IN FUTURE ENDEAVORS.

CONTENTS

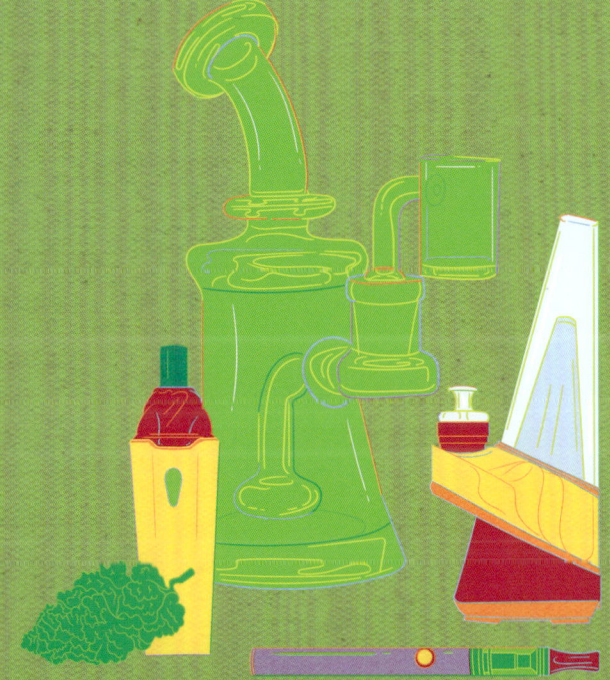

WELCOME!

This book is intended to share fundamental information about the human body and cannabis. For any significant changes to your health and wellness routine, especially those involving medications, always consult with a qualified healthcare professional.

The book that you are holding in your hands represents progress and a new era in cannabis culture—turning the notion of propaganda-ridden "Reefer Madness" upside down as more states legalize the plant, as scientists are freer to study it, and as more and more people turn to it for medicinal and adult use.

Instead of creating hysteria about cannabis, this book is designed to educate you about this complex and unique plant so that you can be comfortable and confident on your own cannabis journey; no matter what point you have reached in it.

I would not have been able to write this book, nor complete my Ph.D. dissertation without the help and brain expanding properties of cannabis. This plant has helped me through loss and hardship, laughs and joy, and provided consistency, reassurance, and spiritual guidance throughout my life. Although the title of this book is a play on the anti-cannabis propaganda film, the goal of it is to reverse some of the propaganda with scientific facts and patient stories. It is time we reclaim the narrative around cannabis from the perspective of the community who loves it.

In 1937, the United States enacted the Marijuana Tax Act, effectively making cannabis illegal. To gain public support, the government launched a major media campaign, including films like *Reefer Madness (1936)*, which portrayed marijuana users as violent and immoral. Harry Anslinger further fueled the fear, declaring marijuana as an addictive drug leading to insanity, criminality, and death.

If you have not seen the movie, it makes for a fun evening—especially with cannabis in the mix! If you have seen it, you will know that the opening of the movie contains a sort of foreword, filled with propaganda. I could not help but want to edit it to reflect what my goals are in this book and to showcase how far we have come as a society to destigmatize and understand cannabis and its many uses.

Mad love,
Dr. Riley Kirk

THE BOOK YOU ARE ABOUT TO READ MAY EDUCATE YOU.

IT WOULD NOT BE POSSIBLE OTHERWISE TO SUFFICIENTLY SHARE THE POWER OF THE COMPLEX MEDICINAL PLANT THAT IS HELPING PEOPLE ALL OVER THE WORLD.

CANNABIS IS THAT PLANT – A COMPLEX AND NUANCED HERB – A REAL BENEFIT TO THE PUBLIC.

THE FIRST EFFECT IS OFTEN A CALM, RELAXING FEELING THAT SOMETIMES CAUSES LAUGHTER. THEN COMES INCREASED INSPIRATION AND PATIENCE. FOCUS MAY RETURN, PRODUCTIVITY MAY SURGE. CREATIVE IDEAS MAY COME NEXT, ALLOWING ONE TO PRODUCE BEAUTIFUL ART.

FOLLOWED BY HEIGHTENED SENSITIVITY, THE TOTAL ABILITY TO BE IN THE MOMENT, THE GAINING OF POWER TO GET ALONG WITH OTHERS LEADING TO ACTS OF PEACE AND UNDERSTANDING – ENDING OFTEN WITH A GOOD NIGHT'S SLEEP.

IN SHARING THE SCIENCE BEHIND THIS TRULY INCREDIBLE AND POWERFUL PLANT, NO ATTEMPT WAS MADE TO EQUIVOCATE.

THE CONTENTS – RESEARCHED, WRITTEN, AND EDITED FOR THIS BOOK – ARE BASED ON SCIENTIFIC FACTS AND STUDIES THAT SHOWCASE THE MANY BENEFITS OF THE PLANT.

IF THE ABUNDANCE OF RESEARCH AND PERSONAL STORIES HELPS TO TAKE THE STIGMA AWAY FROM USING CANNABIS AND ALLOWS YOU TO BEGIN OR CONTINUE YOUR OWN HEALING JOURNEY WITH THE PLANT, THEN THIS BOOK WILL HAVE SUCCEEDED IN ITS GOAL TO EDUCATE AND EMPOWER.

BECAUSE AS CANNABIS LEGALIZATION BECOMES MORE WIDESPREAD AND AS RESEARCH INTO THIS COMPLEX, MIRACULOUS PLANT GROWS, PEOPLE EVERYWHERE WILL BE ABLE TO MAKE THEIR OWN EDUCATED DECISION ON HOW CANNABIS MAY BENEFIT THEM.

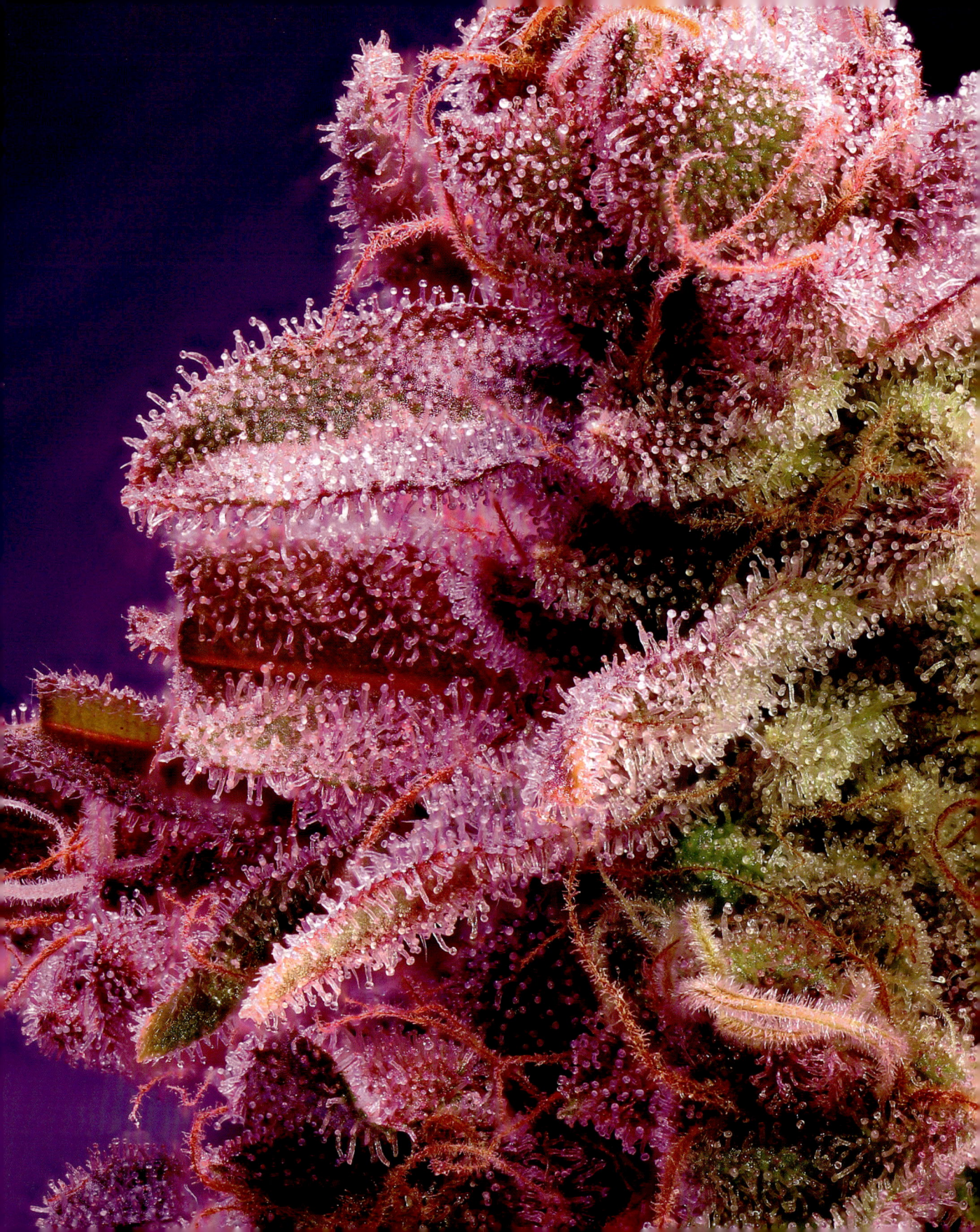

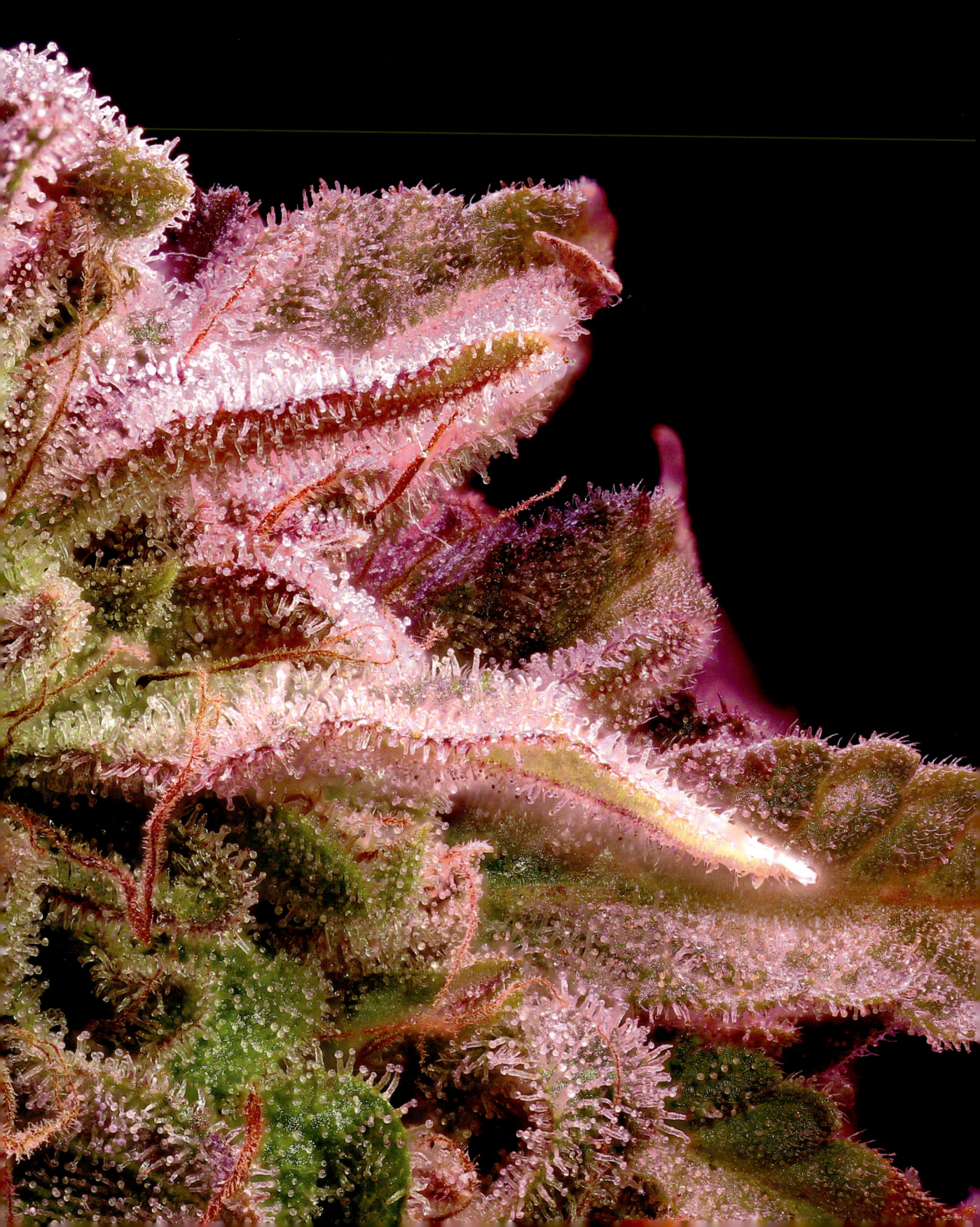

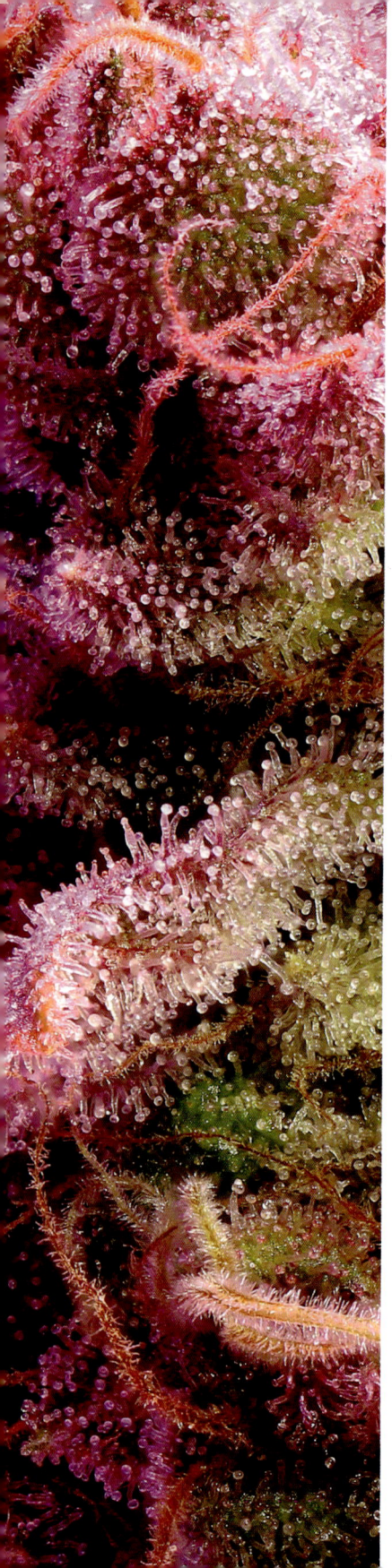

INTRODUCTION

I grew up absolutely fascinated with the natural world, as many children do—but the curiosity never went away for me. As my brain grew and developed, I started to seek more information on the natural substances that we use in our everyday lives, from caffeine and nicotine to ashwagandha, kratom, and kava. It was clear people were taking these substances for their medicinal benefits, or sometimes recreationally, but the more I tried to read up on how they were doing it, the more confused I got. I became a sponge, learning about the traditional practices of herbalists, reading books on natural products, foraging for diverse plants and fungi, growing my own plants, and eventually crafting my own extractions and formulations as well. However, I still struggled to fully understand the scientific papers that were being published on these plants. In journals like *Phytochemistry* or *The Journal of Natural Products*, it seemed to me that the science was written in a language I couldn't understand, and my brain needed to put together the pieces of what I was learning.

Part of what kept my brain curious and outright obsessed with the natural world was cannabis. I am a very nonlinear thinker, and I believe that is due in part to constantly exercising my brain to think beyond the obvious. I found that my brain responded very well to cannabis at a young age when I started using it in high school, and from then I never really looked back. Now as an educated consumer I realize that part of the reason my brain reacted so positively to cannabis is because I have a very hyperactive brain. Hyperactive not only in my thoughts and feelings, but also hyperactive in the form of experiencing seizures from brain hyperactivity when I was young. Looking back, I realize that since starting to be a regular cannabis consumer, my brain has felt at ease, and I have not experienced a seizure as an adult. Later, I learned about the mechanism cannabis works in the brain, and had my own life experiences validated by the scientific literature.

While I always enjoyed consuming cannabis and learning about it, when I started on my journey with it I never thought it would lead to a career. I always assumed I'd be a scientist by trade and a stoner in my off time, because I didn't know you could study cannabis. It was never presented to me in a professional or scientific manner, so I just assumed nobody was doing research on it.

What opened my world was learning about a field of science called pharmacognosy (*pharma-caug-na-see*). This is the science of natural products, the science of natural discoveries, the science of the chemistry of nature—and my obsession. When I learned about this field of study, I pursued it headfirst without looking back. I engulfed myself in research and gave 100% of my time and effort to studying how nature produced such amazing molecules.

What I quickly learned while studying natural products is that we have no shortage of information on cannabis, kratom, kava, echinacea, or any of these other traditionally used herbs. The issue is that we have no mechanism for getting information from the scientific studies to the people actually using the products—**what we were missing was communication.** We weren't missing just the act of discussing the scientific literature, but also the nuance of what it means in the context of life and how we can combine our lived experience as humans with the scientific literature to get a more nuanced look at these medicines.

At the start of the coronavirus pandemic in 2020, I was a scientist who was stuck at home for the first time ever. During this time, much of the world was experiencing increased isolation, depression, anxiety, fear, and loss of community, and many people started to explore cannabis as a result. A new app was starting to take over the world: it was called TikTok. In any other universe I probably would never have started to make videos, but I was home, and I was bored, and I missed teaching students about cannabis and chemistry. I was writing my dissertation at the time and wanted to share some information I knew about cannabis to help others learn about the science behind this plant. The first video I made blew up, then the second, then the third, and my channel quickly grew to more than 400,000 followers. I had no idea so many people wanted to nerd out about the chemistry and pharmacology of cannabis.

Now looking back, years after posting my first video on the internet, I understand a lot better why that content was getting liked and shared so rapidly. The science of cannabis has almost never been presented in a positive and professional way, especially on social media. There was mainly fearmongering especially about daily consumption, or people trying to take a one-gram dab, or smoke out of a fruit. We were missing a focus on the medicinal aspect, on normalization, destigmatization, and most of all, a tool for communicating to parents, physicians, or friends who may not understand why some people gravitate so strongly to this plant. Giving people the information and tools to effectively communicate and advocate for this plant has been the most fulfilling part of my job and the reason I continue to make content. Despite the intense restrictions put on by social media companies, the information persists, and people continue to find value in shared and accessible education around cannabis.

Through building this online community I have learned so much more about the plant and the human brain than I could ever imagine. Some of these comments, stories, emails, etc., have turned into full blown research projects that we now take on

through the cannabis research and education nonprofit that I co-founded called the Network of Applied Pharmacognosy.

From being part of the online and in-person cannabis community I've learned from myself and the people around me that health and well-being is an extremely nonlinear and personalized journey. A single plant can't fix all your problems, but the cannabis plant specifically does have a unique ability to bring us together, help us find similarities, be more open, have more fun, and establish community.

Something that I have noticed in my own life and in many other chronic cannabis users is that cannabis can be a guiding force. It can help you find friends, vet genuine connections, and discover your inner self. Although I haven't always known what path life was going to take me down, I have faith that if I continue to follow what my gut and brain say is good for me, and have faith in the unknown, it will all work out eventually. There are still unknowns in cannabis–we haven't characterized every molecule or every pathway in which it works in the body–but it works, and to get the full benefit of this medicine you must have faith in the unknown. Cannabis has helped me lead a life where I am able to be my true authentic self, and I've seen this plant transform people's lives including my own.

There is not a product type or consumption method that I will discuss in this book that I haven't tried myself. I've read the research, tried the products, overdone it, underdone it, and learned from my experiences over the past decade and a half as a cannabis consumer.

This book pairs my experience with current scientific literature to give you a holistic view of cannabis. It's not going to tell you which way to consume, when to take a hit, or what weed to buy, but it's going to help guide you toward making the right decision for yourself.

Over the past fifty years, the profound and extensive medicinal benefits of cannabis have been well studied and recorded. I distinctly remember a man once asking me, *"There's all these medicinal plants, what makes cannabis so special?"* My answer was short: *"Because it acts on our endocannabinoid system which controls everything in our body."*

I don't want this book to feel like a biology textbook, and you may already be rolling your eyes at the term "endocannabinoid system (ECS)," but hear me out. This system exists IN YOUR BODY. So, learning how to use and respect this plant medicine–which also involves learning about both the ECS and the art of listening to your body–can help you lessen pain, calm your brain, fall asleep, enjoy your favorite foods, prevent mood swings, and so much more!

Cannabis is an incredibly powerful medicine. There are hundreds of compounds in the plant–many with individually robust medicinal properties–and when these molecules are combined, the potential is expansive. **When cannabis is consumed at the right dose, with intention and education, it is far safer and far more efficacious than any other medicine. However, for the same reason that cannabis is such a powerful medicine, failing to treat it with respect can lead to a negative experience and negative relationship with the plant.**

The safety profile of cannabis is exceedingly better than many commonly used substances like nicotine, alcohol, and even some pharmaceutical medications. Cannabis opens the mind and often allows us to be more in touch with our feelings and emotions. Many of its drawbacks come when inexperienced users take the wrong dose of a product and have an unpleasant mental experience. Unfortunately, not everyone is in a good place to have their mind opened with cannabis and should consider seeking other forms of mental health treatment to address any underlying issues before partaking in cannabis or psychedelic medicines.

There are MANY variables that go into consuming cannabis that influence how someone is going to feel, and we can curate that. Cannabis is unlike pharmaceutical medicine; it is a living natural product. This book is your guide through this personal medicine, to explore and learn about the different ways to heal with this plant. **Cannabis is not the easy button. It is not a one-size-fits-all solution and shouldn't be treated like one. To really benefit from this medicine, you need to take the time to learn about both the plant and your self**.

You may have been exposed to a significant amount of misinformation about cannabis from the government, academia, your parents, the news, or many other sources. Propaganda tried to tell us that cannabis was going to make us stupid and lazy dysfunctioning members of society. What we now know is that cannabis is integrated into all social groups; CEOs, physicians, lawyers, and every other profession under the sun enjoys cannabis. The name of this book is *Reefer Wellness* to try to reverse some of the insane propaganda from the Reefer Madness era, with science, facts, and patient stories. I encourage you to have an open mind while you're listening to or reading this book. This book was written in 2023-2024. Currently, cannabis is still federally considered a schedule 1 drug–a category it shares with heroin. Yet, 40 states and the District of Columbia permit medical cannabis. 24 states and the District of Columbia have approved recreational, or adult use of cannabis. The FDA has also approved two drugs derived from cannabis, while the government owns patents such as No. 6,630,507 for the use of cannabis to treat neuroinflammation. Although there are clear and undisputed medicinal benefits, what is still contested is who gets to profit from them.

There are thousands of peer-reviewed literature studies stating the various medicinal benefits of cannabis, and more are published every year as our scientific instruments advance. Scientific studies validate that cannabis use leads to decreases in opiates, alcohol, and pharmaceutical medications. Beyond medicinal benefits, cannabis is an excellent source of happiness and connection to the natural world, both of which society is in dire need of today. The purpose of this book is to combine the scientific literature surrounding cannabis with lived experience and knowledge from regular cannabis consumers– including myself and other members of this community.

Cannabis has profound healing abilities–emotionally, spiritually, and physically. To truly utilize this plant, it is imperative to respect it. We must respect and acknowledge the people who have been incarcerated for growing and dispensing it despite prohibition, respect and listen to our bodies, and respect the hundreds of molecules that are found in this plant. The first step to respecting cannabis is learning about it, and this book can help in that journey.

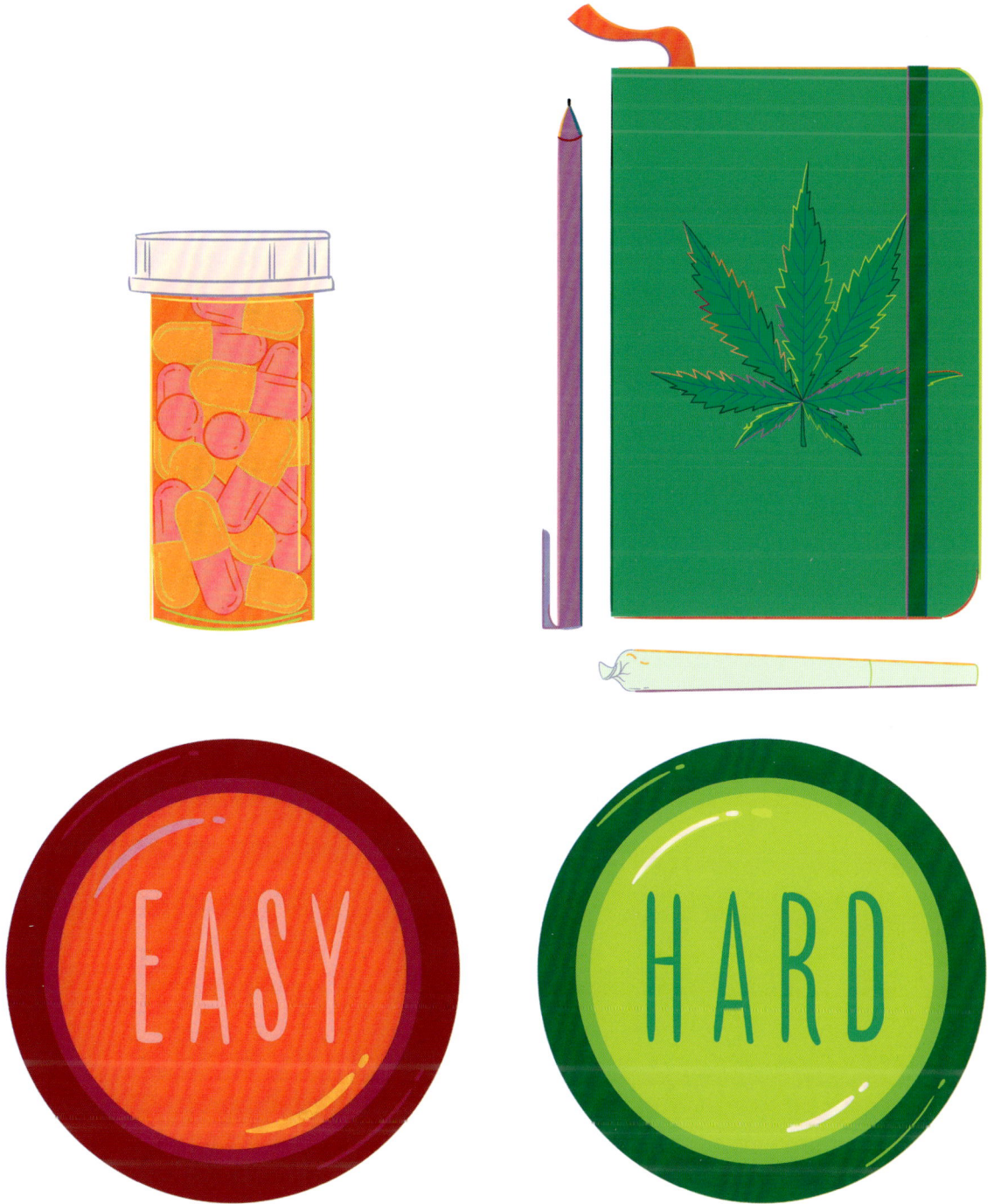

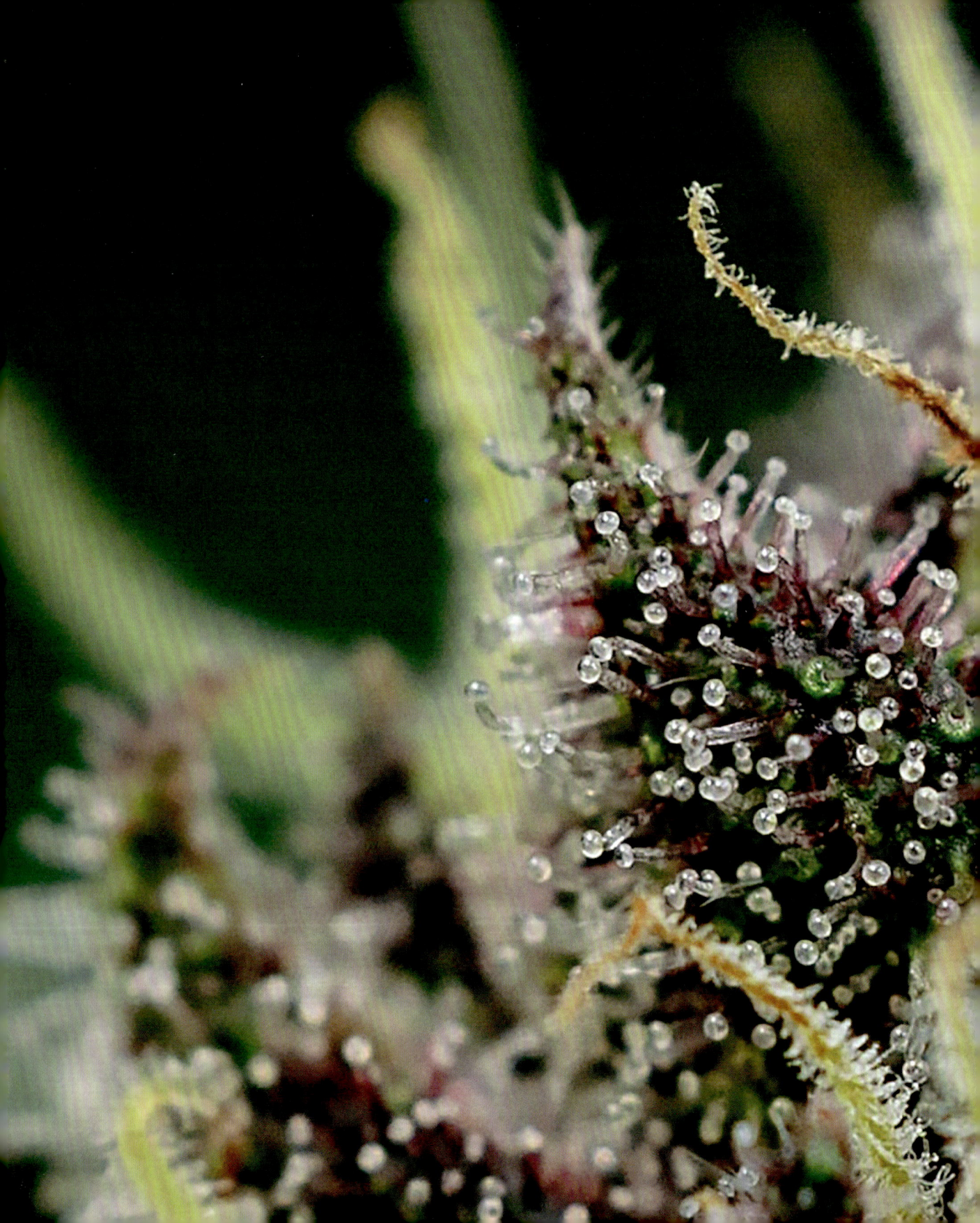

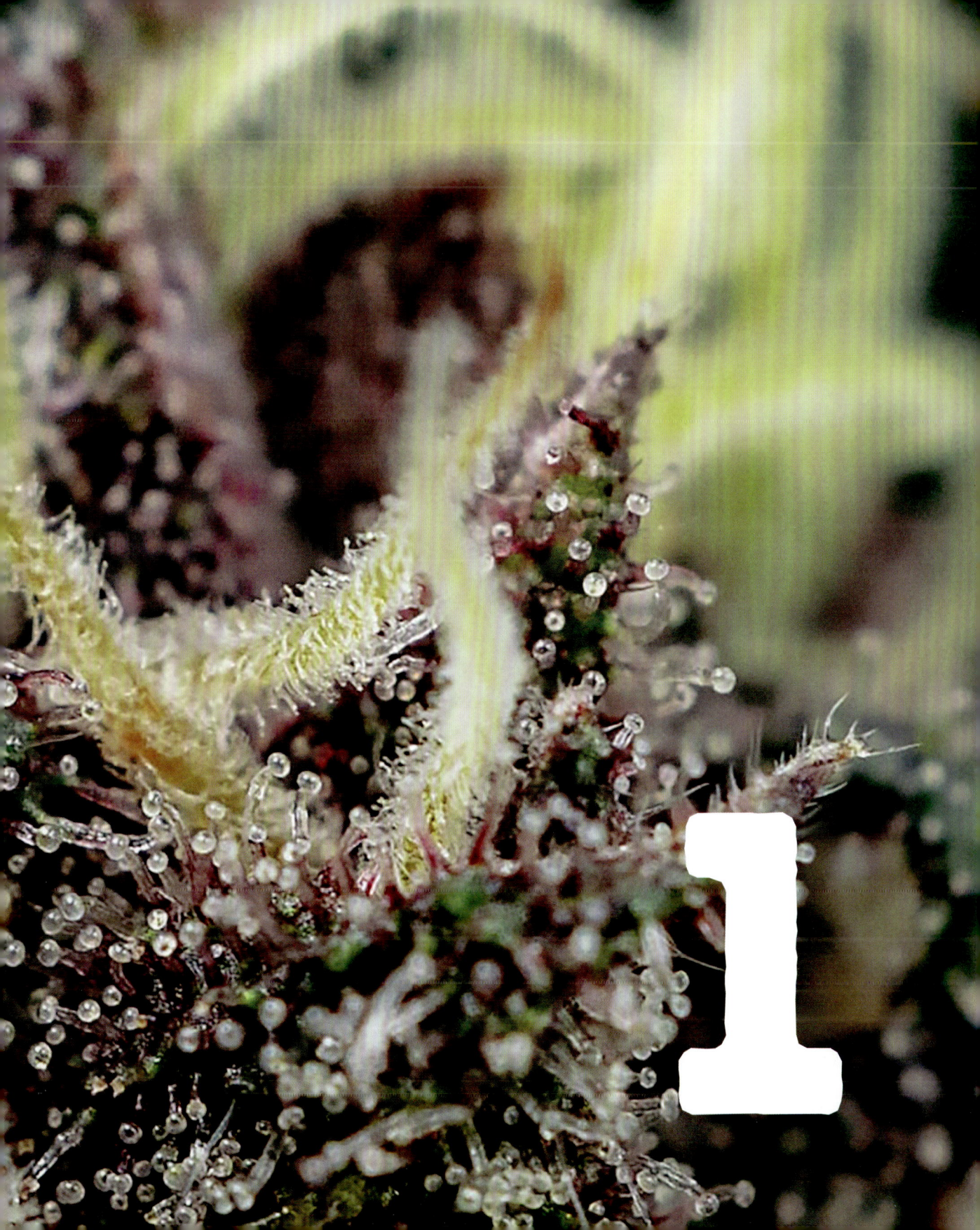

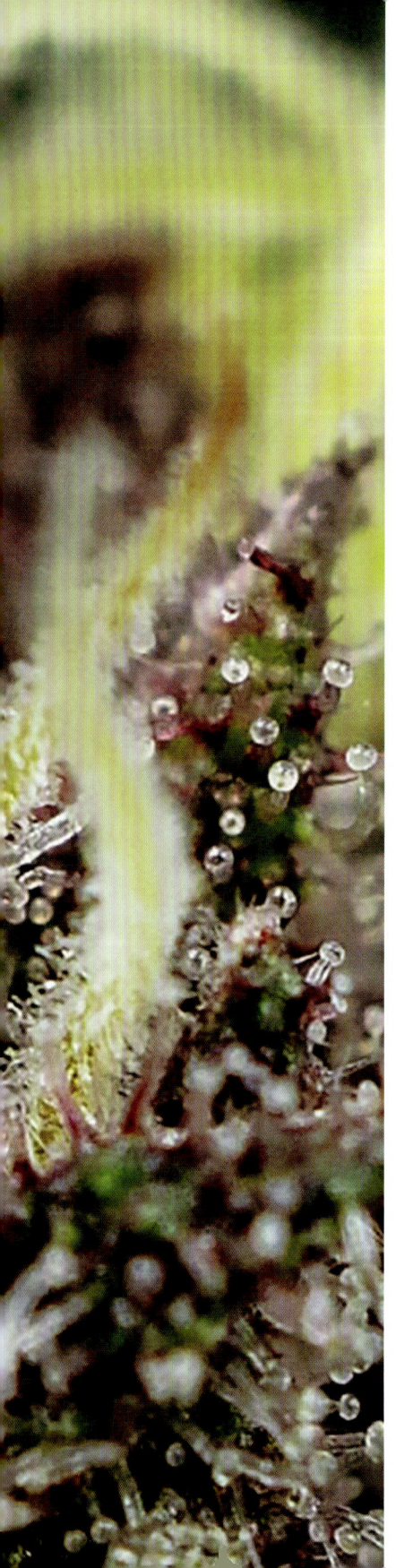

NATURE & DRUGS

Picture a plant in your head—it can be a cannabis plant, a fig tree, a cactus, a dandelion, or whatever your mind wants to produce at this moment. Now picture that plant being eaten by a bug or by a plant-eating animal. How does the plant react? It often doesn't... or at least, not in a way that you can see from the naked eye.

Plants are vulnerable and nature is ruthless, so how do they protect themselves?

A plant defends itself from the environment mainly by producing drug-like molecules. Plants don't have legs to run away, swords to fight off enemies, or voices to scream for help, so they use chemical warfare to protect themselves. For example, if a plant senses an animal trying to eat it, it could protect itself by producing bitter compounds so it tastes bad or a substance that may hurt or kill the animal trying to eat it.

Plants also produce additional chemistry to protect themselves from the intense rays of the sun, prevent bacterial or fungal growth in their tissues, or encourage pollinators to stop by for a visit.

Interestingly, many of these molecules are designed by the plant to act on insects because insects are the biggest threat to the plant's health—but insects are also how the majority of plants spread their pollen and reproduce. The relationship between insects and plants has been developed through millions of years of coevolution. Many of the specialized molecules produced by plants are designed to interact with insect brains to kill them, deter them, incapacitate them, or attract them. But it turns out... the human brain isn't all that different from insects, and we too can feel the effects from these molecules, but in different ways.

Did you just read "The human brain isn't all that different from insects" and almost shut this book in disagreement? If so, allow me to elaborate.

Just like how plants produce all these crazy molecules to protect themselves or signal that they are in danger, our own bodies also produce molecules. These signaling molecules in our brain, often called neurotransmitters or hormones, are responsible for telling us when we're hungry, sad, happy, scared, anxious, etc. We would not be able to think, feel emotions, or really do anything without these signals communicating within our brains. These systems are so important to our survival that almost every animal contains similar systems to keep them alive, and plants have figured this out.

Brains, whether it is an insect brain, a deer brain, or a human brain, operate relatively similarly and therefore a molecule that is engineered by a plant to kill an insect will not kill us often, but it will likely still have some profound activity on our brains—sometimes in good ways, other times in bad ways.

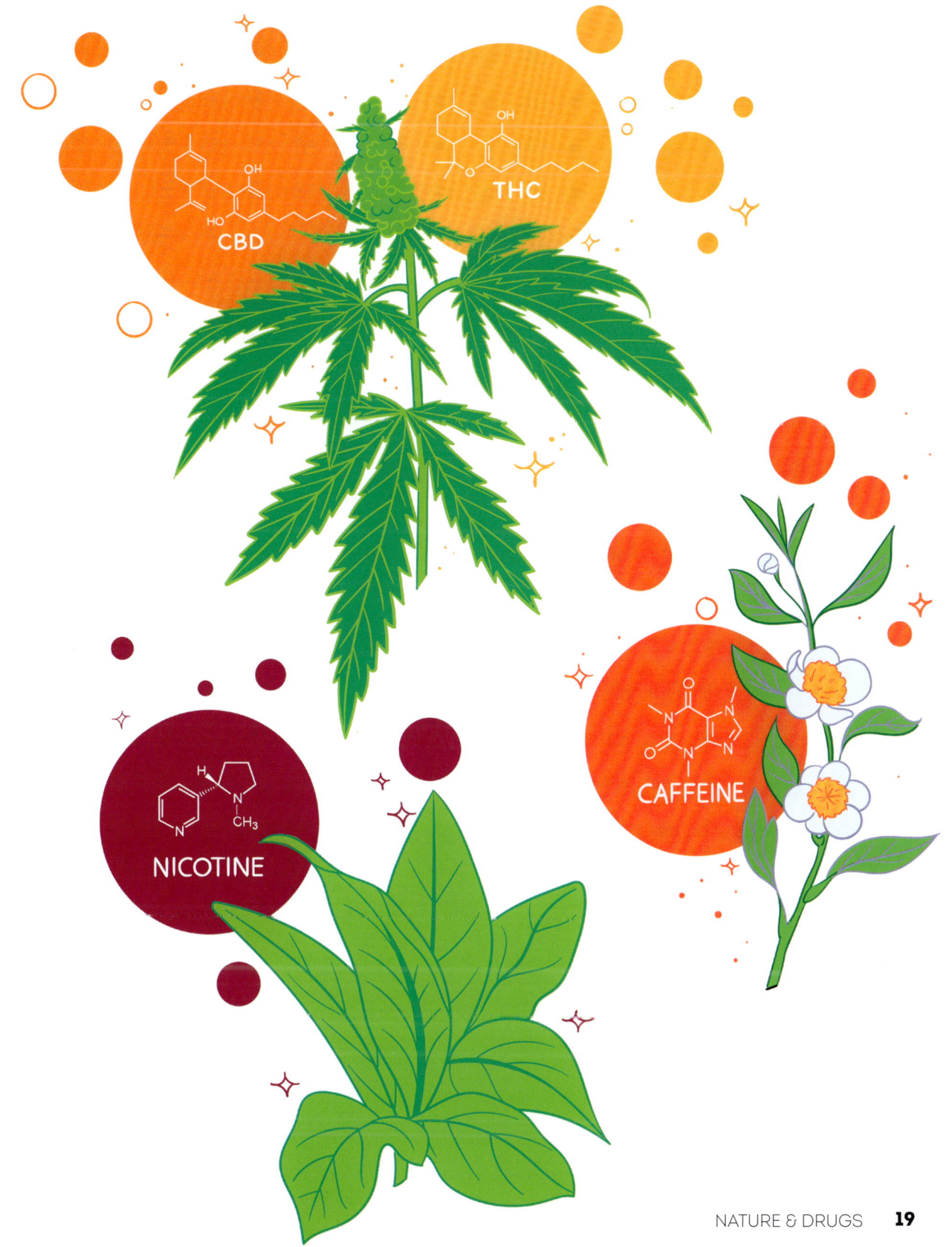

CBD

THC

NICOTINE

CAFFEINE

NATURE IS THE BEST ORGANIC CHEMIST IN THE WORLD

Drugs[1] are all around us. The caffeine we drink in our coffee, the cough medicine we take, and even herbal products like chamomile can all be thought of as drugs. The word drug often has a very intense or even bad connotation. According to the FDA, *"A drug is defined as: A substance recognized by an official pharmacopeia or formulary. A substance intended for use in the diagnosis, cure, mitigation, treatment, or prevention of disease. A substance (other than food) intended to affect the structure or any function of the body."*

But what if, rather than using the word drugs, we used the terms bioactive compounds or biologically active substances? Bioactive compounds have the ability to do something to your body and change the way your body functions, often for good. However, as Paracelsus famously put it, "The Dose Determines the Poison" and too much of anything is harmful.

Prior to industrialization, we didn't have shelves of pharmaceutical drugs, prepackaged in pills for every possible condition. Instead, we had apothecaries, shamans, and healers who would curate a natural remedy for your specific condition. Drugs were synonymous with medicinal plants for a long time, and in some places around the world, they are still one and the same.

Natural products like cannabis were the original "pharmaceutical" medicine; they were all that was available. The modern field of Pharmacognosy (*pharma-caug-na-see*) focuses on finding new drugs from nature. The word pharmacognosy breaks down into the Greek words *pharmakon*, meaning "drug" and *gnosis* meaning "knowledge", because it was the ONLY form of pharmacy and healing we had for centuries.

Although it doesn't seem like it from the outside, the pharmaceutical industry that we see today is still very centered around natural products. In fact, 60% of our current pharmaceutical medications are based on drugs found in nature and produced by plants, fungi, and bacteria. Plants have been engineering and perfecting these molecules for millennia, and even the smartest human brains still can't stack carbons with the same efficiency as mother nature. Nature is the best organic chemist in the world.

Compounds that are initially derived from nature are altered by modern pharmaceutical chemists to be stronger, safer, and more selective—allowing pharmaceutical companies to patent these compounds and make a profit. You *can't* patent natural medicine, but you *can* patent a close derivative to a natural medicine.

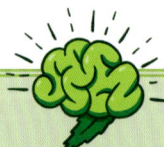

NUGS OF KNOWLEDGE

Did you know that the US government had a patent for the cannabinoid CBG, or cannabigerol, because it was discovered that CBG has antioxidant properties and may help prevent some neurological diseases? This patent, number 6,630,507, stirred quite a bit of commotion in the cannabis world because it was another example of the hypocrisy seen with the government toward cannabis.

NATURE IS ACTIVATING THE BODY

We often consider tetrahydrocannabinol (THC) or cannabidiol (CBD) as the unique chemistry produced by the cannabis plant, but the cannabis plant produces HUNDREDS of bioactive compounds that we can think of as active ingredients in the plant.

Each molecule serves a unique and important purpose to the survival of the plant, and each one has a different effect on our body. The inherent complexity of nature is part of what makes natural medicine so powerful and so contrasting to our current pharmaceutical system. The cannabis plant is composed of hundreds of molecules acting in synergy; some molecules are very similar to each other and some are very different. Additionally, the plant is producing different compounds at different ratios depending on its genetics and environment—adapting, changing, and modifying its chemistry to best protect itself.

This concept of diverse, complex, and dynamic natural medicine is very different from the pharmaceutical model of medicine, which prioritizes one synthetically produced compound at a high dose. Nature works in complex networks, and

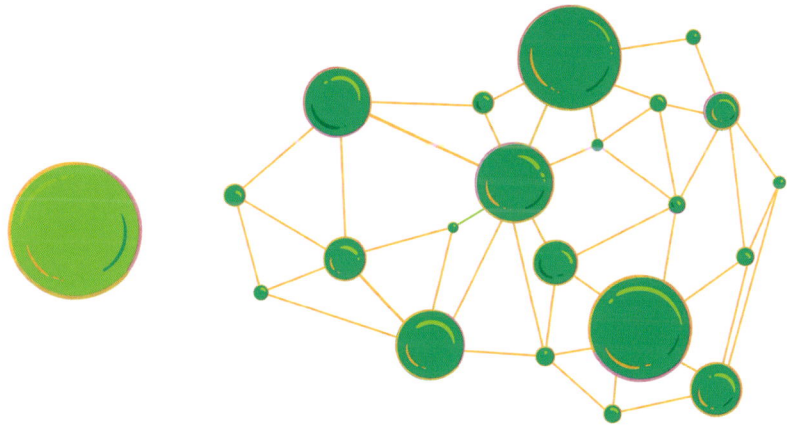

complex medical conditions may require complex natural products that work by tickling dozens of receptors rather than a silver bullet aimed at targeting just one.

When we *feel* something from consuming cannabis, another natural medicine, or a pharmaceutical drug, something profound is happening in our bodies. One, or some, of the molecules in that product are activating receptors in the body. Receptors are essentially little signaling towers present on all your cells and tissues that are waiting for a signal to do something.

Receptors are the basis of all medicine, and to understand how medicines work we must learn about the role of receptors. Some receptors can lessen inflammation when activated, some receptors can make us feel euphoric, some receptors can lessen pain, some receptors can alleviate anxiety, and some receptors allow us to feel touch and heat. Receptors control everything that we feel and experience, and they are imperative to understanding how medicine works and what the potential impact of a medicine will be. Receptors are the basis of how our body talks to itself and how we can turn on and off specific medicinal pathways in the body.

When it comes to pharmaceuticals as medicine, the relationship between the drug and the receptor is usually pretty simple—or it's communicated that way at least. Pharmaceuticals are pure drugs with a targeted effect on the body. While these drugs hope to fulfill the silver bullet theory—where one drug acts on one receptor, and the desired outcome is achieved with little to no side effects—off-target receptors are often activated, leading to unforeseen

side effects. On the other hand, natural products like cannabis have diverse and complex chemistry, often working on multiple systems of the body simultaneously at a range of different doses. They are much more difficult to study because of their complexity and have been notoriously difficult to standardize because of this variability. But to be clear, natural products are not inherently safe—many poisons come from natural products for the same reasons there are so many medicinal compounds.

CANNABINOIDS AND THE ENDOCANNABINOID SYSTEM

One question I often get about cannabis is how it can possibly be good for such a large range of things—like stimulating appetite, lessening pain, reducing inflammation, improving mood, etc. The answer has to do with how cannabis works in the body, and understanding that will help you understand how to cater your cannabis use for your individual needs.

The two most well-known, and the most researched, molecules from the cannabis plant are THC and CBD. Both compounds fall within a larger category of molecules called **cannabinoids**. Cannabis also produces other classes of compounds like the terpenes, flavonoids, flavorants, fatty acids, and more.

Cannabinoids are named after the cannabis plant, because using the plant led to their discovery. In short, knowing that there were some medicinal components inside cannabis through historical accounts and the clear shifts in perception due to smoking cannabis, modern researchers gathered the traditional knowledge and eventually isolated and characterized the main components of the plant like CBD, THC, and a breakdown product of THC called cannabinol (CBN).

Years after the identification of THC from the plant, some of the biggest medical and physiological discoveries of the century occurred. This began with the identification of cannabinoid receptors in the human body, then the identification of the cannabinoids produced by our own bodies, called endocannabinoids because they're produced endogenously, or within us.

It was discovered that THC from the cannabis plant activates the body's cannabinoid 1 receptor (CB1). Activation of the CB1 receptor is what makes us feel high, lowers inflammation, improves mood, enhances appetite, and many more of the infamous effects we get from consuming cannabis. All these effects are controlled via the CB1 receptor, which is the most abundant receptor in the brain and imperative for survival[2].

The cannabinoid receptors exist in our body as part of a larger system of checks and balances. This system is called **the Endocannabinoid System (ECS)**. The ECS is an ancient system that almost all animals on earth contain in their body, not just humans. Everything from jellyfish to slugs, dogs, hamsters, and humans. The purpose of the ECS is to bring balance or **homeostasis** by keeping all the other systems in our body in check.

The existence of this endogenous cannabinoid system in our body may lead you to think that the only way for us to activate these receptors and bring balance to our body is by consuming cannabis, or that our body needs cannabis to survive. But that is not true. In fact, you are able to activate your ECS without cannabis, and people that never use the plant still have healthy, functioning endocannabinoid systems.

The cannabinoid receptors work differently than the other receptor systems in our body—like the dopamine, serotonin, or opiate systems. The ECS is a **retrograde signaling system**, so it works in the **opposite direction**.

Picture a river flowing, it will always flow in one direction, that is the direction that most brain signaling molecules in your body are following. The issue is, if that river is flowing too fast, too slow, or starts to divert in an unwanted direction, there is nothing stopping the river from going completely rogue. The ECS works against the flow of the river—think of it like a beaver swimming against the current, ready to build a dam or cut down a tree when needed. When the ECS is activated, it can bring balance to dysregulated systems throughout the body. **Activation of the ECS from plant cannabinoids (phytocannabinoids) or cannabinoids in the body (endocannabinoids) can bring balance or homeostasis by regulating the other systems.**

THE ENTOURAGE EFFECT

When we smoke, vape, or consume products made with cannabis flower or extracts that show the same complexity as cannabis flower, we are ingesting a cocktail of many different and unique compounds. The interplay of these molecules and potential synergies that may arise from ingesting whole plant medicine is a common phenomenon in the world of natural products or herbalism, but in cannabis it has a special name: **The entourage effect.**

The entourage effect is a theory wherein the different medicinal compounds present in the cannabis plant work together to create profound benefits. So, for example, if we were to isolate THC from the plant, it would feel completely different from—and have fewer benefits than—whole extracts of the plant. Smoking two types of cannabis flower with different levels of active compounds like cannabinoids and terpenes provides completely different effects. I've consumed THC alone and I find the feeling to be hollow and a little disorienting—and a completely different experience to consuming THC with the entourage of other medicinal compounds in the plant, which is often a euphoric, pleasant, expansive feeling.

These chemical synergies are not only present in the plant, but our own bodies also experience this entourage effect as we also produce a diversity of endogenous (within our bodies) molecules to help regulate the different systems. For instance, while our bodies make two main endocannabinoids, 2-AG and Anandamide, a variety of lesser-known molecules also contribute to regulation, producing endocannabinoids that have portions of serotonin, dopamine, or other signaling molecules[3].

Our bodies and the cannabis plant all abide by the laws of nature and do not produce an excess of any single compound. Instead, nature produces diverse molecules that work as a symphony to act on an entourage of receptors. Creating such a range of molecules within our body or the plant allows for redundancy and therefore resilience—**biological resilience is achieved via chemical diversity.**

Cannabis varieties with unique genetics and unique chemical profiles are commonly called **strains**. Some famous strains you may have heard include Gorilla Glue, Pineapple Express, and Blue Dream. However, there are hundreds of unique strains of cannabis that have been bred to produce different effects for the consumer, and often different smells or visual changes like purple nugs or variegated leaves.

The word strain is not a scientifically accurate term for a medicinal plant. Strain is typically used to describe a microorganism like bacteria, something that is evolving so rapidly that we have to have a way to track how it's evolved over time. However, the word strain is a part of cannabis culture, and despite efforts of many scientists to change this term for more botanically correct ones, I believe it is here to stay. What really matters is understanding that different varieties produce different effects. Although, whatever you do, don't call it a strand.

Some other words beside strain that can be used to describe the different varieties of cannabis are cultivar and chemovar. **Cultivar** is a common term in the world of botany and means "cultivation variety," which describes the unique physical characteristics bred from generation to generation of growth. **Chemovar** means "chemical variety" and describes the unique chemistry made by a plant. This is especially relevant in medical cannabis products to help describe the levels and presence of specific cannabinoids, terpenes, and other active compounds. This is most appropriate when describing cannabis based on chemistry, like a CBD-rich chemovar.

Cannabis strains will often be named according to genetic lineage; this is important because it allows us to understand what the effects may be like before ever trying it. For instance, if you really enjoy smoking the strain Blue Dream, but are looking for a new type of flower to try, you may enjoy strains that cross Blue Dream with a different variety.

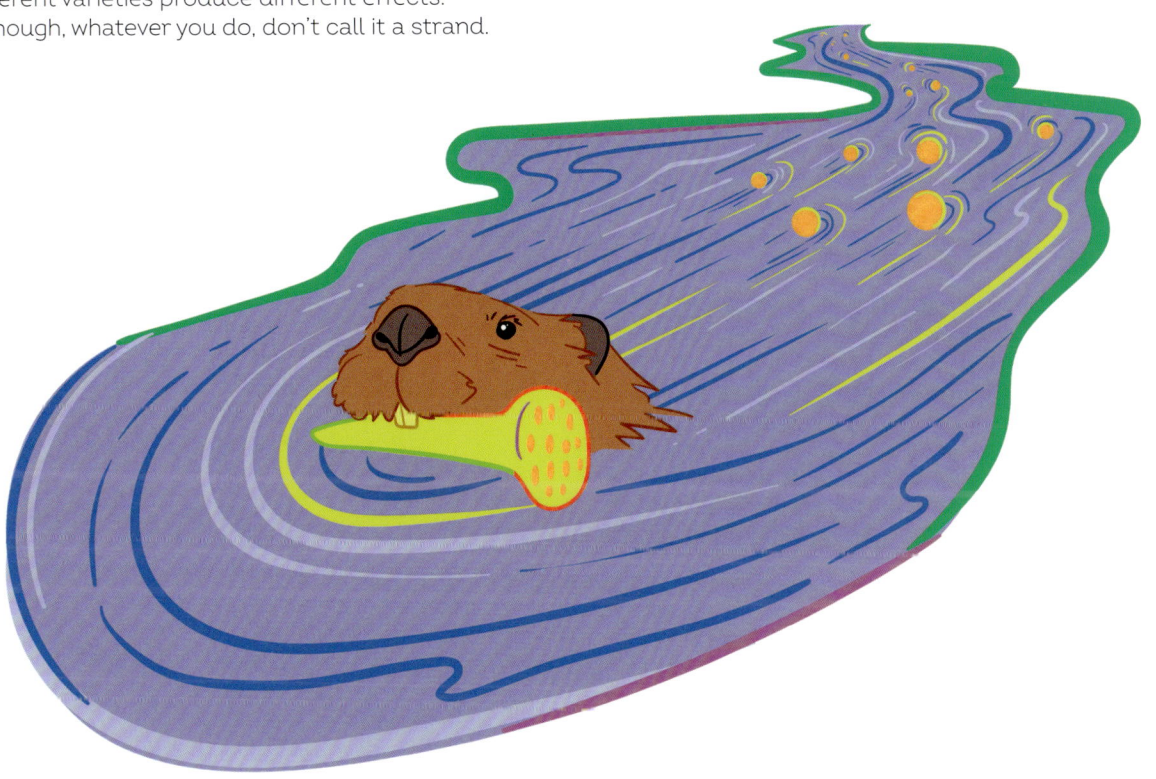

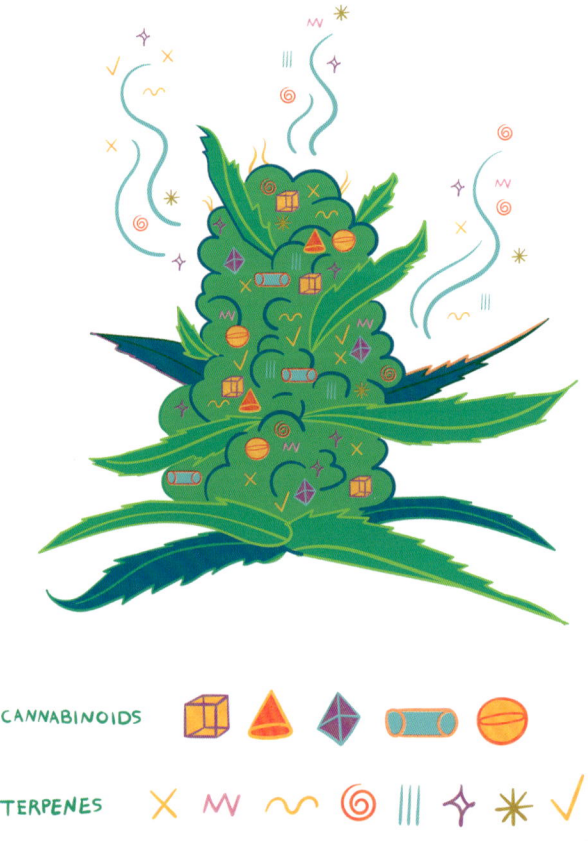

CANNABINOIDS

TERPENES

CLASSIFYING CANNABIS PLANTS

The words indica, sativa, and hybrid are used to describe how a product is going to make you feel. Indica is attributed to the more couch-locking, sedating effects—"in da couch," a play on "indica," is often used to remember this phenomenon. In contrast, sativas offer a more uplifting and energetic high, while hybrids fall somewhere in between both effects.

While there are undoubtedly strain-specific effects that mean some varieties make you feel more hyper and awake while others make you feel more sedated, unfortunately the science shows that most often these words are merely marketing terms. The reality is indica, sativa, and hybrid mean very little as far as predicting how a product is going to make you feel because there is currently no standardization, regulation, or consistency in how brands are labeling products. Science has proved again and again that these terms do not predict the nature of your high,

but that's not to say this won't change in the future. It IS possible to use chemistry to predict and label products based on effects, and many companies are working to refine algorithms to predict effects more accurately in the future. I do think that the terms indica, sativa, and hybrid can be helpful for guiding you to a good place to start, but until these terms are used with scientific rationale or backing, I would recommend a less biased approach to choosing products.

These terms still have a place in the industry to describe the cannabis plants—with sativa-type varieties being tall, airy plants and having long and spindly leaves, and indica-types having fat and wide leaves and being shorter in general. The true "Indicas" and "Sativas" that brought these infamous names to the industry did exist in the past, but with the amount of breeding and genetic mix-up of plant varieties available on the market today, we need new, accurate terms to help describe the effects.

We will discuss a variety of other ways to predict how a product will make you feel. One of the simplest ways to characterize different cannabis varieties is grouping based on the level of THC and CBD. Although there are hundreds of molecules present in the plant, these two are typically the ones customers and growers are most focused on, and therefore base their decisions off of.

This classification system is particularly helpful for differentiating between cannabis that produces more than 0.3% THC, and cannabis that produces less than 0.3% THC. This arbitrary level of THC is the main differentiator when determining if a cannabis product is legally defined as nonintoxicating hemp or intoxicating marijuana. The hemp plant and the marijuana plant are both the exact same plant, *Cannabis sativa*, but are treated with very different regulations for growing, manufacturing, and distributing based on the level of THC present in the final product.

A classification system based on cannabinoid content was first introduced in 1973 by Ernest Small and H.D. Beckstead.

Type I: THC dominant with little to no CBD

Type II: Balanced profile of THC: CBD

Type III: CBD dominant with little to no THC

Types IV & V: Dominant in other cannabinoids like CBG or containing no cannabinoids at all.

Another way of classifying cannabis varieties in more detail based on aroma is a method developed by Napro Research—and adopted by the Emerald Cup, a popular cannabis competition—in 2013. This system applies profiles beyond just THC and CBD, and now includes factors like terpene profiles, flavor profiles, and effects. This six-tier classification system allows the different varieties of cannabis to be grouped into similar categories. The categories include:

- Jacks and Hazes
- Tropical and Floral
- OGs and Gas
- Sweets and Dreams
- Dessert
- Exotics

Each of these categories has distinct effects and aromas and can be a good starting point for someone who is unsure of what cannabis variety to try. Throughout this book we will discuss other ways to home in on which varieties, doses, and consumption methods work best for you.

PARTS OF THE CANNABIS PLANT

Cannabis plants are primarily cultivated for their flowers, which are rich in medicinal compounds. However, over time, we've discovered uses for almost every part of the plant, from the roots to the seeds and buds. Cannabis is typically a dioecious plant, meaning it can be either male or female. Female plants are predominantly grown for cultivation, while males are used during breeding to produce seeds that carry on genetics for future generations. Unlike females, male cannabis plants do not produce flowers but instead have pollen sacs.

BUD (FLOWER)

The cannabis bud, also known as the flower, is the part most commonly smoked. This is because the buds are covered in small resin glands called **trichomes**, which resemble tiny mushrooms under a microscope or appear as sparkles to the naked eye. These trichomes are responsible for producing most of the active compounds, such as terpenes and cannabinoids. Trichomes can also be separated from the plant to create products like hash, or collected at the bottom of your grinder, which is called kief.

The female cannabis plant also features reproductive structures, including **pistils** and **stigmas**. Pistils represent the plant's reproductive organs, while stigmas, which catch pollen, change color from white to amber or brown as the plant matures. The **cola** refers to the main flower at the top of the plant's primary stalk, composed of a dense cluster of smaller buds.

LEAVES

The iconic cannabis leaves are typically serrated, giving them a jagged appearance. They have the general appearance of a hand, and the amount of lobes each leaf has widely varies based on genetics, but is commonly 3, 5, or 7. Cannabis leaves can be classified into two types:

Fan Leaves: These are the largest and most robust leaves, essential for photosynthesis. Although they contain minimal active compounds, they play a crucial role in capturing sunlight to fuel the plant's growth.

Sugar Leaves: These smaller, thinner leaves grow around the flower and are covered in trichomes, giving them a sparkly, frosted appearance. They are rich in active compounds.

STALK

The main stem or stalk of the cannabis plant provides structural support and facilitates the movement of water and nutrients throughout the plant. Cannabis stalks are incredibly strong, and hemp fibers, derived from the stalk, are known for their durability in textiles. The degree of branching depends largely on the plant's genetics, with sativas tending to have more spread-out, airy branches, while indicas are broader and more compact.

ROOTS

The roots of the cannabis plant are vital for absorbing water, nutrients, and oxygen, while also anchoring the plant in place. Healthy roots are essential to the overall well-being of the plant. Sugars produced by the leaves are transported to the soil, where they are broken down by organisms and transformed into energy that the plant can use.

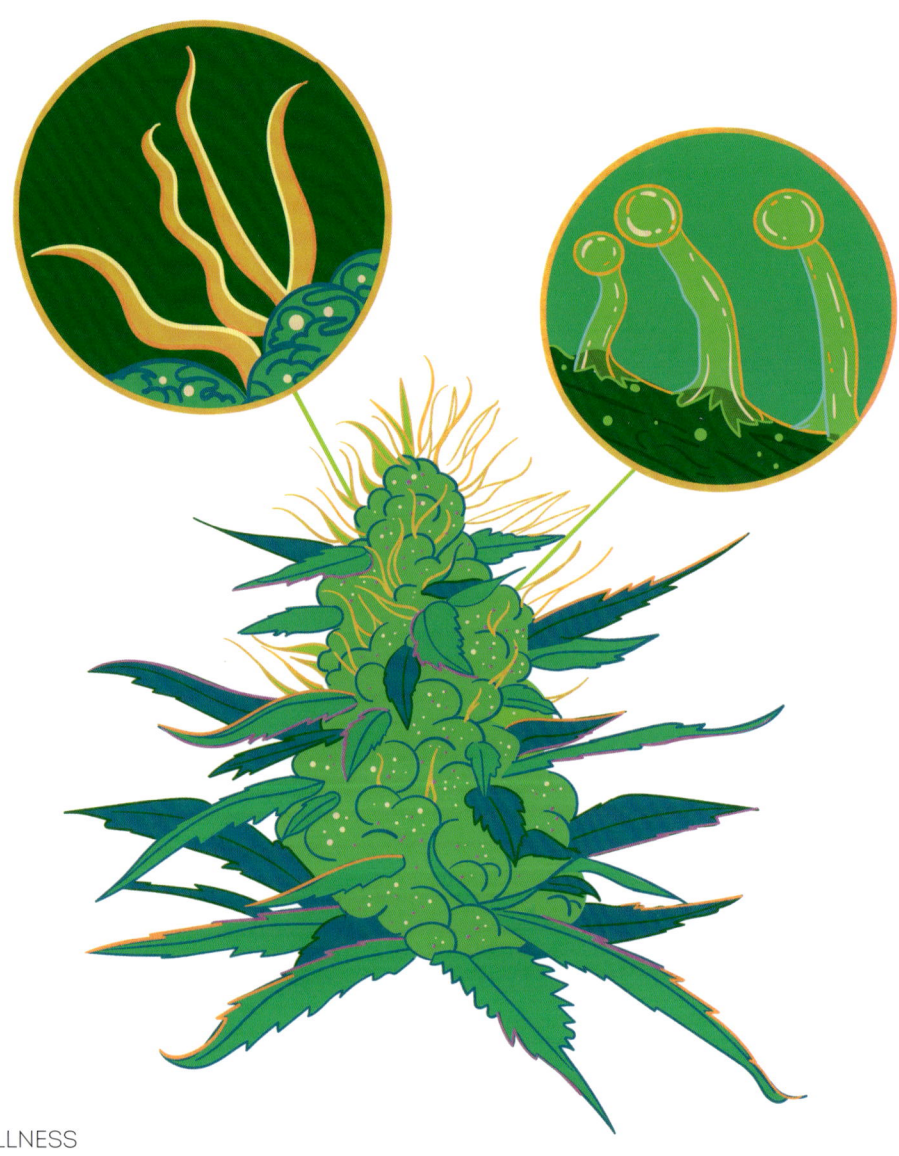

HOW TO IDENTIFY AND EVALUATE HIGH-QUALITY FLOWER

Legal and illicit cannabis markets are filled with cultivators producing high-quality cannabis flower, but there are also products of lesser quality that you'll want to avoid. One key challenge today is that determining quality can be difficult due to various factors such as strict regulations requiring overly dry cannabis, quick turnaround times, limited strain availability, and most importantly, the lack of an industry standard for reporting quality. While quality is largely subjective, depending on the consumer's experience, there are important sensory cues to consider when evaluating your product. Other factors beyond sensory analysis that contribute to quality are the genetics of the plant, the soil it is grown in, and how it was cultivated.

Some people strongly prefer indoor-grown cannabis while others, like myself, feel a special connection to outdoor, or sungrown, varieties. Research indicates that sungrown cannabis tends to offer a broader range of cannabinoids and terpenes, along with lower THC levels, due to the natural spectrum of sunlight and diverse organisms present in nature. Indoor-grown flower, on the other hand, is often more visually appealing with glistening trichomes and higher THC content, but may lack the diversity, spirit, and natural complexity that outdoor cultivation provides.

I encourage you to use all your senses when evaluating cannabis, and always take time to smell the flowers.

SMELL

One of the first indicators of quality is the aroma of the cannabis flower. The scent can help you find the strain that best suits your body while also providing insights into its quality. High-quality cannabis typically has a strong, often pungent smell. While hemp may have a grassy aroma, If flower has not been dried and cured properly it will likely lack nose, or aroma.

APPEARANCE

Visually inspecting the flower can also reveal a lot about its quality. Check for the density of trichomes—the tiny, sparkly structures covering the bud. Many weed connoisseurs and cultivators use a jeweler's loupe to get a magnified look at these small structures. Trichome abundance and integrity are

essential to evaluate because they contain the majority of medicinal compounds. If they are damaged or crushed, terpenes (which contribute to the aroma) will be released, and cannabinoids will degrade more quickly.

TOUCH

When handling the nugs, properly dried and cured flower should have a slight bounce when squeezed. It shouldn't crumble immediately; rather, it should compress slightly and then return to its original form. This elasticity is also apparent when grinding your flower—after grinding, pinch the ground flower to see how well it sticks to itself. When you first open your grinder after adding fresh, properly dried and cured cannabis you will see the flower expand slightly. Whereas dried cannabis will stay lifeless and be difficult to compress into any shape.

ROLLABILITY

"Rollability" refers to how easily the flower can be rolled into a joint. High-quality flower is much easier to work with than dry, brittle nugs. Think of it like building a sandcastle—wet sand holds its shape; just as well-cured flower holds together when rolling. Once the flower is formed into a cylinder, the rest of the rolling process becomes almost automatic.

SMOKEABILITY

When evaluating "smokeability", you'll want to consider factors like smoothness, flavor, harshness, body, and any tingling sensations. The dry and cure process plays a significant role here, as starches are converted into sugars, resulting in a sweeter smoke. Additionally, physical factors like the thickness of the roll can contribute to how smooth and pleasant the smoking experience is.

THE IMPORTANCE OF THE DRY AND CURE PROCESS

The dry and cure process is critical in determining the final quality of cannabis. Many growers can cultivate beautiful plants, but true quality is achieved through patience and precision during these final stages. Once the trichomes turn milky and amber, the plant is harvested and usually hang-dried at 60°F (15.5°C) with 60% relative humidity—this is called the 60/60 method. This process typically takes about a week, depending on the climate, until the branches snap easily, signaling that the plant is ready for curing.

Curing continues the drying process and is key to distinguishing between average and high-quality cannabis. During curing, chlorophyll—which gives the plant its green color—degrades, resulting in a smoother smoke. Starches and other carbohydrates also break down into sugars, further enhancing the flavor and burn quality.

Proper curing preserves the trichomes, ensuring a stronger aroma and better retention of the terpene profile. If your flower smells like ammonia during curing, it's not ready yet—ammonia is a by-product of plant metabolism that is still breaking down.

Lastly, curing redistributes moisture within the bud, maintaining the ideal balance between rollability and low water activity to prevent microbial growth. Cannabis is often cured in glass jars or plastic tubs, which are regularly "burped," aka opened to allow fresh air to circulate, ensuring the bud dries and cures evenly from the inside out.

By engaging your senses—smell, sight, touch, and even the rolling and smoking experience—you can better evaluate the quality of your cannabis and make informed decisions about the products and cultivators you choose.

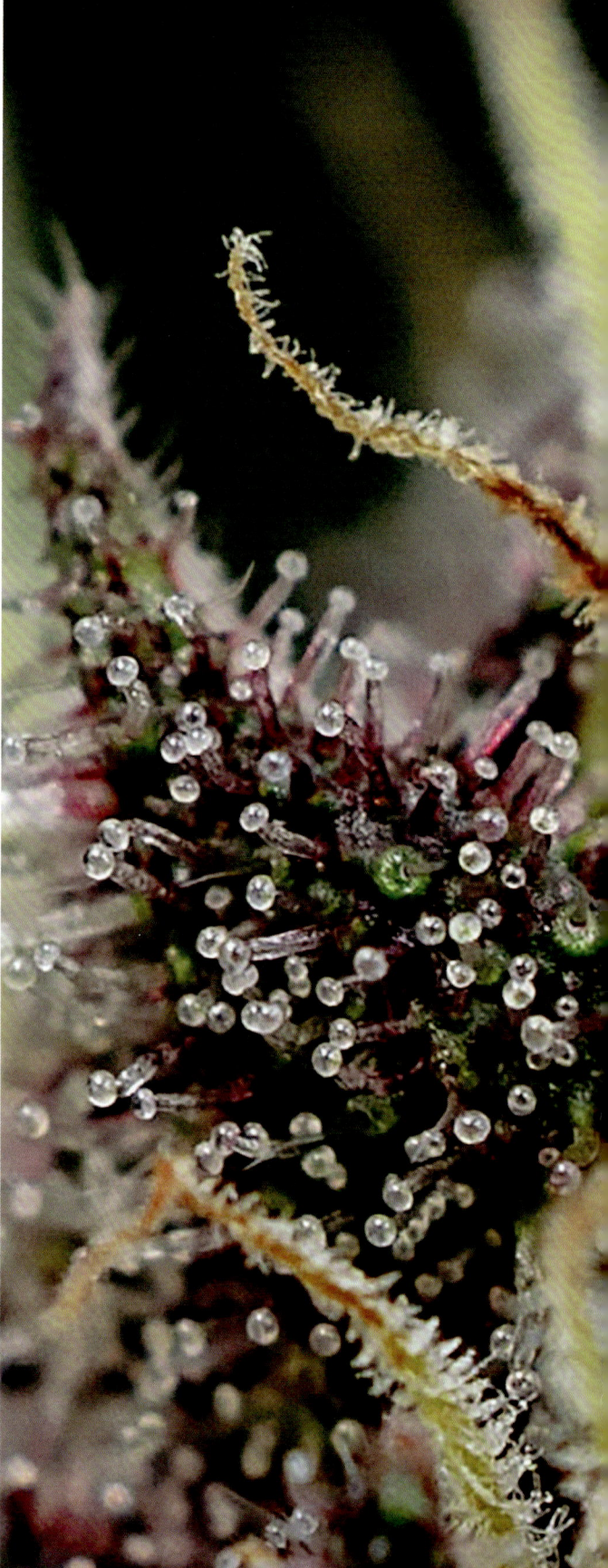

SMOKE BREAK!

LET'S STOP AND RECAP THIS CHAPTER:

⇉ Plants produce awesome drugs because they have coevolved with animals to produce molecules that act on our brains via different types of receptors.

⇉ Humans (and almost all other animals) have endocannabinoid systems.

⇉ The active compounds in the cannabis plant act on cannabinoid receptors to elicit medicinal benefits in our bodies.

⇉ The cannabinoid receptors are part of a larger system in our body called the endocannabinoid system (ECS), which controls almost everything happening in the body and is responsible for maintaining balance within our biological systems.

⇉ We also produce cannabinoids in our body that are called endocannabinoids; these work on the same receptors that the molecules in the cannabis plant act on.

⇉ The hundreds of molecules in the cannabis plant act in synergy to produce profound medicinal effects in our bodies.

⇉ We use the word strains to describe different varieties of cannabis with unique chemistry and genetics. However, newer classification methods separate varieties into categories based on chemistry and effect.

⇉ The drying and curing process of cannabis is essential in producing a quality smokeable flower.

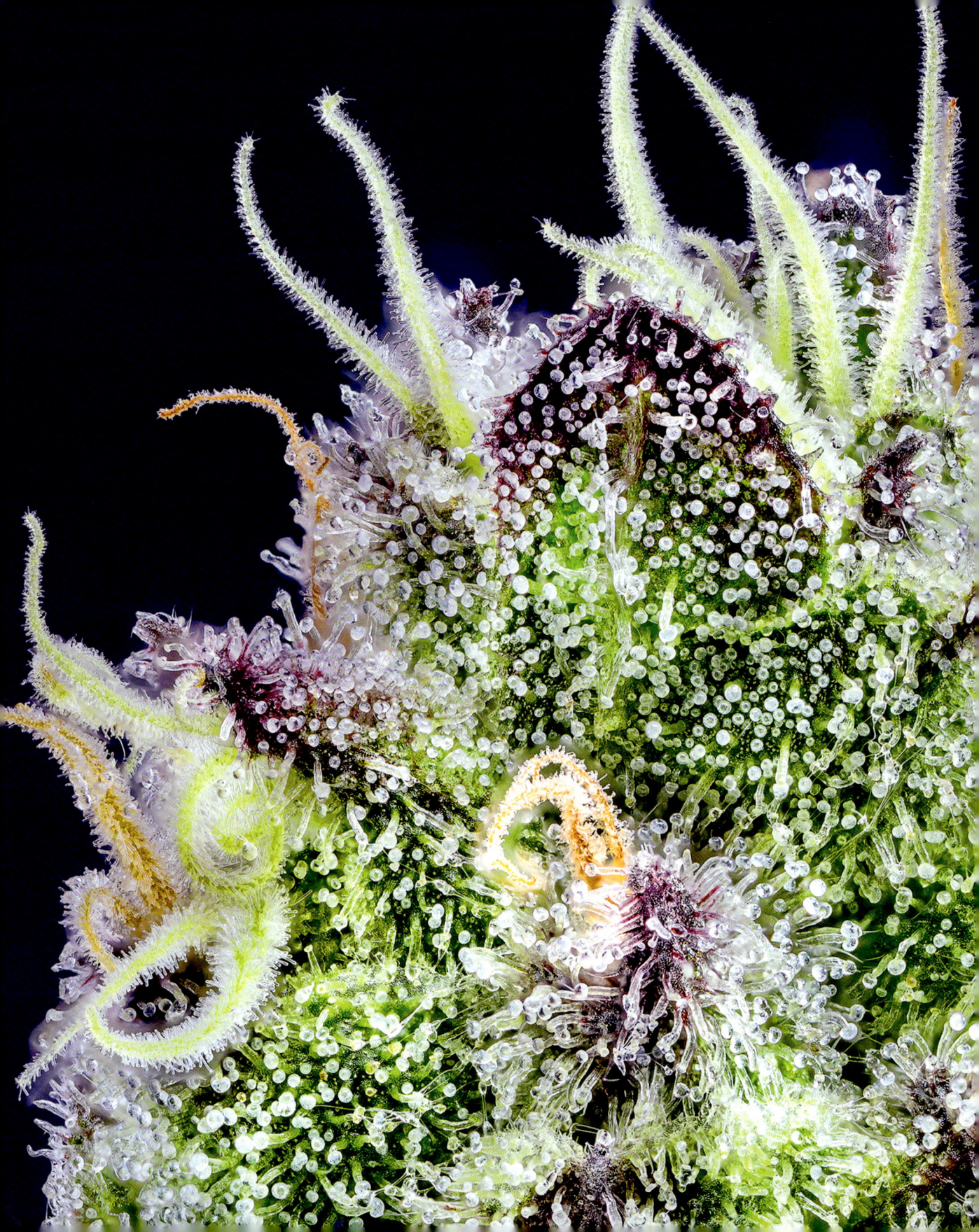

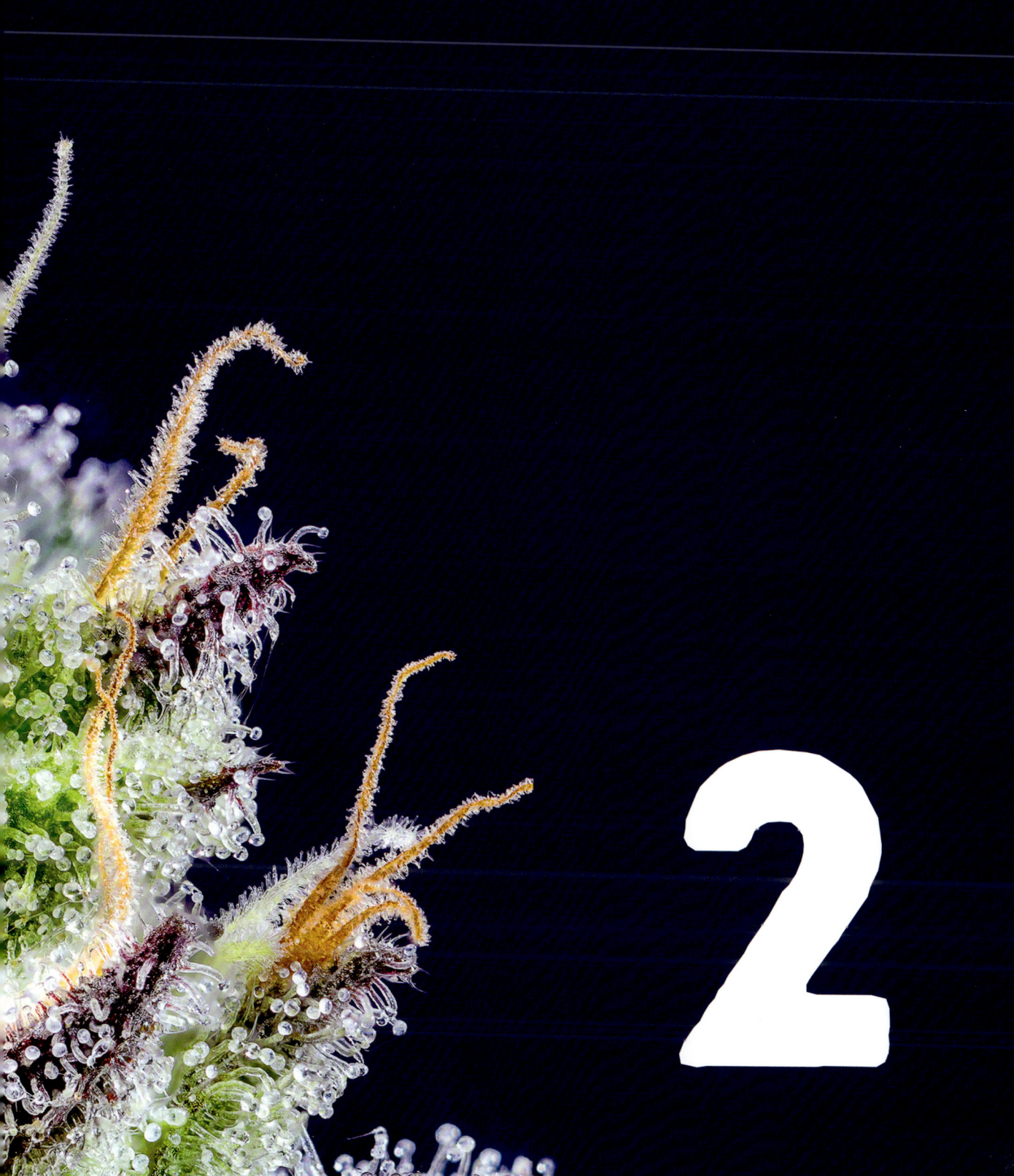

2

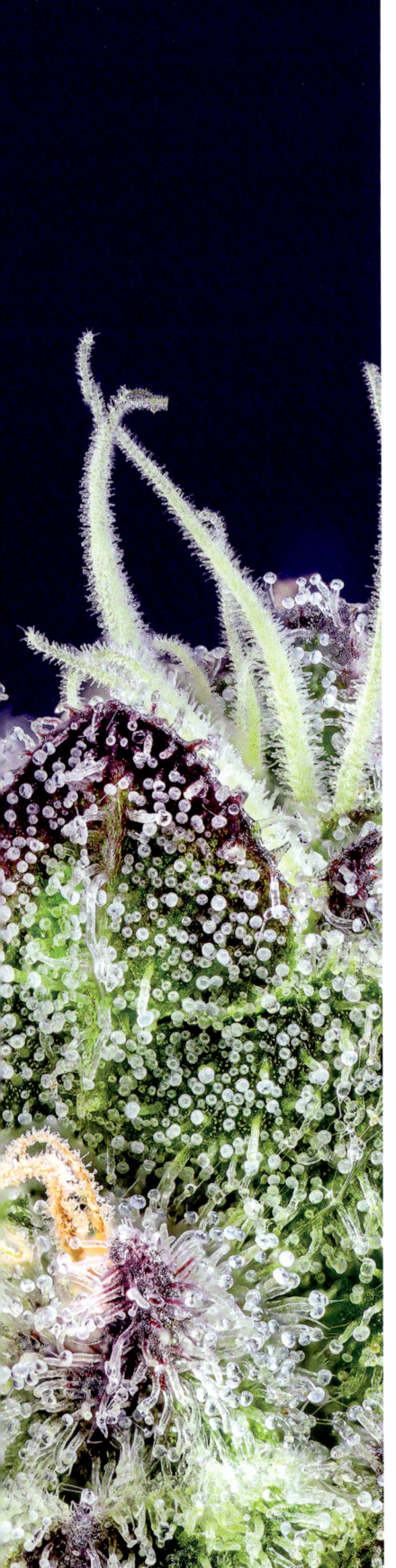

A BRIEF HISTORY OF CANNABIS: GROWERS, SMUGGLERS, HEALERS, & DEALERS

In my medicinal plant garden at home, I can grow the castor plant, which produces the liver toxin Ricin; Datura plants, which produce scopolamine and atropine that act on the muscles of the heart; tobacco, which produces the psychoactive compound nicotine; and many other plants that have killed millions of people over time. Yet I can't grow cannabis, a plant that has never alone killed anyone and has hundreds of documented medicinal benefits.

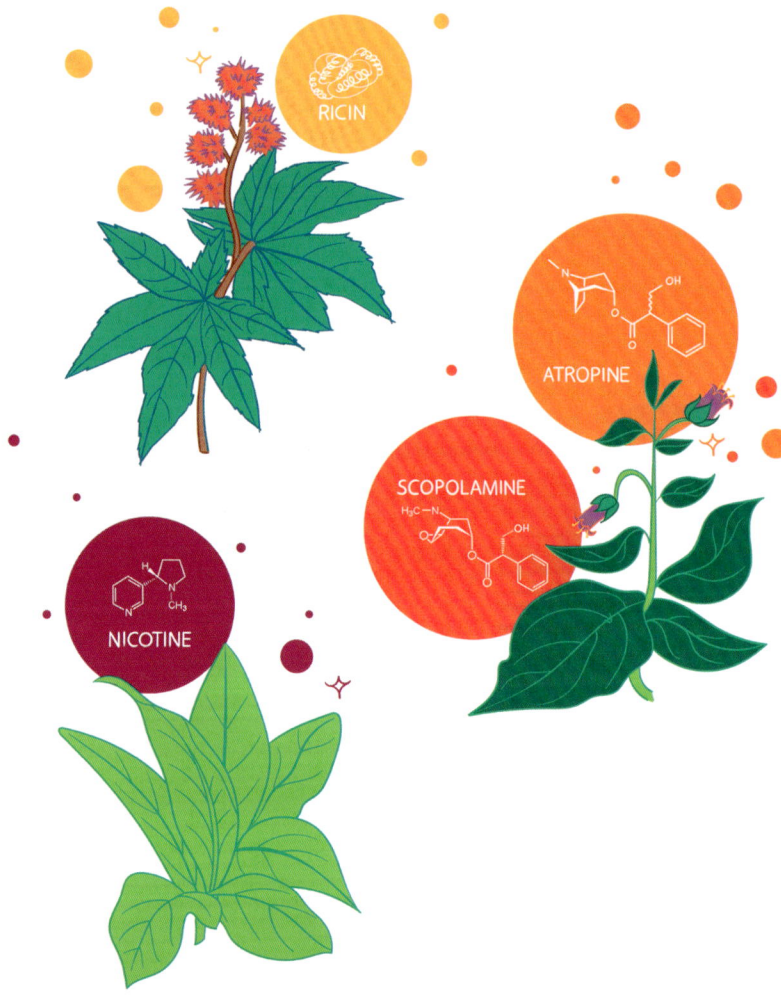

At the time of writing this book in 2024, cannabis is still a schedule 1 drug. The definition of a schedule 1 drug is i) a drug that has no approved medical value and ii) a drug that has a high potential for addiction or abuse. Considering we have two FDA-approved drugs from the cannabis plant–Epidiolex (CBD) and Marinol (THC)–the argument that cannabis has no approved medical value falls short. Cannabis is far less addictive than many regularly used substances like alcohol and tobacco, which are not scheduled at all and are readily available at your local gas station.

The political component of prohibition has been shaped extensively by lobbying from three of the most powerful industries in the world: the tobacco, alcohol, and pharmaceutical industries, who also fund some major political campaigns and are deeply intertwined with many pockets in Congress. Cannabis use marks a steady decline in these mentioned industries and it's no secret that this has been a driving factor of the slow progress toward legalization and heavy amounts of propaganda throughout the years.

Cannabis is a plant. We as animals and members of the natural world have an inherent right to forms of nature, especially to medicinal plants. We have never operated further outside of the natural world than our society is currently living, and it is imperative that we restore our right, globally, to natural medicines. Although we are beginning to have greater access to this plant, it has been a decades-long battle fighting for our right to use and cultivate this medicine–and it is still actively going on. In my opinion, a legal cannabis industry where people don't have the right to cultivation or "homegrow" is not a win for the people but rather another form of government monopoly over medicine. This book will hopefully open your eyes to the level of discrimination that has been aimed at the cannabis community and help you realize that it isn't about safety; it is always about control and whose pockets fill up as cannabis becomes more accessible.

In this chapter, we will briefly walk through how we got to the point where we are now with cannabis. The history of cannabis–and why this plant has remained present for decades despite varying levels of prohibition–is driven by passion, profit, and accessibility. There is no way I will be able to capture the danger, dedication, sacrifice, pain, financial burden, societal judgment, racial discrimination, or

risk that was involved in getting to the point of having a legal cannabis industry in this chapter. There is no doubt that many people who were smuggling, growing, and transporting cannabis may have done so to earn some fat stacks of cash, but many others have reasons far beyond money and have risked everything to provide this medicine, despite what the U.S. pharmacopeia or FDA said was or was not safe and effective. Many men and women have been incarcerated, and still are, for providing cannabis medicine when it was inaccessible to the masses. We stand on the backs of giants, and we can never forget that as our industry matures and develops.

AN ANCIENT MEDICINE

Cannabis is one of mankind's oldest cultivated crops. In fact, the weaving and utilization of hemp fiber from the cannabis plant dates back as long as 10,000 years ago[1]. In China, people cultivated hemp and called it "Ma"; it was thought to have been used for both fiber and medicine. The seeds were often the part of the plant used as medicine, and although the psychoactive effects of cannabis weren't the focus of ancient texts, genetic evidence shows that the plants could produce THC, and likely did produce small amounts. After Chinese cultivation of cannabis began, the plant slowly spread to cultures around the world, from the Southwest Asia to India, Japan, Europe, Africa, and eventually North America.

Some of the ancient Chinese texts have yet to be decoded and still are not fully understood, leaving large gaps in our knowledge of its traditional uses. Cannabis's intimate link to spirituality and religion have been incorporated into religions across the world. With practices like Shintoism binding couples with cannabis to represent a marriage of laughter and happiness, to Hinduism, where the god Shiva was thought to have brought cannabis from the hills of the Himalayan mountains for human enjoyment and enlightenment[2]. Other groups like the Coptic Orthodox Church, Baritus, Sufis of Islam, Early Jewish People, and more used cannabis as a sacrament or spiritual tool[3]. Cannabis is still used today for spiritual and religious purposes, but not often accepted in shared religious spaces. I hope to see this change, as cannabis is one of the most powerful tools in uniting and healing people, while bringing us closer to nature.

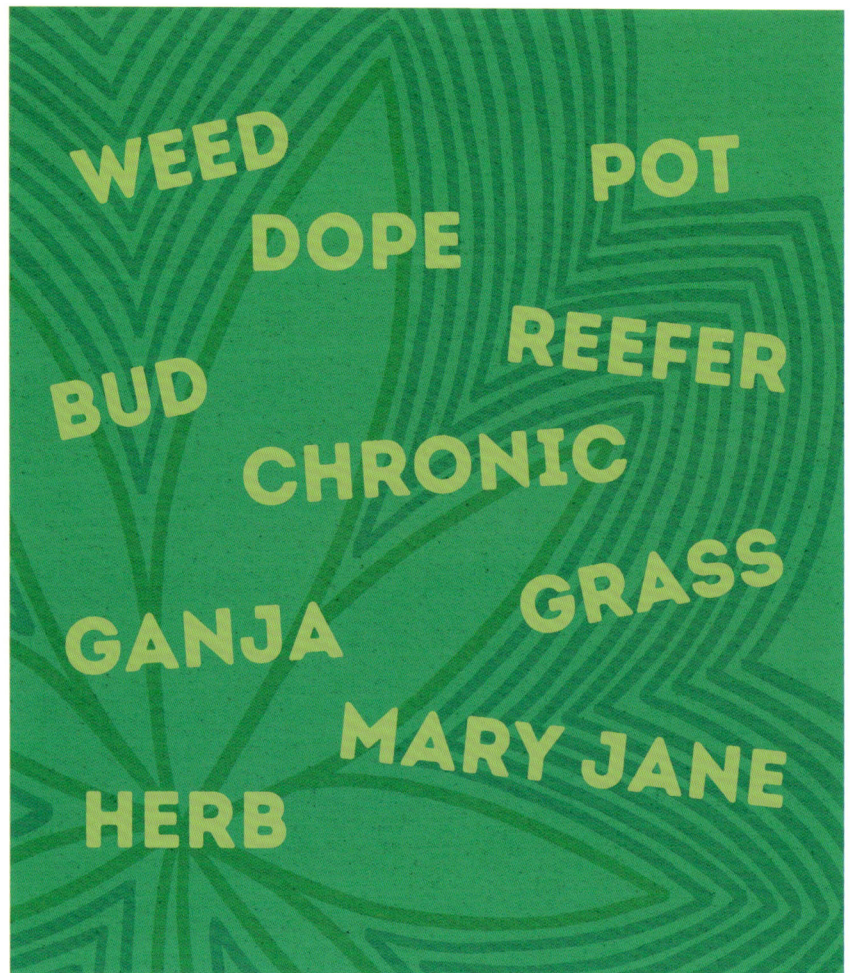

WHAT'S IN A NAME?

Most people do not use the word marijuana to describe cannabis due to the word's racist roots and the amount of discrimination that Mexicans and Mexican Americans have received from using this plant. Even the term "reefer," which is included in the title of this book, has Mexican origin. However, one of the goals of this book is to use science to reverse stigma, as we aim to undo the damage that the propaganda of Reefer Madness caused. While some people are starting to use the term marijuana again to take back the word, personally I choose to use the word cannabis. It is the most accurate description from a scientific basis, and as a white woman I don't feel like I have the historical context to say marijuana.

Other terms that have been regularly used to describe cannabis are hemp from English roots, *hanf* from the Germans, κάνναβις from the Greeks, *canapa* from Italian roots, *konoplija* from the Russians, *qunnab* in Arabic, *kendir* from the Kurkish, and *kanap'is* from Georgian routes. There are also several slang terms for cannabis.

So, you have quite a few options that don't have racist roots, and I'd highly recommend picking one of these.

THE EVOLUTION OF CANNABIS LEGISLATION

It is thought that people started to really smoke cannabis "bud" in the mid 1800s in areas like Jamaica and Barbados from flower brought over from India. By the late 1800s sailors continued to spread the plant through the West Indies and to Mexico. It wasn't until 1903 that the first documented use of what we think of as cannabis was recorded in Brownville, Texas. That same year, the first cannabis prohibition law relating to Mexican use of the plant was passed.

As jazz exploded in New Orleans in the early 1900s, white Americans were worried that the "voodoo" music was a threat to get white women dancing, and cannabis began to be associated with good music, free thinking, and straight up vibes.

Interestingly, as racist white leaders began to make legislation to limit the use of cannabis across the United States, most had no idea that they had been taking cannabis in their medicinal concoctions for decades before. From 1850 to 1937, cannabis had been used as the first-line treatment for more than 100 different medical conditions outlined in the U.S. Pharmacopeia—including as a marriage saver, working as a powerful aphrodisiac.

Reefer Madness and reefer racism continued through the early 20th century. During prohibition, people continued to use cannabis, but it was not safe to grow, smoke, or sell products. Cannabis is stanky and loud, and using cannabis was dangerous in most areas. Cannabis was smuggled into the United States from areas across the world including Thailand, Mexico, and Jamaica. Quality cannabis was scarce and smuggled herb sold for big money. Some of the most notorious smugglers were California surfers. Some rural communities even grew cannabis if they could get their hands on some seeds.

The population of people who were exposed to the insane propaganda from Reefer Madness saying that cannabis makes you stupid and lazy are now the politicians running the country, and the propaganda is strong, although sometimes less obvious to this day. When communicating about cannabis with grandparents, politicians, or elders, I always start by encouraging people to start with a blank slate of knowledge on cannabis: act like you have no preconceived notion of the plant and listen to the facts in the most unbiased way possible. **Because if there was a pharmaceutical drug that could relieve pain, heighten mood, and reduce inflammation with almost no side effects like cannabis does, it would be prescribed to everyone over 40.**

The people most affected by prohibition were the Black and brown populations, as they were targeted so the state could lock them up and remove them from society. This has not changed today; the majority of cannabis-related arrests are people from Black and brown communities. The American Civil Liberties Union concluded in 2020 that Black people are 3.64 times more likely than white people to be arrested for cannabis possession.

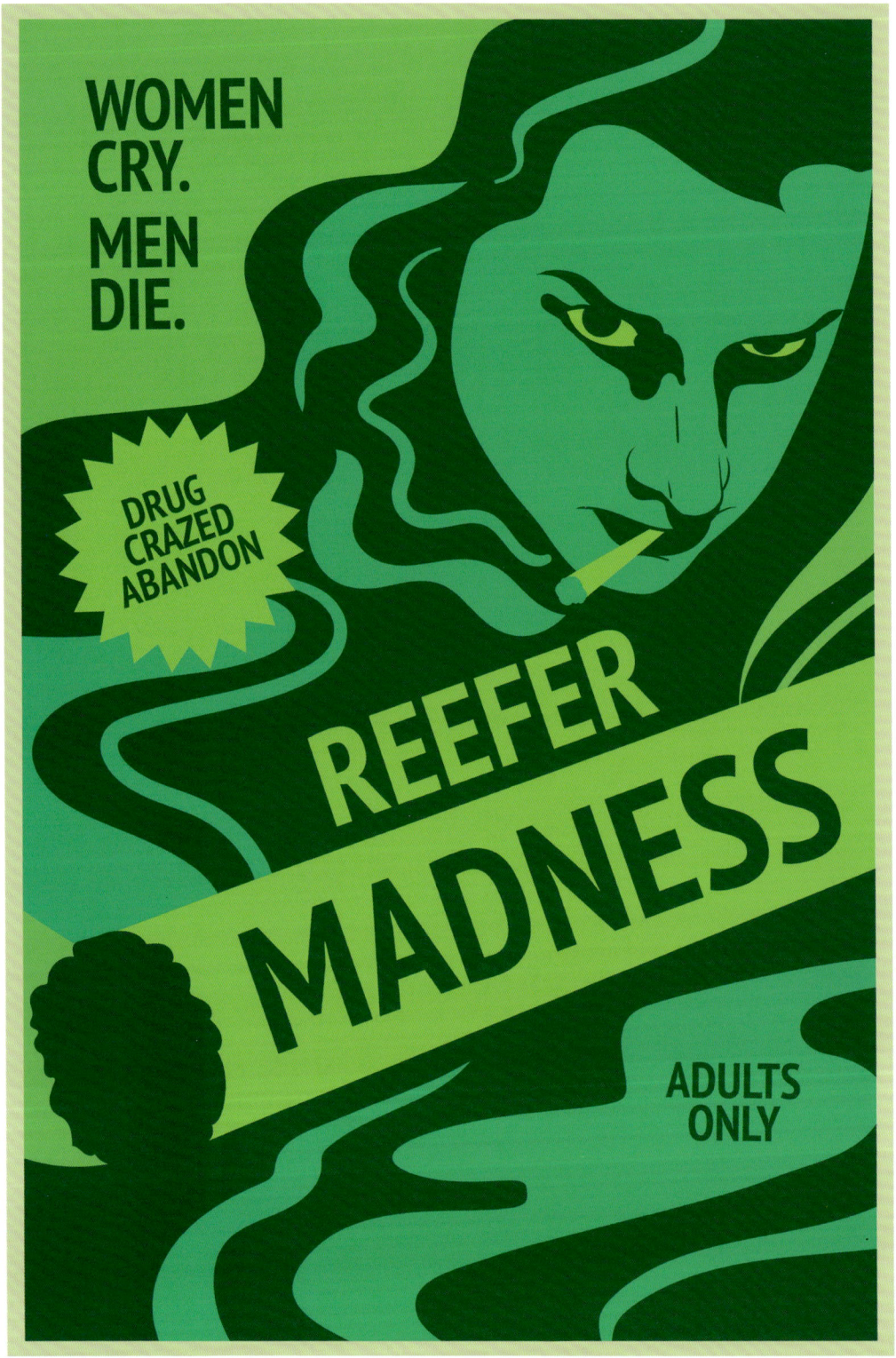

CANNABIS AND THE LAW

Henry Anslinger, the first commissioner of the Federal Bureau of Narcotics (which would later be turned into the modern-day DEA) and the main coordinator of the war on drugs, said to the U.S. Congress that there were "between 50,000 and 100,000 marijuana smokers in the U.S.," mostly "Negroes and Mexicans, and entertainers." Anslinger's goal was to rid all drugs from the U.S. However, as he had no evidence to support his claim that cannabis was dangerous, he contacted 30 scientists asking for their advice. Of the 30 scientists, 29 said cannabis was not dangerous, and only one said it was—leading to a swarm of press releases and hysteria.

The blatant discrimination toward cannabis consumers began with the Marijuana Tax Act during Franklin D. Roosevelt's presidency in 1937, but things got worse with President Richard Nixon and the Passing of the Controlled Substances Act of 1970. This act erroneously classified cannabis as a schedule 1 drug in the United States alongside heroin and other highly dangerous pharmaceutical drugs. The passing of this act limited research and increased the penalties for possessing cannabis and was rooted in absolutely zero scientific rationale, but it remains implemented to this day.

During the 1970s and 1980s, cannabis became increasingly mainstream and was often in the forefront of hippie and rock culture. The counterculture movement of the '70s and distrust in the U.S. government led to cannabis use often being a symbol of freedom, rebellion, and community. The normalization of cannabis use began conversations about drug policy and reform which are still being discussed and amended today.

In 1996, the state of California was the first to have legal medical cannabis when voters approved Proposition 215, also known as the Compassionate Use Act. After this, other states began slowly voting for medical programs, and eventually Washington and Colorado were the first states to approve adult-use (recreational) programs in 2012. States continue to slowly adopt medical and adult use programs across the U.S., and countries across the world are slowly beginning to legalize and become more accepting of cannabis.

Some countries like Thailand and Germany are now using their leniency toward cannabis as a means of getting more canna-tourism with resorts and social clubs opening liberally.

In 2024, as this book was being written, the United States Food and Drug Administration (FDA) just accepted that cannabis has medicinal value—after more than 30,000 peer-reviewed publications on cannabis and the endocannabinoid system, and 4 million patients with medical cards, two FDA-approved drugs, and not one single death attributed to cannabis use alone. Because of the FDA's acknowledgment of cannabis's medical value, it is being proposed for rescheduling from a schedule 1 to a schedule 3 drug. Although this is a step in the right direction, it is difficult to celebrate; because of the safety profile and efficacy of cannabis medicine, it should absolutely be descheduled rather than rescheduled.

KEY PLAYERS IN CANNABIS RESEARCH

The cannabis plant has been consumed for more than 1,000 years across many cultures, ethnicities, and religions. However, physicians were naive to the medicinal uses for much of this time, because traditional knowledge was not shared or communicated to physicians of the modern age. It wasn't until William O'Shaughnessy, a British physician serving in India, shared a 40-page paper revealing the medical use of cannabis that some of cannabis's traditional uses were finally unveiled and began getting utilized.

Toward the end of the 19th century, the first efforts toward isolating compounds from the cannabis plant began. A group at Cambridge University processed Indian charas (hand-rolled hashish) into a rich red oil, which was later consumed by one of the lab technicians, producing a cannabis-like high. This first compound isolated from the plant was named cannabinol, now commonly abbreviated as CBN. CBN is typically produced as a breakdown product of THC, but still has similar effects on the body and can produce the classic high feeling from cannabis. It is thought that the scientists were trying to isolate THC from the charas, but during the extraction and purification procedures in 1896—when we didn't have sophisticated lab equipment, and everything took a lot of time and exposure to heat and oxygen—the THC they were trying to isolate ended up converting to mainly CBN. The molecular structure of CBN was later determined during the 1930s in the United Kingdom by other scientists.

During the mid-20th century, new technology was being developed in laboratories to allow easier purification of molecules from plant material. Cannabis contains more than 400 unique active compounds, and it is very difficult to separate them out, isolate them, purify them, and then characterize them. With the invention of modern chromatography (separation technology), scientists were now able to start isolating pure cannabinoids in higher amounts to study and identify.

In 1964, at the Hebrew University of Jerusalem, two chemists, Dr. Yehiel Gaoni and Dr. Raphael Mechoulam, isolated and characterized THC for the first time. This was a massive discovery that finally placed a molecule with the enchanting properties of cannabis, but it was still unknown what was happening in our body and why cannabis made us feel differently. It was great that we finally identified the molecule responsible for the effects, but HOW it was causing these effects in our bodies was the next mystery to uncover.

Something unique about THC, and other cannabinoids, compared to other drug-like compounds that have been discovered in nature is that THC is a very fatty molecule. Most compounds in our body that bind to receptors are not super fatty. So at the time, researchers assumed that THC and other fatty compounds from the plant acted rather indiscriminately or nonspecifically in the body—potentially interacting with the fatty membranes to cause some changes. However, it appeared that the natural compounds and some of the synthetic compounds being produced in laboratories showed very high levels of stereospecificity, meaning the configuration of the molecule matters A LOT to the level of effects it would induce in the body. Because of this specific nature, it was later hypothesized that it MUST act on some sort of target or receptor within the body—and that hypothesis was correct.

It wasn't until Dr. Allyn Howlett's laboratory at St. Louis University Medical School discovered a receptor in our body that was activated by THC and named it the cannabinoid-1 receptor (CB1). This was a MASSIVELY important finding proving that THC acts on a specific class of receptors called a G-protein coupled receptor (GPCR). GPCRs make up about 40% of drugs currently on the market (although this number may decrease as we see more biologic drugs produced) and have immense therapeutic value because of their specificity and drugability[4].

Energy is the currency of life. Our body would not produce cannabinoid receptors to the extent that it does if it didn't have a reason to. The cannabinoid 1 receptor is the most abundant type of receptor in the brain and is necessary for survival. This would lead a lot of people to think that maybe our bodies are designed for THC, but that is not the case. The vast majority of people and animals will never interact with the cannabis plant during their life, but they still have cannabinoid receptors in the body.

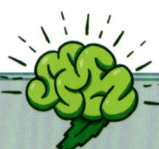

NUGS OF KNOWLEDGE

Cannabis is not the first instance where the traditional use of a plant has led to the discovery of a system within our body. Another well-known example is the case of the opium poppy plant or Papaver somniferum. *The milk or latex from the poppy plant was used for centuries both therapeutically and recreationally, and researchers were able to identify the main active compounds in the plant as morphine and codeine. Years later, the opiate receptors in our body were identified, as well as the forms, of these compounds produced by our own bodies: the endorphins, aka the endogenous morphine compounds.*

In 1992, Dr. Raphael Mechoulam's research group in Israel was the first to identify endocannabinoids, cannabinoids produced within our own bodies. Mechoulam's group first published on Anandamide—named after the Sanskrit word *ananda*, meaning "happiness, joy, or bliss"—in 1992, then 2-arachidonoyl glycerol or 2-AG (a much less sexy name for some reason) in 1995. Around this same time another cannabinoid receptor, the cannabinoid 2 receptor, was identified primarily in the immune cells (as opposed to the CB1 receptor, which is mainly in the brain).

Today, discoveries continue to be made, whether it is new cannabinoid or terpene molecules, or completely new classes of compounds in the plant. One such example is the flavorants, described by Abstrax Tech for the first time in 2023, which are smelly compounds from cannabis that are not terpenes but provide unique aromas like skunky or sweet. As the legal landscape relaxes for studying cannabis, we will continue to make discoveries that change how we dose and consume this medicine.

I do think it is a little silly how tight the regulations are on cannabis and testing animal models for cannabis because there are millions of people consuming this plant every single day. We spend millions on animal models and test tube experiments but haven't even begun engaging the community of daily consumers to understand the tangible benefits of using this medicine.

FURTHER SCOPE FOR CANNABIS RESEARCH

We are still struggling to understand the vast use of cannabinoid medicine and the importance of the endocannabinoid system in modern medicine and research. Because the ECS plays such a vital role in brain function, immune function, inflammation, metabolic health, pain, cancer, and so many other biological processes, **the potential for this medicine is unparalleled.** Most research that is done is still focusing on a singular molecule and the potential therapeutic value, a reductionist approach taken in almost all pharmaceutical studies because it allows us to create potential new drugs via the pharmaceutical pipeline. However, this is not how people are using cannabis, nor is it how people have traditionally used cannabis. Most side effects that we've seen from cannabis come when we isolate THC and other active components, raise the dose, and decrease the complexity of the medicine.

Although it is more difficult, we need to start studying cannabis in the context of complex plant medicine to fully understand the value of synergies in nature, molecular redundancy, and the benefits of chemically diverse medicine. Nature works in complex networks, not isolated systems. Once we fully release the shackles that have been at the feet of researchers for decades, we will start to understand this medicine in a modern context and use data to advocate for patient rights.

One such shackle that has been prominent in cannabis research has been the lack of access to the plant material for researchers to study. There currently is no avenue for cannabis research scientists funded through the government in the United States to study the products that are available on the legal market. Rather, a select few universities and companies can cultivate cannabis for research purposes. This is an improvement from where we were five years ago, when only the University of Mississippi was able to cultivate cannabis for research purposes. Later research found that the cannabis grown at this university was not representative AT ALL of the products available to consumers—the university's plant genetically resembled hemp much more than the THC-dominant cannabis used by most consumers.

Despite the massive scientific progress, there are still many unknowns in cannabis as there are hundreds of compounds in the plant—and the amount and type of molecules differ based on what strain or chemotype it is. Additionally, our bodies are very complex, and have different levels of receptors, endocannabinoids, metabolism, brain chemistry, etc. There are still many unknown molecules in this medicinal plant, just like there are unknown molecules in the tea you drink before bed, or unknown pathways to how pharmaceutical medications work in the body; but an unknown in cannabis is much different than an unknown in a synthesized pharmaceutical drug.

Unknown compounds in a pharmaceutical or synthetic cannabis product were made in the laboratory and have only been used for a short amount of time. The unknowns produced in the plant are molecules we have already been consuming for decades at least. We don't fully know the chemistry of most natural products including other medicinal plants, fungi, and bacteria. Having faith in the unknown, and understanding that we do not currently have the scientific tools to evaluate the complexity of this plant medicine combined with the complexity of the human body, can be part of the spiritual connection to this plant. People knew of cannabis's medicinal benefits long before modern lab equipment because of the way it has healed our mind and body.

The molecules Skatole and Indole were just identified in cannabis in 2023 for the first time. These molecules highly resemble psychoactive compounds like DMT, and it is hypothesized that they contribute to the feeling of mysticism when consuming some varieties, a feeling consumers have been aware of despite lacking the molecular evidence for a long time. **What else haven't we discovered scientifically that may contribute to our unique experience? Do we have to isolate it to know it exists, and can we even detect it with our current tools?**

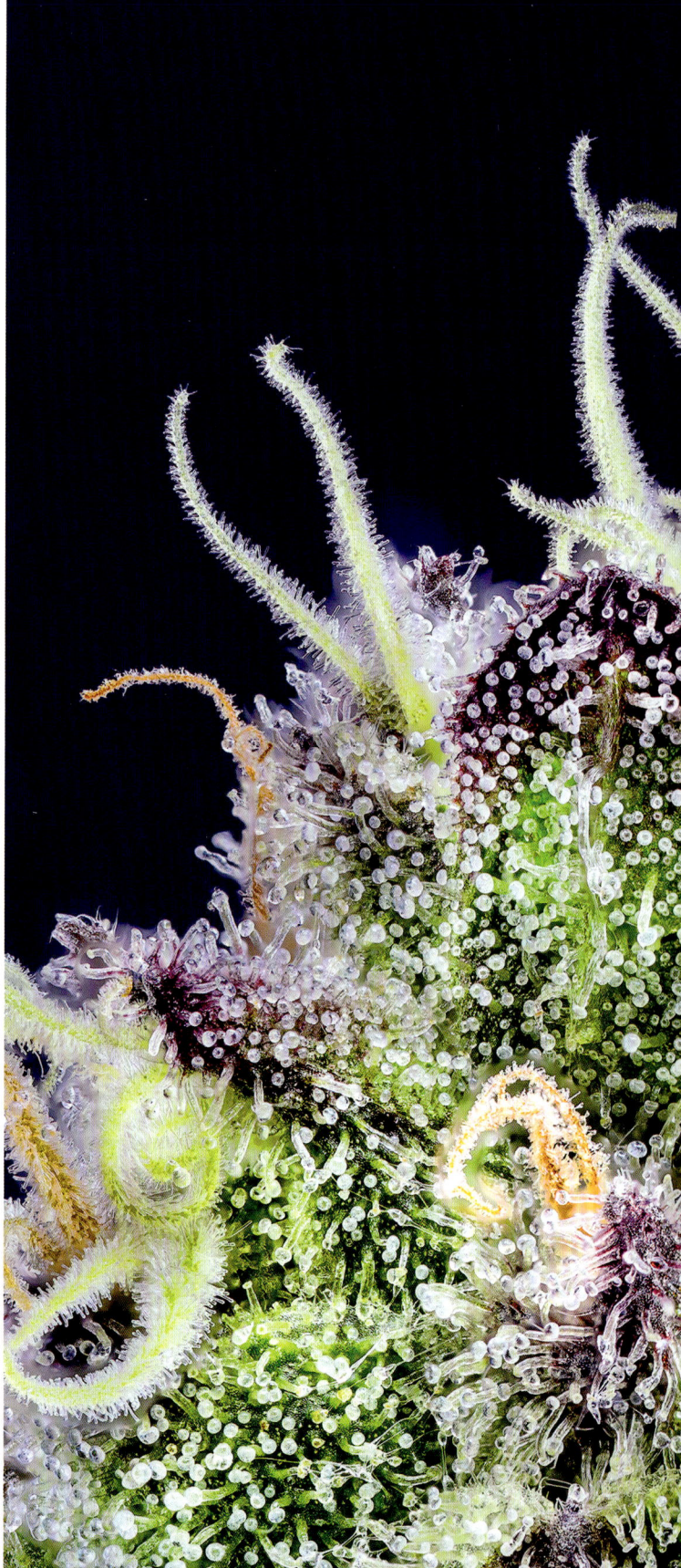

SMOKE BREAK

LET'S RECAP WHAT WE LEARNED:

⇄ Despite cannabis having hundreds of medicinal benefits and no recorded deaths, it remains a schedule 1 drug—categorized as having no medical value and a high potential for abuse—while alcohol and tobacco, which are more addictive, remain legal.

⇄ The prohibition of cannabis is strongly influenced by political lobbying from powerful industries such as tobacco, alcohol, and pharmaceuticals, which see cannabis as a threat to their market share.

⇄ Cannabis has been cultivated and used for thousands of years, with historical records showing its use for fiber, medicine, and spiritual purposes in cultures from China to the Southwest Asia, Africa, and Europe.

⇄ The war on cannabis has disproportionately affected Black and brown communities, with arrests for cannabis possession being significantly higher among these populations, even though usage rates are similar across races.

⇄ Despite significant scientific discoveries proving cannabis's medicinal properties, regulatory barriers continue to hinder research, and the fight for full legalization and the right to home cultivation remains ongoing.

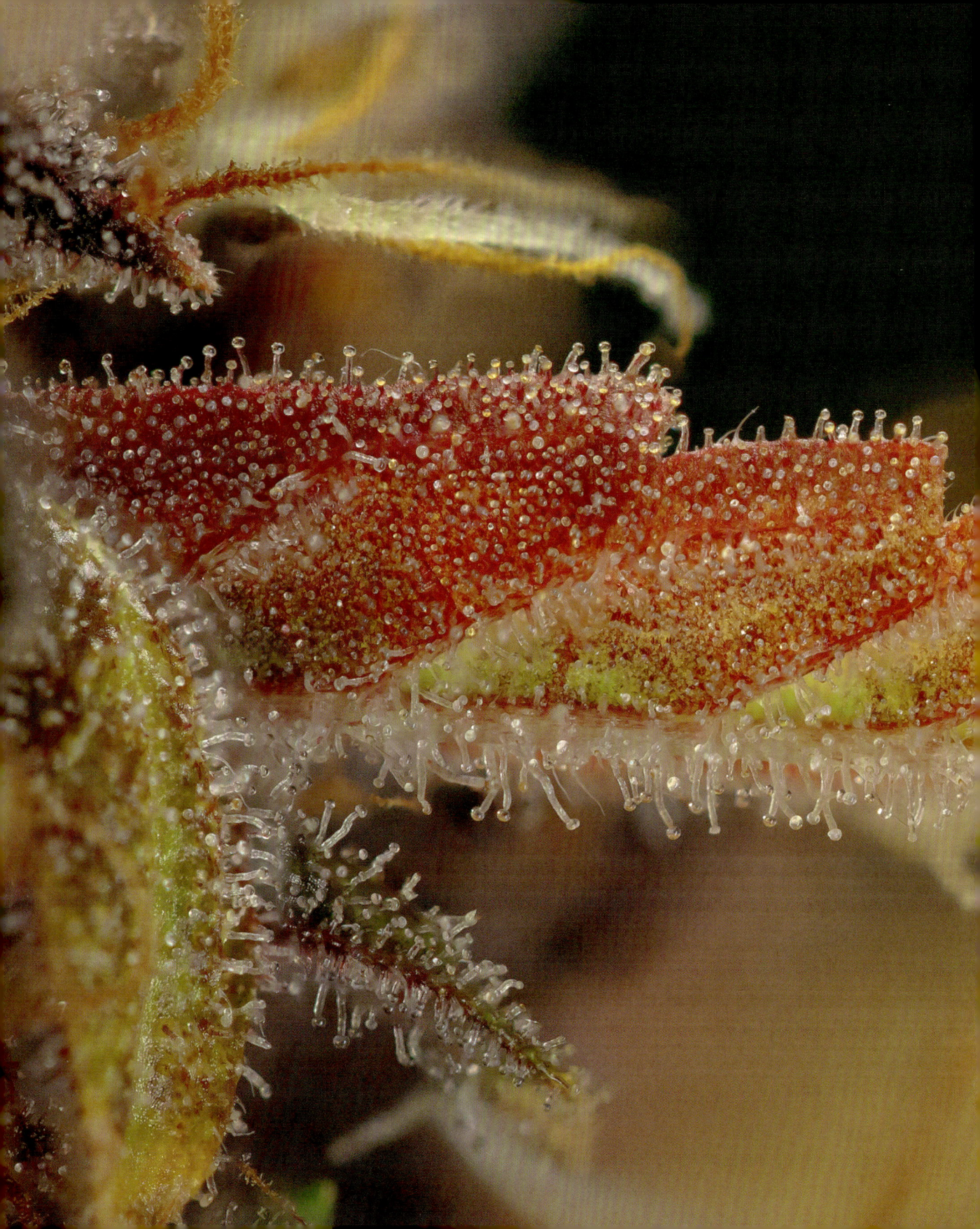

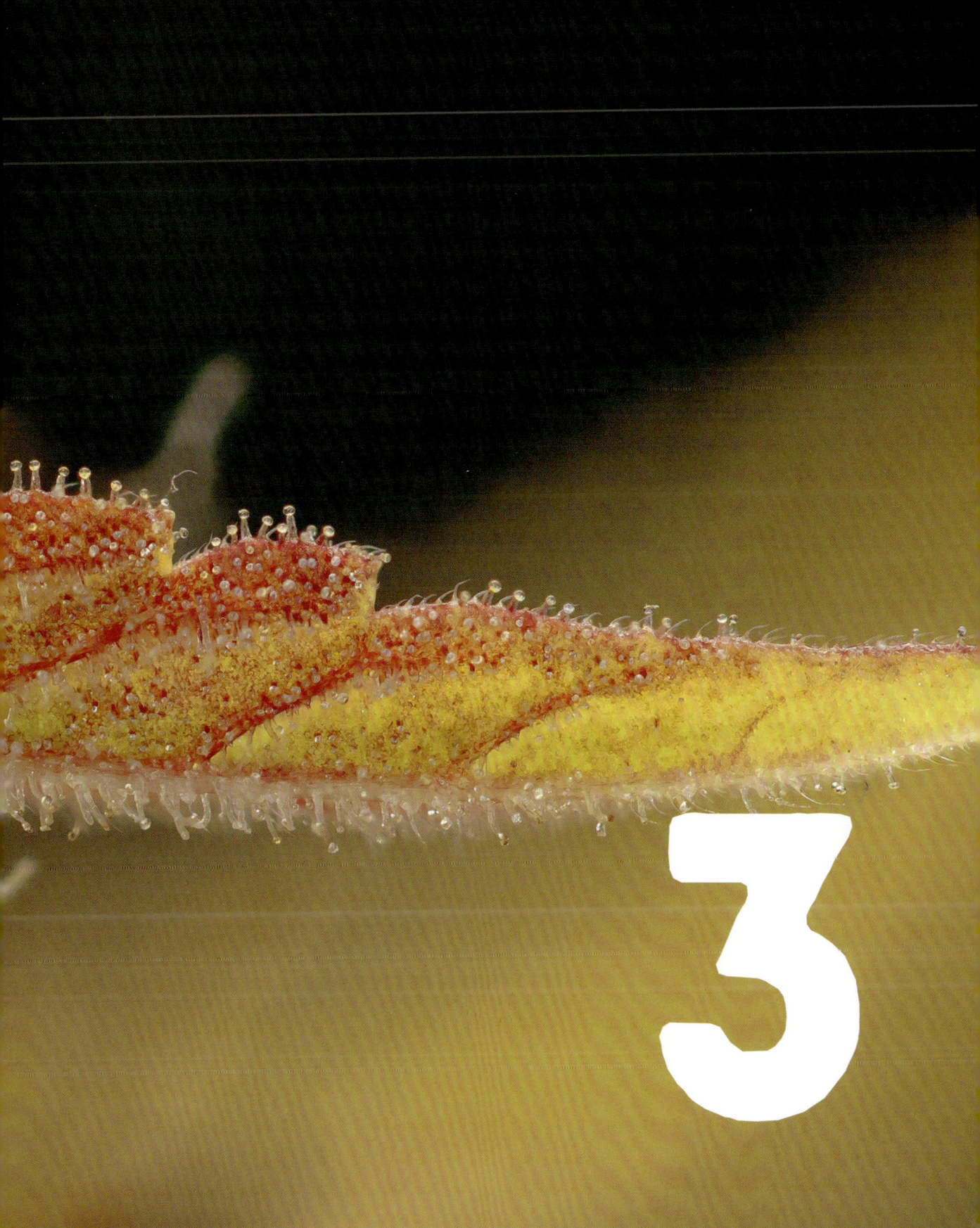

3

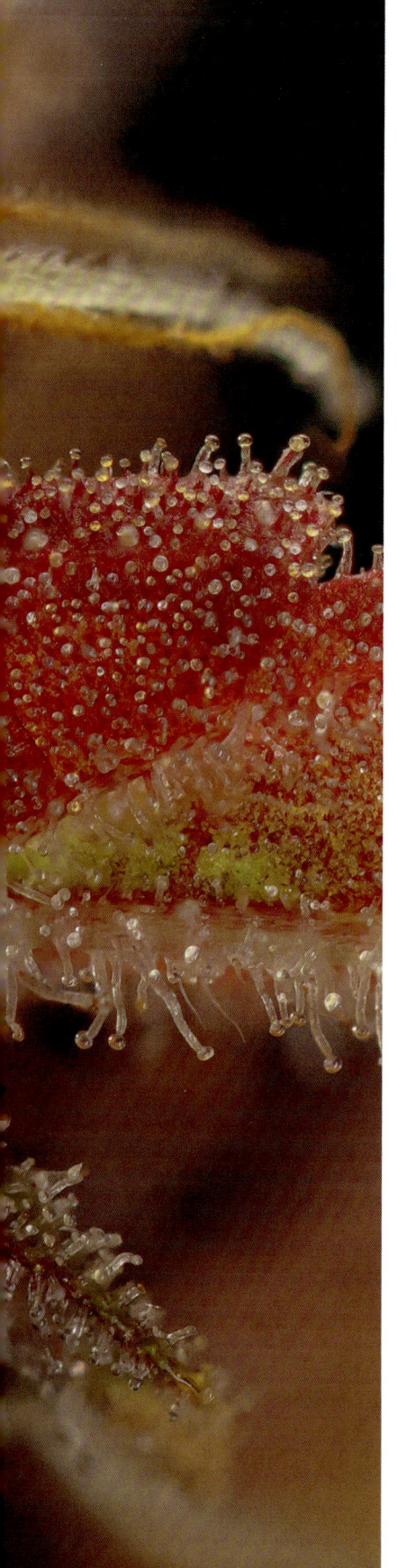

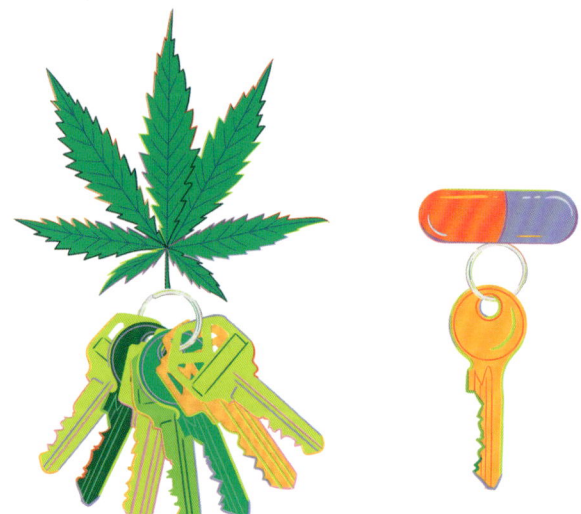

MOLECULES, RECEPTORS, AND THE ENDOCANNABINOID SYSTEM

It's no secret that cannabis is good for... everything. Do you have a headache? Gut issues? Sore knee? Weed might help. Yet, while cannabis offers solutions for many, not everyone's dosing will look the same. Our bodies are dynamic, and our dosing of cannabis products should also be.

Learning to use cannabis—and figuring out how to gauge your body's needs and sense patterns in your health—is a practice of learning your body.

Throughout this chapter, we will be looking at some of the science behind how weed works with our body In doing so, we will be referencing many different molecules found within the plant and/or our own body. Think of each individual molecule that we discuss as a very specific key to the locks, or receptors, located within your body. When we look at a whole plant extract of cannabis, with hundreds of different molecules, there are hundreds of different keys present. Not every key can unlock every lock in the body—each one leads to a very specific interaction.

On a molecular scale, the amino acids that make up a receptor (lock), have specific polarity and configurations that attract or repel certain types of molecules. If the right key is present, it will activate the receptor and unlock the lock—allowing the molecule to engage in a series of interactions, and eventually open the door to medicinal possibilities. Other factors like the physical size of the molecule and the location of the receptors in the body are also important, and we will continue to discuss.

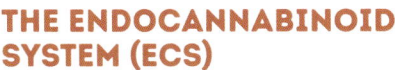

THE ENDOCANNABINOID SYSTEM (ECS)

The interaction of cannabis with the endocannabinoid system is the basis of how this medicine is good for so many different things. The ECS is in every organ of the body and intertwined from your eyeballs to your sweat glands. Some cannabis products target specific areas of the ECS—for instance, if you apply a topical lotion on your skin, you are activating the cannabinoid receptors on that specific part of your body—while other means of consumption, like taking edibles or smoking, have a more widespread and less localized effect.

The endocannabinoid system (ECS) is made up of three main components:

> **1. Cannabinoid receptors:** The targets that cannabinoids bind to in the body.
>
> **2. Enzymes:** Molecular machines that build and break down the endocannabinoids.
>
> **3. Endocannabinoids:** Molecules or signals your body makes that act on cannabinoid receptors.

RECEPTORS

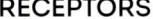

Receptors are long threads of amino acids folded to create a specific binding pocket for their molecules of choice, and these are the reason you feel any sensation in your body. They are small satellites sitting all over you—in every organ, every tissue, every cell of your body—waiting for a very specific key or signal.

Receptors are the way that your body talks to itself. If your leg needs to communicate to your brain that it's in pain, it is going to use molecules and receptors to get that message across. If you accidentally place your hand near a hot stove, your thermoreceptors will be activated to quickly let your brain know to move your hand. You have specialized receptors for touch, temperature, smell, vision, inflammation, and literally everything else your body does.

A receptor can tell when the right or wrong molecule is present depending on how the molecule interacts with it. If the shape of the molecule can perfectly interact with the binding pocket, the receptor can be turned on or activated.

Binding Sites

This isn't the first book to use a lock and key metaphor to describe pharmacology. The classic lock and key example is a good way of describing what is referred to by pharmacology nerds like myself as the **orthosteric binding site**, or the main keyhole.

My friend Evan uses the term "molecular cargo pants" rather than locks to describe receptors. He says it better explains how complex receptor-drug interactions can be. In the way that cargo pants have one pocket perfectly shaped for your phone, another for your wallet, a third for your tater tots, and so on, some receptors offer additional binding potential as well. Each key or molecule has the potential to bind to multiple different locks, and there can even be multiple different key holes on the same lock. These other places that a molecule could bind to a receptor are called **allosteric binding sites**, and they are relevant for how you may dose your cannabis products.

If a molecule binds to the allosteric site (secondary site), it may slightly change the shape of the receptor in a way that doesn't allow other molecules to bind to the main site, or it might alter the way they interact with the receptor. In some cases, an allosteric compound can enhance the way something else binds—this is called a **positive allosteric modulator**. In others, it can negatively affect it—this is a **negative allosteric modulator**. A negative allosteric modulator on the CB1 receptor can balance out the effects of THC, and CBD is one of the best known examples[1]. **This is why combining CBD with THC often leads to less anxiety and paranoia.** CBD can help prevent overstimulation of the cannabinoid receptors, which can be critical for people who are prone to anxiety or are extremely sensitive to the effects of THC.

Interestingly, our bodies produce both positive and negative allosteric modulators of the cannabinoid receptors, which work to fine-tune the effects from our endocannabinoids. A compound called lypoxin A has been shown to be a positive allosteric modulator on the CB1 receptor, and pepcan-12 and pregnenolone are negative allosteric modulators[2]. Pregnenolone has even been trialed as a potential antidote to cannabis overconsumption and a possible addiction treatment for other substances.

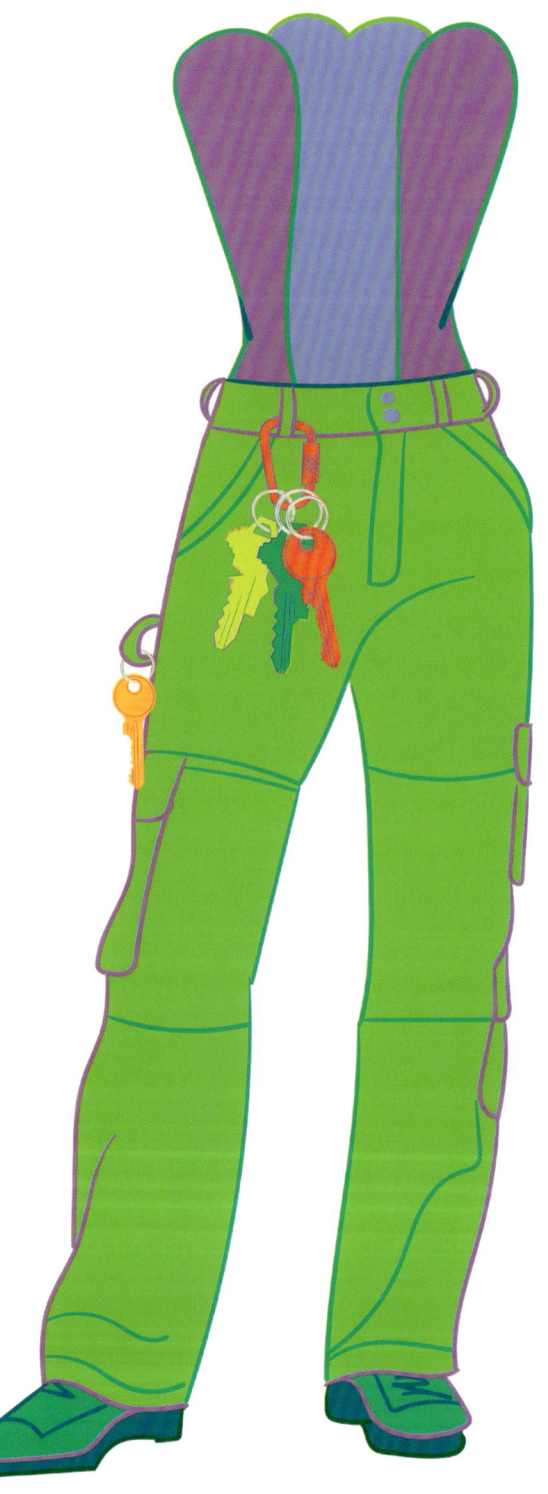

Types of Receptors

We are going to discuss two different types of receptors in relation to cannabis and the body:

1. G-Protein-Coupled Receptor (GPCR)

GPCRs are the most common type of receptor that drugs bind to, and the targets of most pharmaceutical drugs. GPCRs are shaped like a ribbon that is intertwined throughout a membrane with seven ribbons going back and forth–the odd number 7 is important here. One end of this receptor is on the outside of the cell and one is on the inside of the cell, allowing molecules that are floating around the outside to bind and initiate a reaction on the inside of a cell–sort of like a phone line from the outside world to the inside world.

The two main receptors in the ECS are the cannabinoid 1 (CB1) and cannabinoid 2 (CB2) receptors–these are both GPCRs. Because the purpose of the ECS is to bring balance or regulate the other systems in the body, one could argue that every receptor in the body is technically part of the ECS, **because there are no isolated systems in the body**, but we will be focusing on the ones that compounds in cannabis directly act on. Although these other receptors are not the main players in the ECS, they are pieces of the puzzle that is cannabis medicine. Examples of receptors that are part of the larger endocannabinoid-ome are GPR55, another type of G-protein coupled receptor, and the serotonin receptors 5HTXX–which are named after the chemical name of serotonin: 5-hydroxytryptamine (5-HT).

2. Ion gated channel

When a molecule binds to this receptor, a channel opens through the membrane, allowing specific ions, like sodium or magnesium, to pass through TRPV channels are a type of ion gated channel involved in the therapeutic actions of cannabis and cannabinoids, especially for pain management.

Agonist or Antagonist

There are multiple ways a molecule can interact with a receptor beyond just "unlocking it." Some molecules can turn off a receptor, some turn on a receptor; some just sit on top and prevent other things from binding to the receptor, like shoving bubblegum in a lock; and some bind to the side of the receptor, slightly changing how the receptor works.

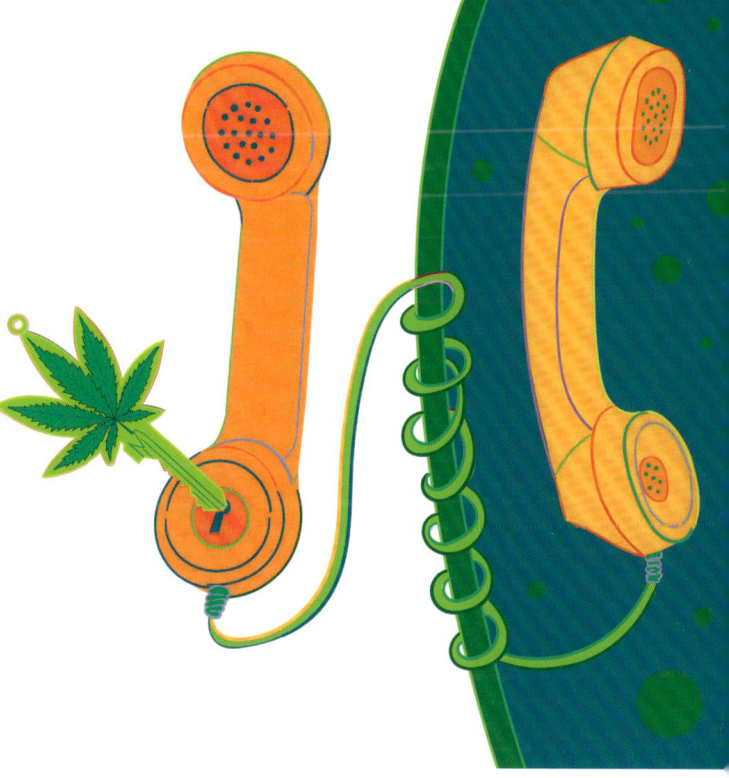

In general, if a drug or molecule turns on the receptor, it is called an **agonist**. If it turns off the receptor, it's called an **antagonist**. Some drugs are agonists at specific doses and antagonists at other doses; some drugs can act as an agonist on one receptor and an antagonist on a different receptor.

The Cannabinoid Receptors
1. The Cannabinoid 1 (CB1) Receptor

The CB1 receptor is one of the most abundant receptors in the brain, and it's critical for our survival. The CB1 receptor is located on the presynaptic neuron, which produces, stores, and sends the neurotransmitters like serotonin, dopamine, GABA, and glutamate to the next neuron. This is unique, because other receptors are located on the postsynaptic neuron, which typically receives the signals, as most of these other receptors are waiting to receive the brain signals and then carry on that message in the form of an electric signal called an action potential. In Chapter 1 we discussed these molecules flowing like a river–for typical neurotransmitter signaling the messages flow down the river from neuron 1 to neuron 2.

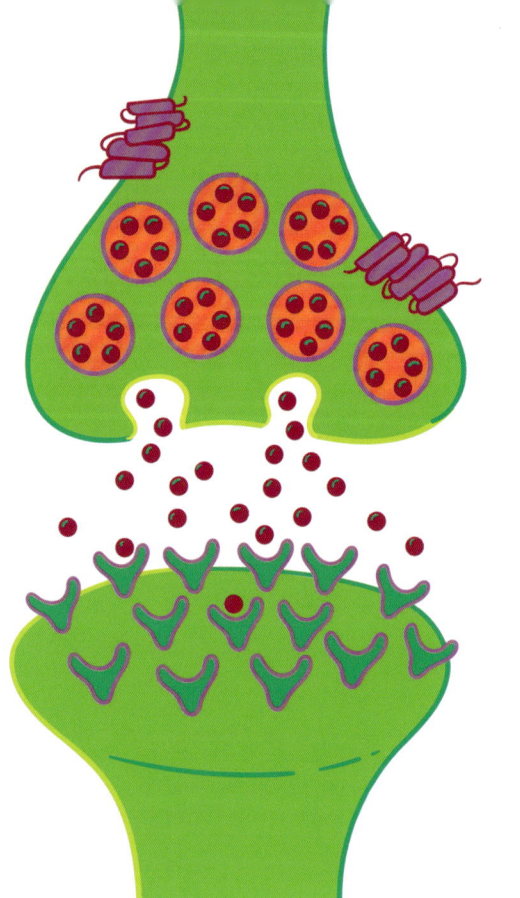

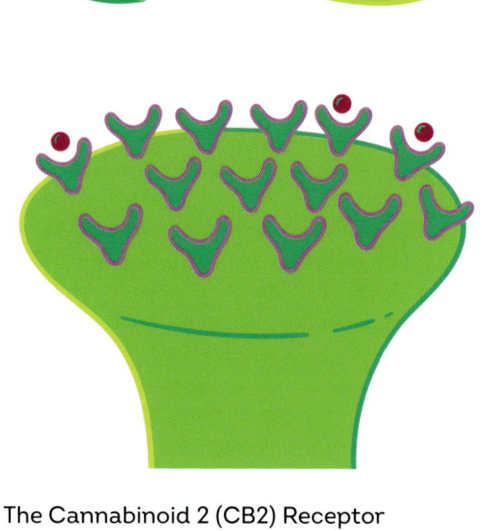

However, the main goal of CB1 is to control the release of OTHER neurotransmitters in the brain, not to send action potentials. As the CB1 receptors are located on the opposite neuron compared to the other signaling systems, **it is operating in the opposite direction**. This is called retrograde signaling. **The ECS is the only retrograde signaling system, which is why it is the master regulator in the body.** Therefore, endocannabinoid signals are traveling upstream to the CB1 receptor, against the current of the other brain messages. Think of the CB1 receptors as cops on our brain cells: if one of the neurotransmitters is speeding and acting erratically, the CB1 receptor is activated to stop the signal before it causes too much damage.

CB1 receptors are widespread throughout the brain, but they are the most abundant in the frontal cortex, the hippocampus, cerebellum, basal ganglia, solitary tract, and cingulate gyrus[3]. These areas are the parts of our brain responsible for nausea, memory, creativity, balance, social behaviors, and many other of the distinct changes that we associate with cannabis use.

2. The Cannabinoid 2 (CB2) Receptor

The CB2 receptor has a very different role in the body compared to the CB1 receptor. Rather than regulating neurotransmitter release, it is heavily involved in inflammation and the immune system. Although the CB1 receptor is mainly found in the brain, and the CB2 receptor in other areas of the body, there is still considerable overlap between the two. After all, our brains still have an immune system, and the CB2 receptors can be found on some of the brain's immune cells—such as microglial cells—and the other immune factories in our body like the spleen, thymus and tonsils. The CB2 receptor on the brain's immune cells has been speculated to be involved in a variety of brain conditions caused by chronic inflammation like Alzheimer's disease, Parkinson's disease, multiple sclerosis, stress, and addiction[4]. Although both the CB1 and CB2 receptors are cannabinoid receptors, they share only 44% similarity between the two receptors. They are activated by different compounds, located in different areas, and serve different roles in the body.

ENZYMES

Nobody likes to talk about enzymes because they're not sexy and they don't have sexy names, but they are incredibly important components of the endocannabinoid system. The main role of the enzymes in the ECS is to build the endocannabinoids when needed and then immediately break them down after. Enzymes are like little molecular machines. Each enzyme has a job, and the job in this case is to either build endocannabinoids using the fats in our bodies, or to break them down into fatty building blocks to be recycled and used later.

Because endocannabinoids are made from fatty molecules in our body, taking supplements with healthy oils like fish oil or hemp seed oil can help supplement our ECS and provide the necessary building blocks for synthesizing more endocannabinoids. Hemp seed oil contains high amounts of omega-3 fatty acids like alpha-linolenic acid (ALA), which are naturally present in a 3:1 ratio to omega-6 fatty acids—a ratio shown to be optimal for human health and utilization.

DRUG TARGETS

The enzymes in the ECS responsible for synthesizing and breaking down endocannabinoids have been a focal point for the development of some clinical drugs. This approach parallels that of selective serotonin reuptake inhibitors (SSRIs), aiming to prolong the presence of endocannabinoids in the synapse by preventing their enzymatic breakdown and enhancing their effectiveness. These prolonging effects have been studied for social anxiety, pain, and PTSD.

For example, inhibiting the enzyme responsible for breaking down anandamide, called FAAH, has been studied extensively. A French clinical trial for a new drug called BIA 10-2474 that targeted FAAH was even tested on humans. However, there were very severe side effects to this drug, leaving one person dead and others hospitalized. This isn't the only story about pharmaceutical drugs that manipulate the ECS going very wrong and should be a lesson to scientists moving forward.

Additionally, there are other enzymes called fatty-acid binding proteins (FABP) that help transport our bodies' endocannabinoids to the proper enzymes for metabolism. These represent another potential drug target to increase endocannabinoid activity. In fact, both THC and CBD bind to FABPs[5]. This mechanism is thought to be part of how CBD works for epilepsy, as it affects endocannabinoid levels.

These enzymes are also "drug targets" for natural products beyond the cannabis plant. Other plants also have compounds that inhibit these enzymes, such as a compound from the red clover called Biochanin A that has been shown to be a potent FAAH inhibitor, or kaempferol found in broccoli.

NUGS OF KNOWLEDGE

The way we know whether something is an omega-3 versus omega-6 fatty acid is where the first double bond is located from the end of the molecule. Omega-3s have a double bond three carbons in, and omega-6s have a double bond six carbons in.

kaempferol

Biochanin A

Endocannabinoid	Make (synthesize)	Break (degrade)
AEA	NAPE-PLD (N-arachidonoyl phosphatidylethanolamine phospholipase D)	FAAH (Fatty Acid Amide Hydrolase) and COX-2 (Cyclooxygenase-2)
2-AG	DGL (Diacylglycerol Lipase)	MAGL (Monoacylglycerol Lipase)

ENDOCANNABINOIDS AND ENZYMES

Because endocannabinoids are produced on demand, utilized, and then immediately recycled, they can act very **locally** in the body. This ability to specifically act on one location, even one cell, is unique to the cannabinoids produced by our body. When we smoke or eat cannabis products, the cannabinoids from the plant, like THC, don't selectively activate some cannabinoid receptors. Instead, they hit your body like a wave and activate receptors in multiple areas of the brain and body–globally not locally.

Some components of the ECS are relatively constant and broad; this is called "basal signaling." Other signals that are more targeted and specific are known as 'phasic signaling'. Although both main endocannabinoids are thought to have significant overlap for their role in the ECS maintenance, it is generally believed that AEA works more in a constant manner and 2-AG more as a reactive response[6].

In our body, both major endocannabinoids, AEA and 2-AG, activate both the CB1 and CB2 receptors at different levels. 2-AG is a full agonist, meaning it is capable of fully activating the receptors while AEA is a partial agonist and can partially activate the receptors[7].

CANNABINOIDS

Cannabinoids are a class of compounds defined as molecules that activate cannabinoid receptors in the body. But there are different types of cannabinoids, classified based on where they are made.

Something that makes cannabinoids unique is that they are fat signaling molecules, whereas most other signaling and drug compounds are much less fatty.

NUGS OF KNOWLEDGE

The fatty nature of all cannabinoids is why we infuse THC into other fatty things like butter and oil, rather than non-fatty things like water–because "like dissolves like" meaning a fatty base will dissolve a fatty substance. This is also why we can use water filtration in bongs and bubblers and not lose any of the active compounds- cannabinoids won't dissolve in water but some of the other junk in smoke will!

ENDOCANNABINOIDS

Endocannabinoids are molecules that are naturally produced within our bodies. They act as signals that send messages through cannabinoid receptors. Endocannabinoids are involved in regulating many things in the body including memory, pleasure, movement, time perception, appetite, and pain. Sound familiar? These are also many of the ways that THC affects the body. The main endocannabinoids and THC act in very similar ways in the body. It is likely that the cannabinoids in the plant evolved to mimic the role of cannabinoids in the body of other animals like insects or herbivores.

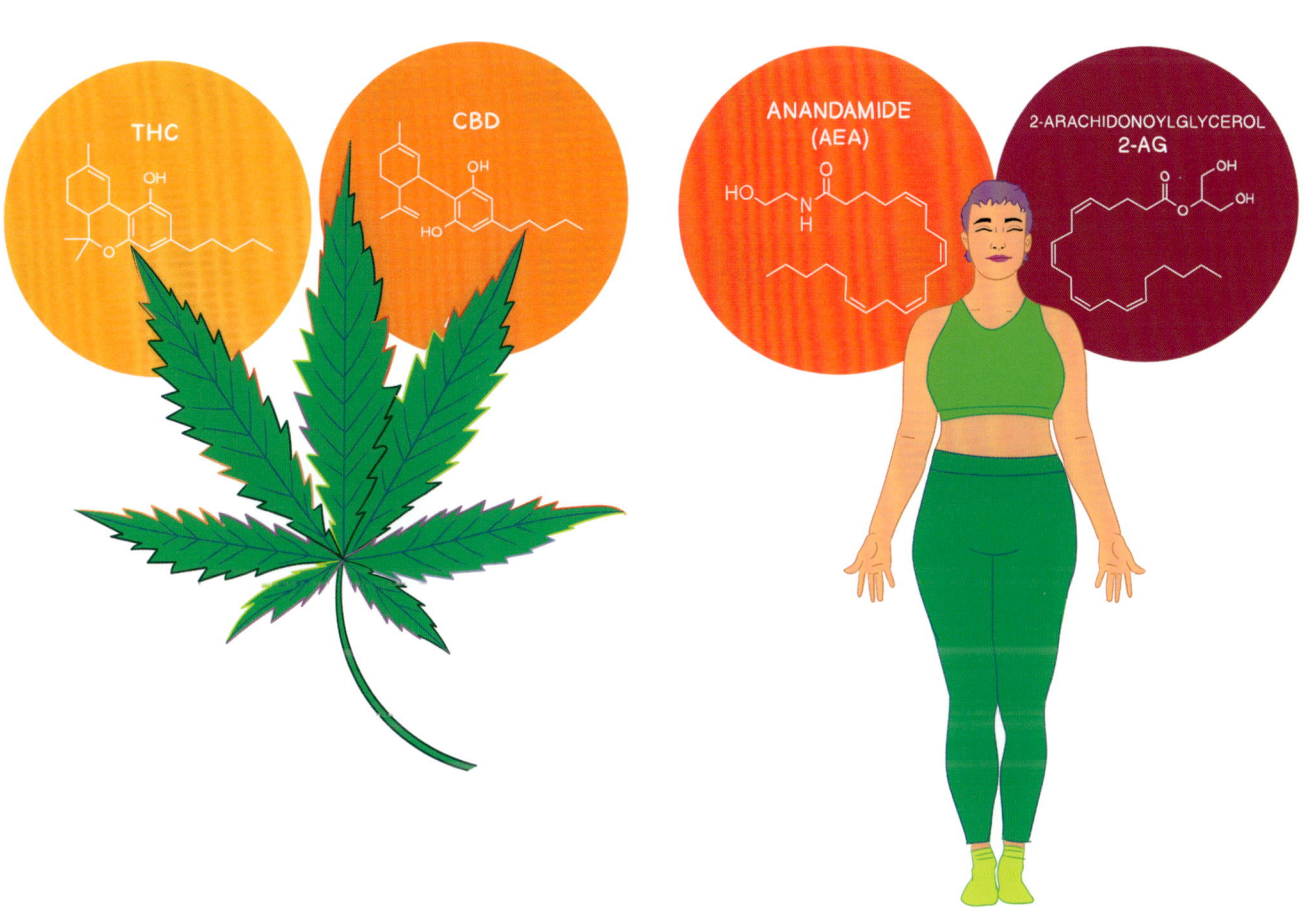

Structure

Endocannabionids are really long and really flexible. Their spaghetti-like structure allows them to be twisted and folded in different ways—the molecule lacks rigidity. It is a long, thin cord with some kinks in it. Because of this, these molecules can take a variety of shapes, wiggle through cell membranes, and bind to a variety of receptors in different ways, acting like flexible keys.

In contrast, THC is much less flexible. It contains rings in its structure that allow it to hold itself together. One of those rings is broken in the structure of CBD—which is the only structural difference between THC and CBD—making it much less rigid. Losing that ring frees the CBD molecule to twist and fold in new ways, allowing it to conform to different shapes and be more promiscuous on different receptors.

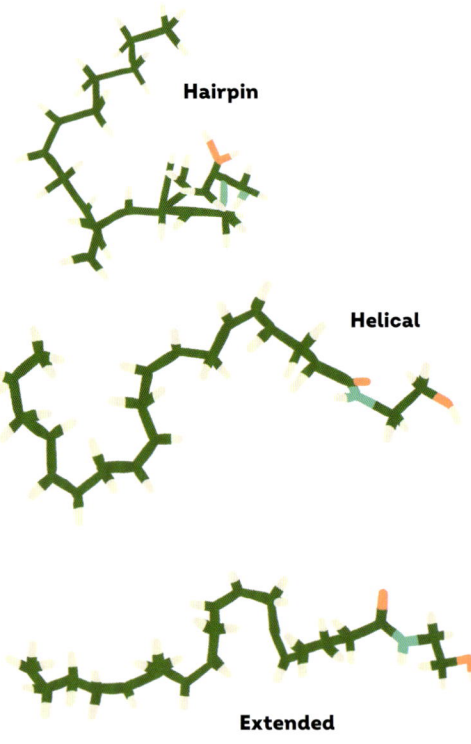

Hairpin

Helical

Extended

Some endocannabinoids are interesting combinations of neurotransmitters, like dopamine or serotonin, paired with arachidonic acid—the base skeleton of most endocannabinoids—but we still aren't fully sure what each molecule does in the body.

Endocannabinoid Tone

Endocannabinoids are used to regulate important functions like memory, sleep, and inflammation. The levels of endocannabinoids change throughout the day as well as throughout months and years as our body develops and changes. **Endocannabinoid tone** refers to an individual baseline level of endocannabinoids in the body, the rate they are being made and broken down by enzymes, and the level of cannabinoid receptors. Together, the ECS tone is how well your ECS is currently working to maintain balance in the body.

Now what would theoretically happen if your endocannabinoid tone was off, or low? **Clinical Endocannabinoid Deficiency (CED),** a theory developed by Dr. Ethan Russo in 2015, considers why people with chronic migraines, irritable bowel disease (IBD), fibromyalgia, and other treatment-resistant conditions react so positively to cannabis. It posits that these conditions, and likely many others, are caused by a reduced production of endocannabinoids, leading to a dysregulated state which can be inflammatory and often painful.

The Endocannabinoids Anandamide (AEA) and 2-Arachidonoylglycerol (2-AG)

Anandamide (AEA) and 2-Arachidonoylglycerol (2-AG) are the two main endocannabinoids that act on the cannabinoid receptors in our bodies. Anandamide, also known as N-arachidonoylethanolamine, or abbreviated as AEA, was the first endocannabinoid to be discovered. Much like THC, AEA works as a partial agonist on both the CB1 receptor and CB2 receptor.

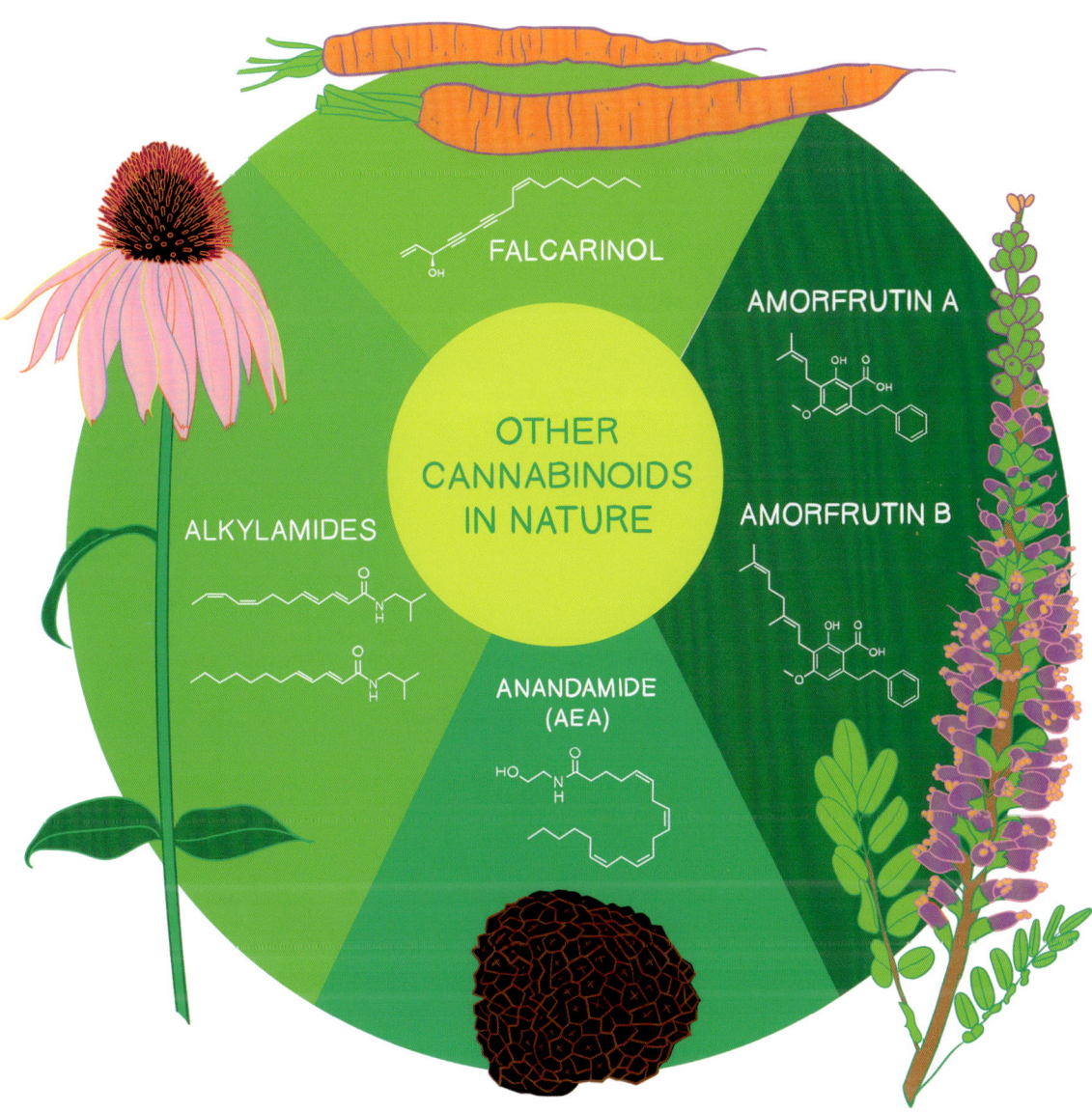

OTHER CANNABINOIDS IN NATURE

FALCARINOL

AMORFRUTIN A

AMORFRUTIN B

ALKYLAMIDES

ANANDAMIDE (AEA)

Although AEA and 2-AG look remarkably similar to each other, they are made and broken down by different enzymes, found at varied concentrations in the brain, and act on the receptors in distinct ways. As mentioned earlier, 2-AG can fully activate the CB1 receptor, acting as a full agonist, whereas AEA works as a partial activator or partial agonist of the CB1 receptor. 2-AG not only acts stronger on the CB1 receptor, but it is also found in much higher concentrations in the brain, estimated more than 100x higher than AEA[8]. Interestingly, some molecules found in the plant like CBD have been found to trigger the production and release of 2-AG, which is sort of like your body releasing a version of THC when we consume CBD[9]!

PHYTOCANNABINOIDS

Phytocannabinoids are produced by a plant—the prefix phyto- refers to something coming from a plant. When we discuss phytocannabinoids they are almost always coming from the cannabis plant, although there are other plant species capable of making compounds that activate the cannabinoid receptors and which are therefore cannabinoids.

Some examples are the purple coneflower (Echinacea sp.), which produces a class of compounds called the alkylamides that have strong activity on the CB2 receptor. Additionally, compounds found in carrots act on the CB1 receptor as antagonists, causing inflammation on the skin[10]. Various species of the flowering plant Rhododendron produce cannabinoids that are similar in structure to cannabichromene (CBC) or cannabicyclol (CBL) found in the cannabis plant. Some legumes like *Amorpha fruticosa* contain amorfrutins, which have cannabinoid activity, and various fungi have even been shown to produce halogenated cannabinoids like 8-chlorocannabiorcichromenic acid with activity on cannabinoid receptors.

Producing Phytocannabinoids

There are more than 150 cannabinoids produced in the cannabis plant, but not every cannabis plant produces every phytocannabinoid. A plant's production of specific phytocannabinoids depends on a few factors:

1. Genetics: Is the plant genetically capable of producing the molecule? Some plants are bred over time so that they gain or lose the genetic code for the enzymes to produce the molecules. If they don't have the blueprint, they can't build the compound.

2. The environment: Genes for producing specific molecules are "turned on" by specific environmental factors. For instance, THC amounts are directly related to light exposure because one of the roles of THCA is to protect the plant from UV damage. Therefore, if we give it more light, it produces more light protecting compounds. Other molecules in the plant have different triggers to create them, like the amount of bacteria, or animal predation, and if the environment is not correct it won't be produced, or will be produced at a limited level.

3. Energy is the currency of life: The cannabis plant has a limited amount of energy and a finite amount of molecules it can make. When evaluating the profile of a plant, you can often see the energy distribution through the molecules. For instance, a plant that produces 30% THCA typically produces very little other compounds like CBDA or CBGA because it has used the majority of its energy to make THCA. With balanced varieties, you may see 15% THCA and 15% CBDA, because the plant is able to increase the diversity of molecules but reduce the amount of each. What you don't see is 20% THCA, 20% CBDA, and 30% CBGA because this isn't feasible for the amount of energy the plant has for producing cannabinoids.

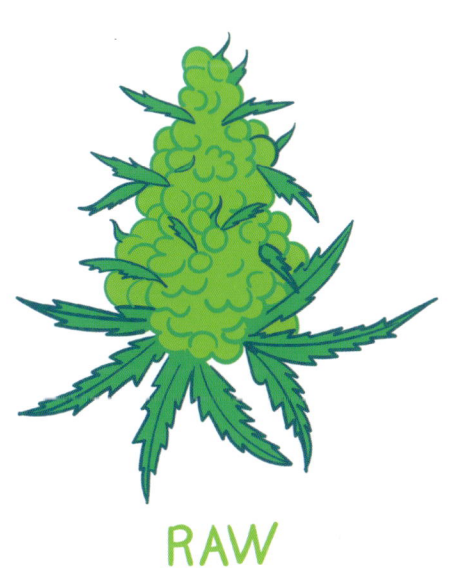

RAW

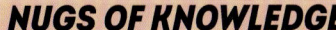

NUGS OF KNOWLEDGE

Varieties grown outdoors typically contain lower amounts of THCA, the precursor to THC, but a higher diversity of compounds. The plant's energy is used to protect itself from a variety of environmental stressors unique to outdoor growing, and can't funnel all of its energy toward THCA. Indoor cultivation of cannabis is often catered towards producing very high levels of THC, and in turn, often produces a lower diversity of other compounds.

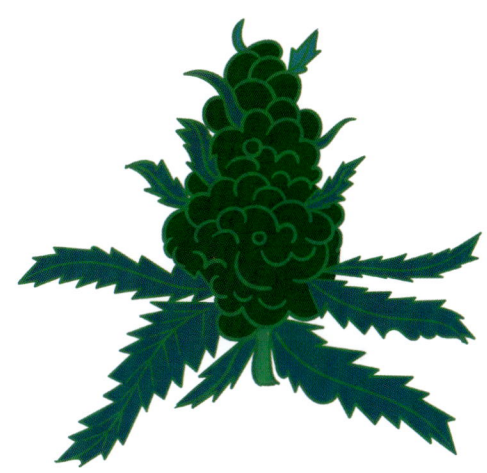

TRANSFORMED

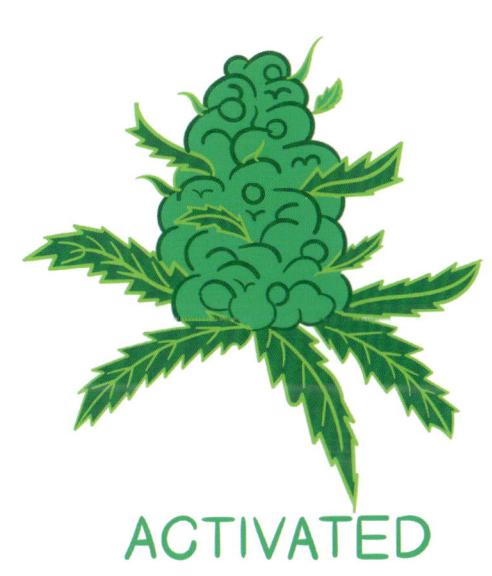

ACTIVATED

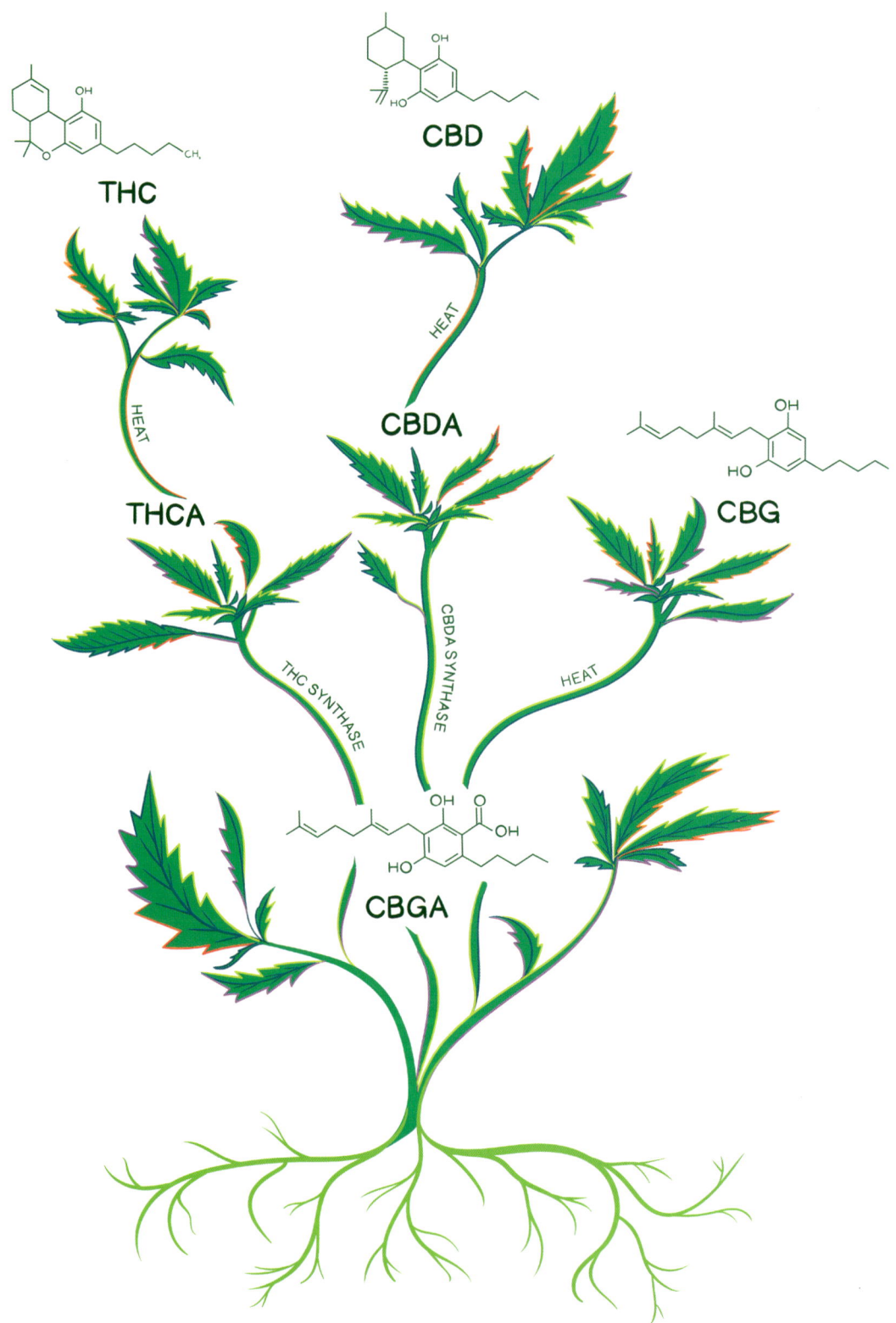

THC

CBD

THCA

CBDA

CBG

HEAT

HEAT

THC SYNTHASE

CBDA SYNTHASE

HEAT

CBGA

Acidic Cannabinoids

Phytocannabinoids go through varying levels of change throughout their life from when they're synthesized within the plant to when they tickle the CB1 receptors in our brains. When the plant is growing and producing the cannabinoids, it is producing them in the acidic form, meaning the actual molecular structure has an acid group on it in the form of a carboxylic acid, or CO_2. So, rather than CBD, the plant produces CBDA (acid), and rather than THC, it produces THCA. The reason all cannabinoids contain this same acid group is because all cannabinoids are built from the same starting materials, or the same mother cannabinoid.

The acidic cannabinoid cannabigerolic acid or CBGA is referred to as the "Mother of all cannabinoids" because it is the starting material that the plant uses to build other cannabinoids. Essentially CBGA is produced by combining two different molecules in the plant, then the plant uses a variety of enzymes to twist, fold, and modify the molecule to create unique structures. CBDA is produced from CBGA using the enzyme CBDA synthase, THCA is produced from CBGA using the enzyme THCA synthase, CBCA is produced using the enzyme CBCA synthase, and so on.

The acidic version of THC, THCA, does not get you high, but research suggests it may be a great option for anti-nausea or vomiting, chronic inflammation, and seizure disorders[11]. Although THCA does not have direct activity on CB1 receptors, it reduces inflammatory signals via other mechanisms and may also allow THC to interact with the receptors longer[12].

CBDA, the acidic precursor to CBD, has also been shown to reduce inflammation, and is much more bioavailable in the body compared to CBD. Interestingly, much of the research into CBDA points to it being a stronger and more efficacious compound compared to CBD. CBDA reduces inflammatory pain, anxiety, and nausea better than CBD does. Many of these benefits are likely due to CBDA's stronger ability to bind to serotonin receptor 5-HT1A. While CBDA shares CBD's ability to enhance 5-HT1A receptor activation, the acidic compound does not interact efficiently with CB1 receptors as either an agonist or antagonist[13].

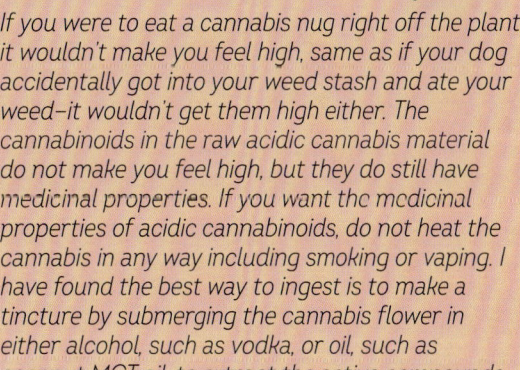

NUGS OF KNOWLEDGE

If you were to eat a cannabis nug right off the plant it wouldn't make you feel high, same as if your dog accidentally got into your weed stash and ate your weed–it wouldn't get them high either. The cannabinoids in the raw acidic cannabis material do not make you feel high, but they do still have medicinal properties. If you want the medicinal properties of acidic cannabinoids, do not heat the cannabis in any way including smoking or vaping. I have found the best way to ingest is to make a tincture by submerging the cannabis flower in either alcohol, such as vodka, or oil, such as coconut MCT oil, to extract the active compounds.

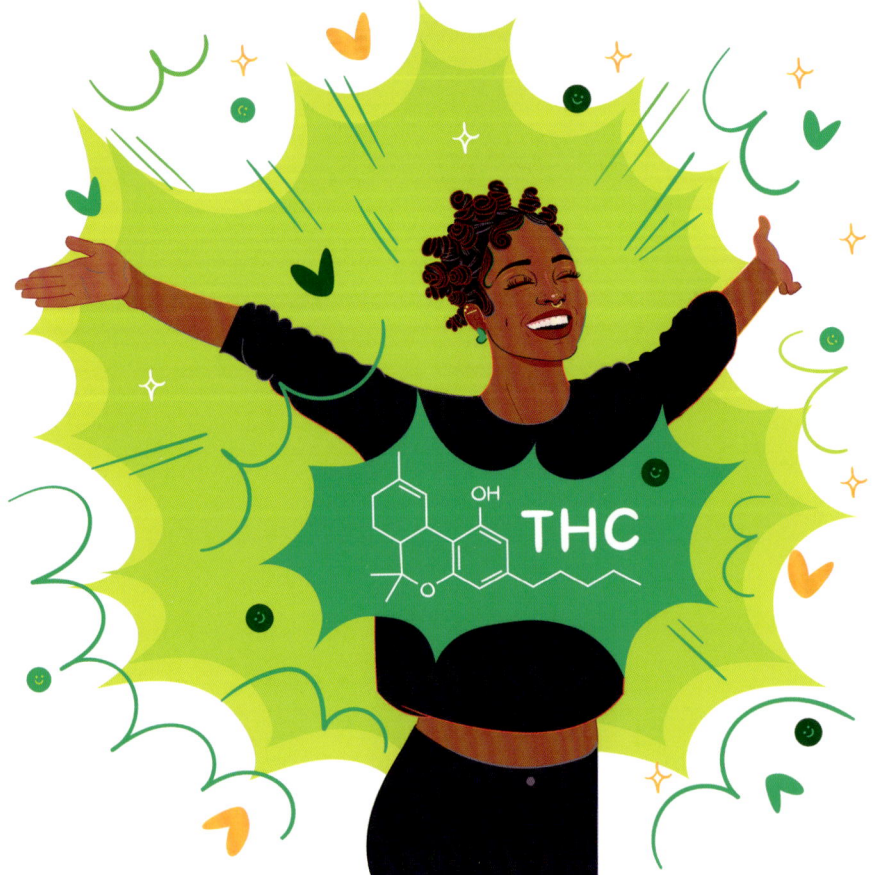

Activated Cannabinoids

The creative, funny, pain-free feelings we associate with cannabis are attributed to activated, non-acidic cannabinoids like THC and CBD. To activate the compounds, and remove their acid group, we simply heat the plant material which releases the acid. This is the process of **decarboxylation, because we are removing a carboxylic acid group**, but most of us just call it smoking weed. Anytime you smoke or vape cannabis, you are decarboxylating the herb and activating the compounds by removing the carboxylic acid. However, if you prefer to eat cannabis as edibles, you will need to heat the flower ahead of time to activate the compounds and feel the effects.

THC is the molecule in cannabis mainly responsible for many of the therapeutic and euphoric effects. However, the cannabis plant does not produce THC, it produces the acidic version THCA, which we activate by heating (smoking/vaping/cooking) to turn it into THC. THC is commonly referred to by its scientific name which is delta-9-tetrahydrocannabinol or just delta-9 THC because there is a double bond, or a delta, on the 9th carbon position of the molecule.

THC has known benefits for a variety of conditions such as reducing pain, increasing appetite, and enhancing mood. It also has antioxidant effects in the brain, anti-itch (think topicals) effects, and is a potent anti-inflammatory agent. THC acts on CB1 receptors as a partial agonist, or partial activator of the receptor, similar to how the endocannabinoid anandamide works.

THC is one of the best-known anti-nausea drugs ever discovered and can work for anything from gnarly hangovers to intense migraines. Marinol, a pharmaceutical drug that is pure THC, was approved for weight loss among AIDS patients, as well chemotherapy induced nausea.

THC often causes vasodilation—or expansion of the blood vessels. This is part of the reason why **many people use THC products before working out because it gets you ready for a good pump**, and why chronic cannabis consumers tend to have lower blood pressure. However, it can lead to some adverse effects like feeling dizzy or lightheaded, which is ESPECIALLY concerning for older people who may be at risk of falling.

THC acts in a biphasic manner, meaning at low doses it causes one reaction but at high doses a completely different response, which is really important for dosing if you are prone to anxiety. At low doses it can help relieve anxiety, but at high doses it can cause anxiety. So, if you're already having a rough day, have a stressful event coming up, or are simply an anxious person–keep the dose low and use products balanced with other compounds like CBD or THCV.

If you are using a THC product for the first time and don't know how or where to start, I would recommend starting low and slow. You may not even feel the effects at first, but at least you'll be able to tell how intensely your body reacts. If you're taking an edible, start as low as 1 or 2 milligrams. I like to take a 5 mg gummy or chocolate and cut it in half, giving a 2.5 mg dose. For flower, just one or two puffs. If you can, for both edibles and inhalables, look for balanced CBD:THC products when you are new to cannabis. Adding CBD is a form of harm reduction, especially for brains that are not used to the effects of cannabis. Some people are low responders to cannabis and may require higher than normal doses. Other people are high responders and may require a smaller dose. Until you understand your body's reaction to cannabis, play it on the safe side.

There are more than 100 peer-reviewed publications on THC and THC-related products; however, we are still missing a significant amount of relevant data on product types and doses as it is still virtually impossible to study products straight out of a dispensary with our current research landscape. Community knowledge is a treasure trove of expert knowledge from decades of self-experimentation. If you want to try cannabis for the first time, your best tool is going to be a seasoned cannabis consumer.

Delta 9 THC vs. Delta 8 THC

You may have seen a new cannabis market emerge in the past decade, with the birth of delta 8 THC products. Delta 8 THC (D8THC) is a naturally occurring compound from the cannabis plant. However, if you were to purchase a D8THC product online or at your local gas station or smoke shop, that D8THC is not from the cannabis plant. The cannabis plant does produce this compound, but it produces very little D8THC; most found within the cannabis plant is a breakdown product of the "regular" delta 9 THC (D9THC) from exposure to light and oxygen and is not produced in sufficient quantities to be extracted.

There are two main differences between D8THC and D9THC: the location of a single double bond in the chemical structure, and the fact that D9THC typically comes from the plant while D8THC typically comes from a laboratory. However, some companies are also producing synthetically made D9THC by converting it from CBD as well.

From a chemistry perspective, D8THC is more stable than D9THC because the electron's dense areas are more evenly distributed, leaving it less likely to be changed. This increased stability has led to researchers wondering if it may be a better drug candidate compared to the more common D9THC for some therapeutic purposes. However, I would argue that the best drug candidate is the one naturally produced in the plant which has an extremely wide safety profile, and has experienced millions of years of coevolution with animals.

Delta-9-THC

Delta-8-THC

Because the cannabis plant mainly produces D9THC (in acid form), which has clear activity on the brain, the compound is highly regulated and deemed a schedule 1 substance. Hemp-derived products remained legal because the hemp plant produces very little D9THC. However, the definition of a hemp-derived product is quite vague. So, hemp companies began taking pure CBD, and with a few steps in the laboratory involving heat and acid, converted the CBD to D8THC, or other synthetically made compounds similar to THC (they can also make hemp-derived D9THC). D8THC is about ½ to ⅓ less potent than D9THC, so it often takes more D8THC to feel comparable effects to D9THC.

The issue with D8THC isn't that its lab made; the issue is that it is lab made and is not regulated, while governing agencies overregulate and limit access to the natural product. With D8THC, or other synthetic hemp cannabinoid products like HHC or delta-10 THC products, there are no means of checking the safety before it reaches consumers' hands. In the legal cannabis market, plant products go through extensive lab testing before reaching consumers to ensure there are no residual solvents, pesticides, heavy metals, etc. There is no way to know which products are tested and which are not on the unregulated hemp market.

What bothers me more than anything about this market is that many consumers also don't know that these products are made synthetically. When they see THC on a label, they immediately assume it is from the plant and are not aware of what they are ingesting. Unfortunately, synthetic hemp-derived cannabinoid products are most abundant in places that do not have access to naturally occurring plant products due to prohibition. The limited access to the plant has led to consumers ingesting synthetic cannabinoids in place of safe, naturally occurring compounds.

THCV is your short friend–this molecule is literally shorter than the other cannabinoids and best known for helping **stop the munchies**. THCV has activity at both the CB1 and CB2 receptors but has a stronger affinity for the CB2 receptor[14]. Structurally, THCV's zigzag-like chain is similar to regular THC, but shorter by two carbons. This small change makes a massive difference in the role it plays in the body, leading to THCV acting almost opposite to THC at the CB1 receptor. At low doses, THCV works as an antagonist on the CB1 receptor or can effectively turn it off or down. At high doses, it is an agonist[15] (but not a strong one).

THCV has garnered the most interest as a compound to help with **weight loss**. Because THCV acts almost opposite to THC, at low doses–around 10 mg/day–it can help to suppress appetite[16].

Some THCV-rich varieties of cannabis can get as high as 16% THCV and likely even higher with more advanced breeding. Popular cultivars rich in THCV include Durban Poison, Tangie and Girl Scout Cookies.

THCV is also being researched as a tool to help take away the high feeling from too much THC. As THCV acts in the opposite way as THC it may be helpful in counteracting some of the negative effects such as paranoia and anxiety.

Other "short" cannabinoids also exist in lower concentrations, such as CBDV which is a potential treatment for nausea and vomiting as well as seizures via its activity on the TRPV1 channel[17].

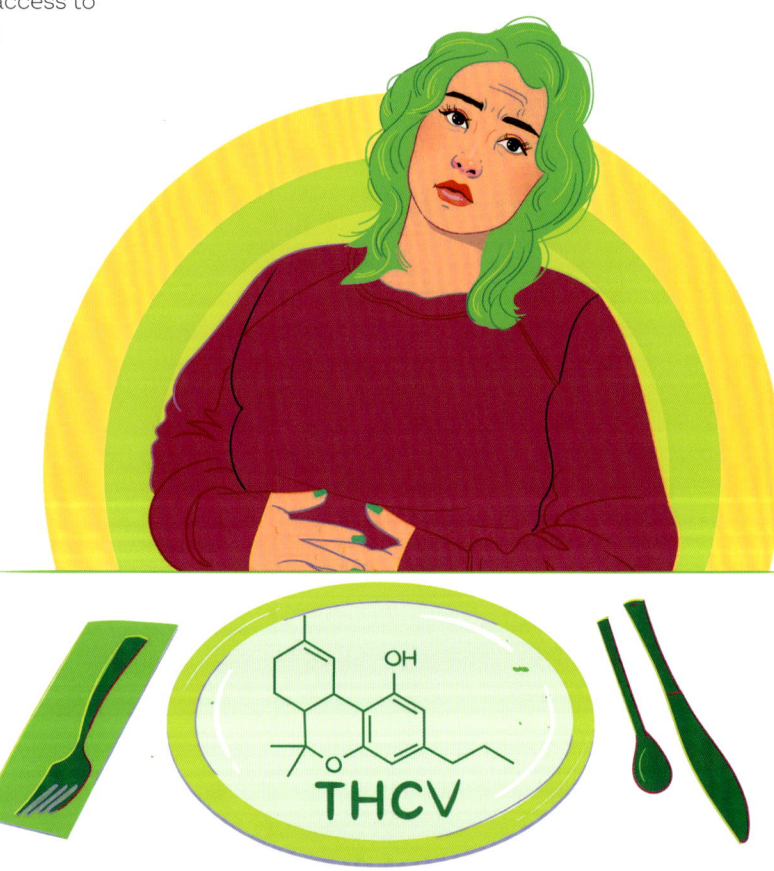

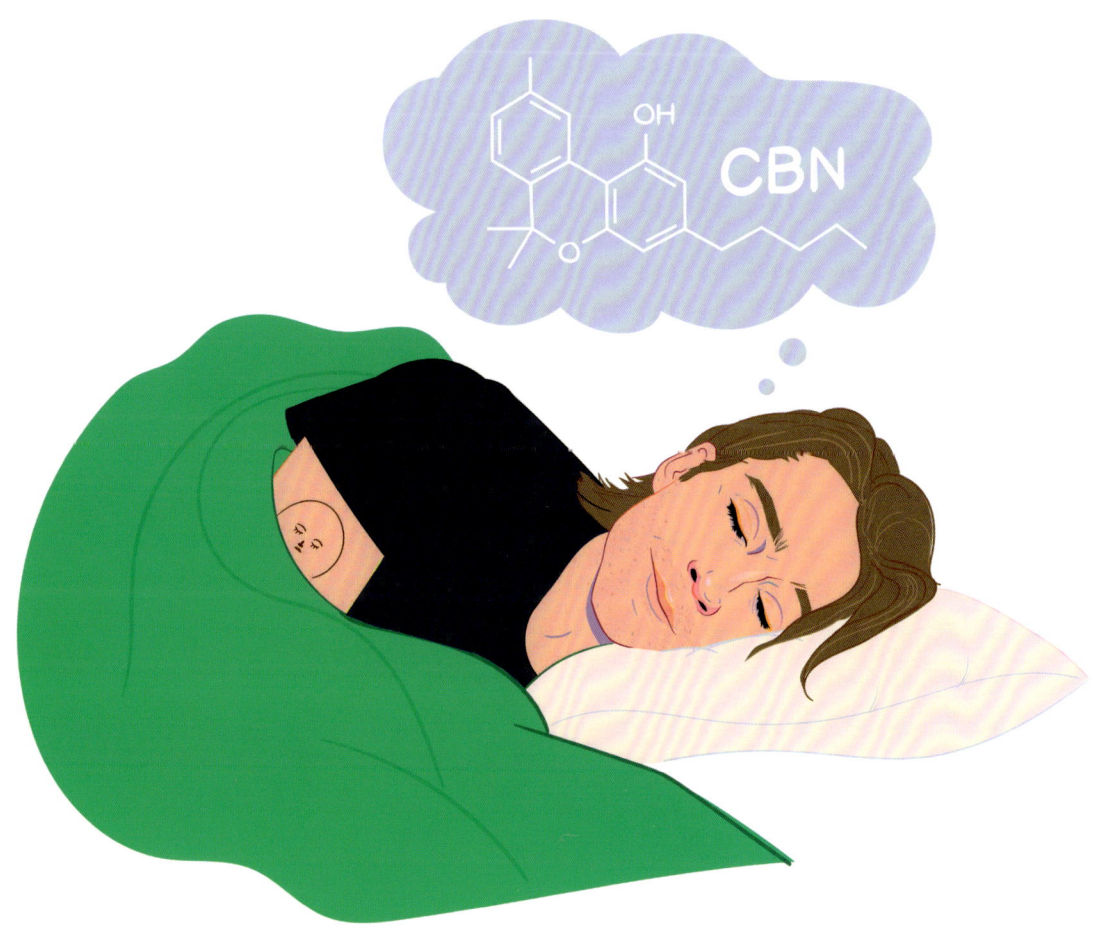

Cannabinol (CBN) is the main breakdown product of THC. Even though we often associate breakdown products as negative things, in this case, CBN is an important compound best known for helping people with sleep.

If you were to leave your THC products out, exposing them to oxygen, heat, and light, some of the chemistry would slowly begin to change. Although breakdown products don't always look like their parent molecule, CBN acts and looks very similar to THC. CBN is about ¼ as potent on the CB1 receptor in comparison to THC. This means it is still capable of making you feel high, but it takes higher doses and has less of an effect. CBN products are great for people who want the benefits of THC but are very sensitive to the effects. CBN has sedative, anti-inflammatory, antibiotic, and anticonvulsant properties[18].

Sleep is by far the most common effect that CBN is formulated for. Although the clinical data is lacking, one study found that 20 mg of CBN reduced the number of times someone awoke during the night and lowered sleep disturbance scores[19]. Another study in rats reported that CBN had sleep enhancing effects as long as four hours after administration[20]—but this study needs to be repeated in humans. These studies also indicated that CBN contributes to less of a groggy or "weed hangover" type feeling that many people get from THC, and I can attest to that. Those who wish to use cannabis for sleep but can't afford to feel the lingering effects in the morning, or need to still be ready and responsive if their child or loved ones need help during the night, may find CBN to be a nice, less-intoxicating alternative to THC.

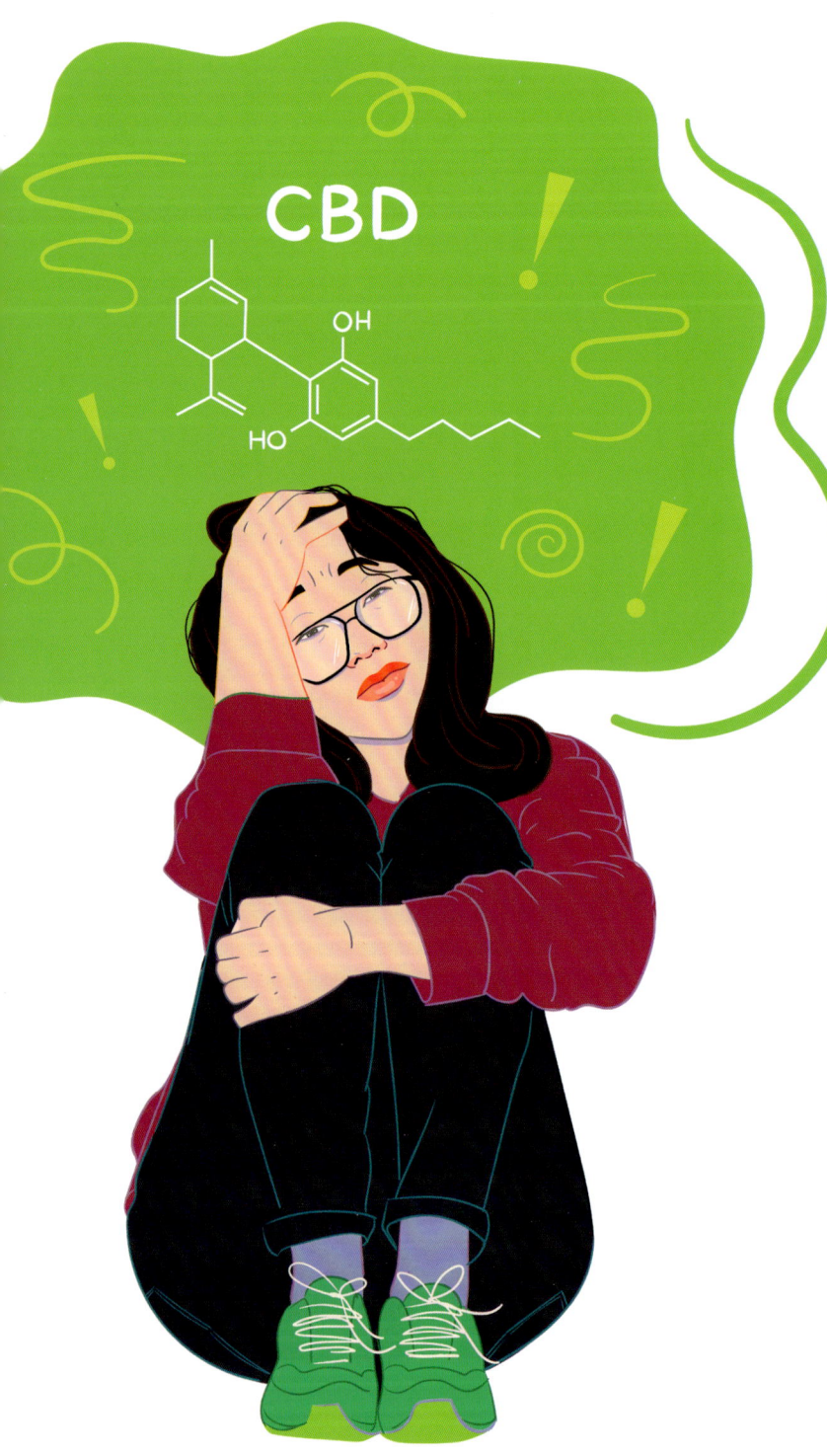

Because CBN is not being readily synthesized in the plant, you will not (or shouldn't) find high amounts of CBN in cannabis flower products. CBN-forward vapes, tinctures, topicals, and edibles are readily available because they are formulated with CBN isolate. The CBN isolate is typically made in a laboratory, but tested legal products are safe to consume and work very well for many people.

In topical formulations, CBN can help prevent excessive skin cell growth[21]. It is also being investigated as a solution to epidermolysis bullosa—a series of skin conditions that cause excessive itchiness—as well as topical burn care—because of the agonistic activity of CBN on the TRPV2 receptor, which is involved in high temperature sensing.

CBD does not produce a euphoric or high feeling when consumed. It is best known for helping with inflammation and is much more promiscuous than THC—CBD is not loyal to one receptor or even a few; it interacts with a myriad of different receptors in the body. In fact, **we still don't understand the exact mechanism by which CBD exerts all its benefits because it is very nonlinear.** CBD is a much more flexible key compared to THC, which is quite rigid. Because there is no middle ring in the structure of CBD like there is on THC, it can twist and turn and contort itself in different forms to fit unique receptors or locks.

CBD is best known for helping with seizure conditions, which led to the development of a pharmaceutical medication, Epidiolex, which is used to treat rare and severe forms of seizures. CBD is thought to help with seizures from a variety of mechanisms, such as by working on the GPR55 receptor located on neurons in the brain. CBD acts as an antagonist on this receptor and essentially blocks it from being activated, which in turn prevents the neuron from getting too excited, firing, and contributing to a seizure[22].

CBD is also used for a myriad of conditions such as pain, migraines, insomnia, anxiety, depression, and autoimmune conditions. Research has shown that CBD can essentially switch the body from producing pro-inflammatory compounds to anti-inflammatory compounds, altering immune responses and inflammation, which affects most conditions[23].

Furthermore, many pharmaceutical drugs for anxiety and depression target serotonin receptors. CBD is thought to help with mental health conditions like anxiety and depression by affecting the brain's response to serotonin, specifically through partial activation of the serotonin 5HT1A receptor–much like how pharmaceutical drugs for anxiety and depression target serotonin receptors–although the exact mechanism of CBD on this receptor is disputed.

Beyond this, CBD is thought to help with pain by acting on the TRPV1 channel as a potent agonist or activator. Activation of the TRPV1 receptor can help with pain and reduce inflammation associated with pain. Studies have shown that CBD not only contributes to less pain perception, but also an increase in pain tolerance[24]. TRPV1 receptors are found throughout the body including the skin, which is one way that CBD topicals work for pain.

Dosing CBD

In my opinion, the best use of CBD is to balance out the effects from THC and enhance the medicinal value of your cannabis. CBD can bind to the same receptor as THC, the CB1 receptor, but in a very different way. CBD acts on the receptor in a separate location, which does not activate the receptor, but changes the way that THC can interact with the receptor. This interaction with CBD and the CB1 receptor is called a **negative allosteric modulator**. This type of activity is especially important in conditions like seizures where it is important that our brains aren't overstimulated from THC, which can also cause seizures in high doses, and for preventing some adverse effects of THC like that on short-term memory or anxiety.

Dosing CBD can be difficult because most studies that research the effective dose of CBD are either conducted on animals or using pure CBD, which doesn't always represent the products people are taking. Different doses of CBD may be necessary for different effects, but I tend to believe most people are not taking enough CBD, as the research indicates you need 100mg or more to receive many of the therapeutic benefits. CBD, similar to THC, acts in a biphasic manner, so low levels have very different effects from high levels. For example, when taking CBD for sleep, many people respond best to a higher dose around 200 mg-600 mg because higher doses tend to have sedating effects whereas lower doses have stimulating effects and may be better for daytime use[25].

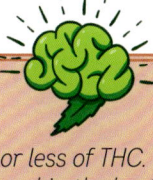

NUGS OF KNOWLEDGE

A hemp product must contain 0.3% or less of THC. However, when heat is applied to cannabis, the heat acts as a catalyst, transforming some molecules into completely new compounds, which in turn have unique action on our body. When you heat hemp flower, the heat changes some of the CBD into THC, and both D8THC and D9THC are produced. This means if you choose to smoke hemp flower you may feel more of an effect compared to taking a CBD tincture or gummy that is not exposed to heat. This additional formation of THC is likely received as a positive addition for most people, but it is good to be aware of. If you are incredibly sensitive to the effects of THC and don't want to be intoxicated, other consumption methods such as edibles or vaping at lower temperatures, may be the best for daytime use.

If you are taking CBD isolate, or pure CBD, it is safe to take it in relatively high doses. For example, studies on CBD and anxiety have shown a minimum of 200 mg to be effective[26]–Epidiolex for seizures is typically dosed between 300 mg to more than 1 gram (1,000 mg) per day. Although this is shown to be safe, that is a lot of CBD for your liver to process, and CBD does have some drug interactions. Studies have shown that even small amounts of THC combined with CBD can help lower the dose of BOTH compounds needed. In general, starting with at least 20 mg of a full spectrum CBD product and working your way up until you feel the desired relief is a good plan. Remember you won't feel "high" with CBD products, but you may feel the absence of pain or inflammation, enhanced mood, more flexibility, etc.

Cannabigerol (CBG) is a cannabinoid that comes from the acidic precursor in the plant CBGA or the mother of all cannabinoids.

Because CBGA is the starting material for so many other compounds it is often found at low concentrations as THCA is prioritized in breeding. However, new advances in cannabis genetics paired with new interest in CBG have led to selective breeding leading of cannabis that is very high in CBGA.

The molecular structure of CBG is very flexible, allowing it to take up more space on the active site of receptors. CBG has been reported to help with a wide diversity of ailments including glaucoma, bone diseases, neuroinflammation, inflammatory gut conditions, focus, and skin treatment for psoriasis[27]. CBG products, just like CBD products including flower, tinctures, gummies, etc., can be purchased legally online as many are classified as hemp that contains less than 0.3% THC. **These hemp products may be difficult to find in dispensaries because they are available online and therefore retailers don't need to pay the extra fees and taxes associated with cannabis-specific dispensaries.**

Topical formulations containing CBG can help reduce the inflammatory skin conditions of psoriasis by preventing the overgrowth of skin cells[28].

Beyond the skin, CBG and derivatives of CBG activate PPARγ receptors, act as an antagonist on serotonin 5-HT1A receptors, and act as a potent competitive inhibitor of anandamide–all of which can have neuroprotective effects. The activity on PPARγ could reduce the severity of several conditions like Huntingtons disease (HD), Parkinson's disease, and multiple sclerosis[29].

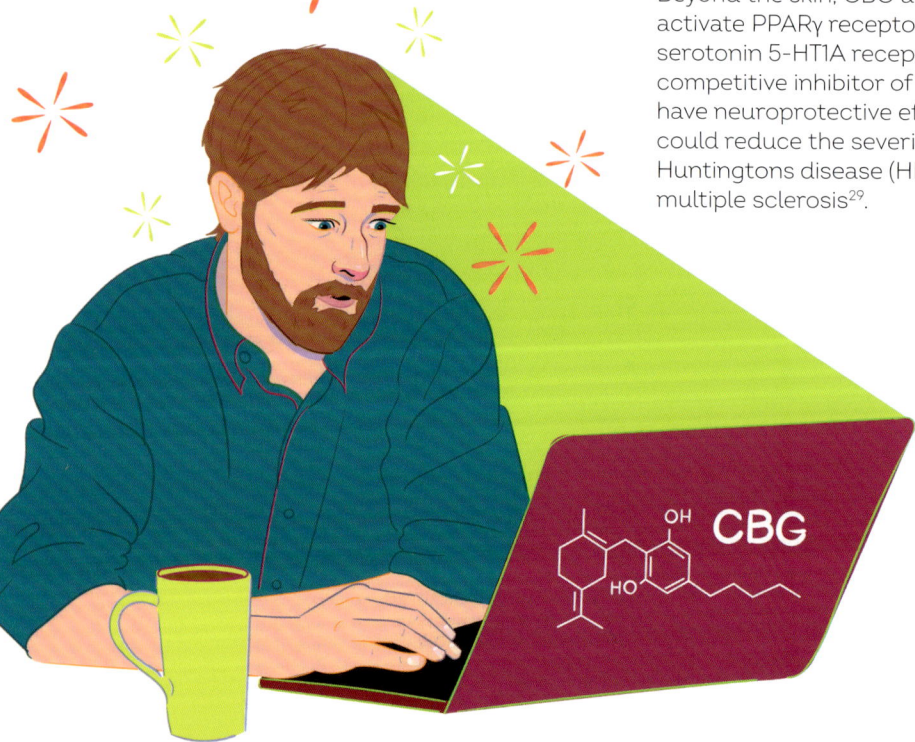

In cell and rat models of gut inflammation and colitis, CBG administration has significantly reduced inflammatory activity, prevented colitis-associated damage, and reduced tumor activity in colorectal cancer[30].

CBG also has antimicrobial activity against antibiotic resistant strains of *Staphylococcus aureus*, the bacteria responsible for staph infections[31]. Systemic studies in mice have shown CBG to be as effective as vancomycin at reducing growth.

Currently CBG is the only known cannabinoid that activates the α-2 adrenoceptor–this is likely why so many people use **CBG products during the day.**

Other drugs that activate the α-2 adrenoceptor like clonidine and guanfacine are used as antihypertensive (help lower blood pressure) agents, and to treat ADHD and issues with executive functioning. However, much of the details of CBG's activity on these receptors are still unknown so it is difficult to determine the true role of this receptor in CBG's wide pharmacology.

From personal experience, CBG does cause noticeable changes in the brain. My favorite way to consume CBG is in tincture form as I find a lot of CBG-dominant flower to be harsh to smoke, but the effects are fantastic. For daytime focus, while putting the brain at ease, it is my go-to cannabinoid.

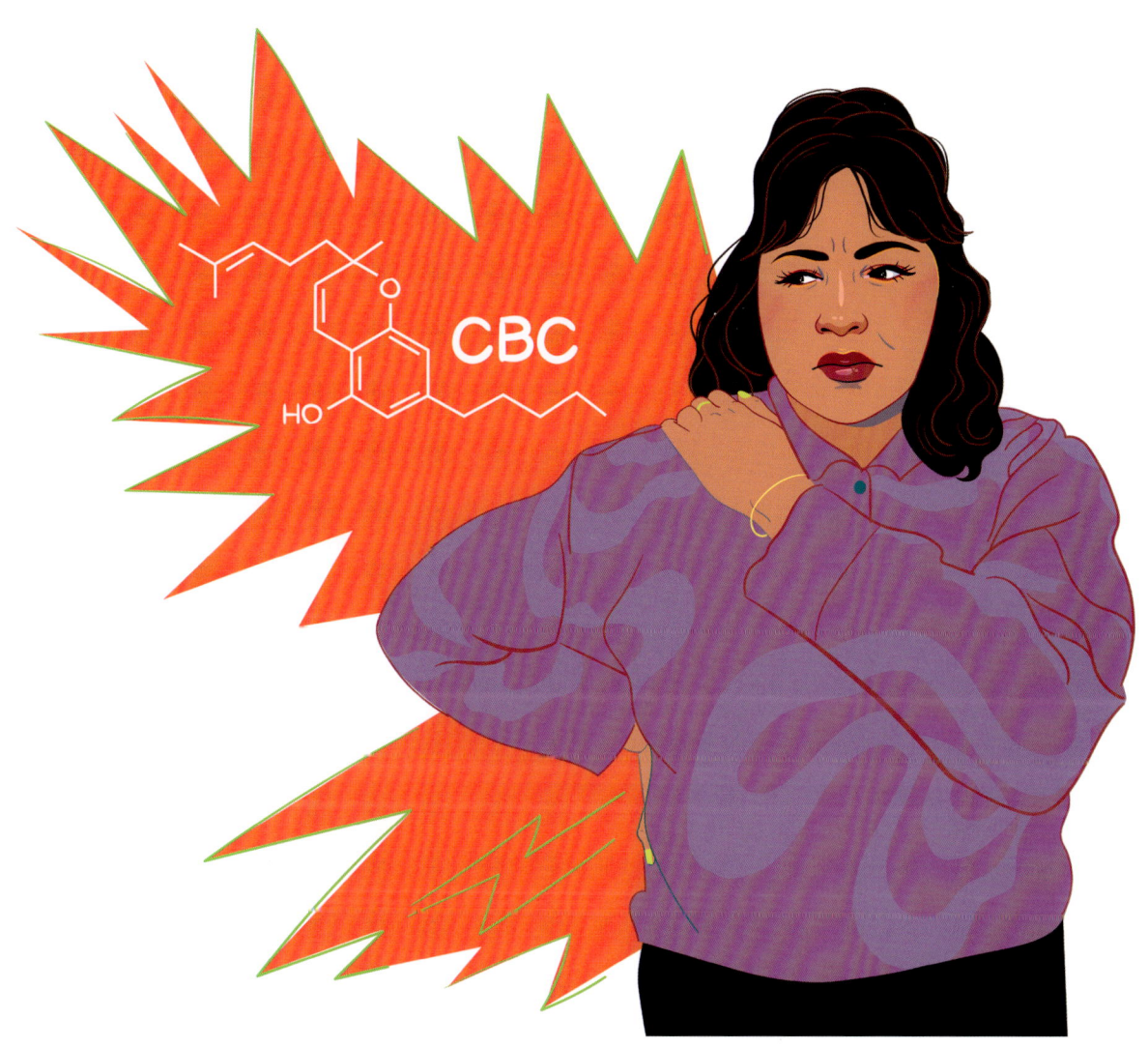

Cannabichromene or CBC comes from the acidic precursor in the plant cannabichromenic acid (CBCA), and some varieties of cannabis have relatively high amounts of cannabichromene. Varieties rich in CBC have been selectively bred for a recessive gene that produces this compound, and similar compounds to CBC have been isolated from other plants like the Rhododendron bush.

CBC is also easy to synthesize in the laboratory. Many products entering the legal market may have CBC that is not plant-derived but synthesized in the laboratory from precursors olivetol and citral. CBC products are currently rare on the legal cannabis market. However, I predict this will quickly change as more people become aware of CBC and the many benefits.

Evidence shows CBC can directly activate the CB2 receptor—but not the CB1 receptor—and inhibit the reuptake of anandamide[32]. Activation of the CB2 receptor may be beneficial for inflammatory conditions like pain, arthritis, neurodegenerative diseases, and cancer to name a few. Additionally, CBC has shown to have a positive effect on stem progenitor cells, which are essential in brain function[33]. As a CB2 agonist, CBC also lacks the CNS-related effects of 'getting high' or disoriented while still helping relieve symptoms. **Maybe more exciting, data suggests that CBC and THC have synergistic effects, especially in regard to pain, and may be used best in combination[34]—getting for pain relief from the anti-inflammatory CBC mediated through the CB2 receptor and pain relieving effects from THC mediated through the CB1 receptor.**

As far as dosing CBC products, one study found that CBC doses of up to 25 mg are generally well accepted. Although we don't have great data on how CBC is metabolized in edible form, it appears that CBC is better absorbed into the bloodstream compared to other cannabinoids like CBD and THC[35]. CBC breaks down into another cannabinoid called cannnabicyclol (CBL) when exposed to light or excessive heat during smoking. CBL is also found in aged hashish, but little is known about its activity in the body.

THE SMELLS OF CANNABIS

Cannabis is one of the stankyest plants—it is always obvious when people have cannabis on them or when they have just consumed. The smell of cannabis comes from a variety of stinky molecules but is most associated with terpenes.

TERPENES

Terpenes are small compounds that all plants produce, but cannabis specifically has been bred to produce high amounts of terpenes and a large variety. In general, when shopping for cannabis at a dispensary, the terpene levels in flower will be between 2-3%, but that can vary greatly depending on the cultivar, date of harvest, indoor vs outdoor grown, etc.

A molecule is classified as a terpene if it is a hydrocarbon (made of strictly hydrogen and carbons) and if it's made of a specific type of building block called an isoprene unit, which is a small five carbon chain. Interestingly, humans also produce isoprene and it's the second most dominant volatile compound in human breath[36]. In the plant, these isoprene units are combined by the plant's enzymes and folded in different ways to create the unique terpenes that we smell. If a terpene does contain oxygen as well as carbons and hydrogens, it's called a terpenoid not a terpene.

Many of the terpenes produced by cannabis are the same terpenes produced by other common plants and are the compounds responsible for their signature scent. For example, pinene is a common terpene and it is the main terpene in pine trees. Linalool is the signature scent of lavender and limonene is a common molecule in citrus plants. Humans have emotional connections to smells, and the smelly molecules can have direct bioactivity in our bodies, expanding the medicinal benefits and personalized medicine beyond cannabinoids.

The flowers of plants typically contain the highest amount of terpenes because the terpene's role in the plant is to attract or repel specific animals, usually insects. Terpenes are very light molecules, so they evaporate and float up our noses or into the air easily, sending their signals far and wide, attracting the right pollinators and hopefully repelling some hungry herbivores.

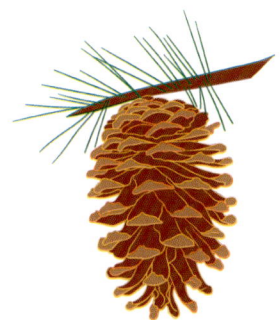

**PINENE
(PINE)**

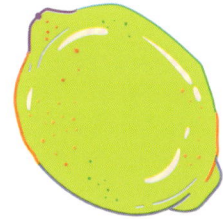

**LIMONENE
(LEMON)**

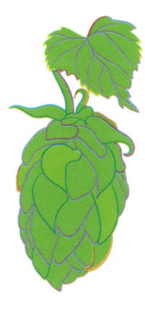

**HUMULENE
(HOPS)**

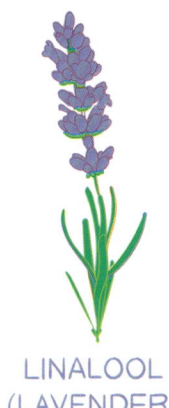

**LINALOOL
(LAVENDER)**

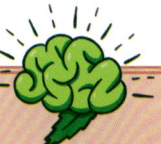

NUGS OF KNOWLEDGE

The leftover portion of a joint is often called "the roach"; one experiment that I was involved with researched the chemical composition of roaches and found that there were significantly higher levels of CBN (breakdown product of THC known for making people tired), and these heavier sesquiterpenes, also known for making people feel tired. Is this why smoking roaches feels different than smoking a fresh joint? One way to find out is from smoking a century joint, which is all the leftover flower from your roaches added together in one roachy, toasty joint.

The Mechanics of Smell

Different people have different affinities towards specific terpene smells. It is similar to the reaction that people have to specific perfumes.

Each person has more than 400 smell receptors in their nose that contribute to how we perceive scents. An individual's smell receptors provide them with a preference toward specific aromas as our sense of smell is more closely linked to our memory than any other sense. Think of grandma's spaghetti sauce, fresh cut grass, pool chlorine, that one specific sunscreen, etc. The way someone gravitates towards a smell could be a product of anything from a memory of the past to genetics involved in your smell genes. Small changes in the genes that code for how we smell can affect how strong someone finds an odor and how pleasant or unpleasant it is to them.

Smell changes as products age. When the plant is growing, it is producing a variety of different terpenes and other smelly molecules that have different sizes. The smallest of the terpenes are the monoterpenes that are made from two isoprene units added together. Because these are physically the smallest, they often evaporate the fastest. This is especially important when considering what happens to the cannabis plants after harvest. Post-harvest, the flower is typically dried and cured. During the dry and cure process, the plants often are in areas with good airflow and moderate temperatures, which causes some of the terpenes to be lost to the environment. The heavier terpenes like sesquiterpenes, which are made from three isoprene units, are heavier, and therefore evaporate slower so less is lost to the environment.

Many in Number

In cannabis, the signature smell is not attributed to one singular terpene, or two, or three—it is created by a complex mixture of many terpenes and other compounds. Some varieties or strains have different dominant terpenes, some have different ratios of terpenes, and some have the presence or absence of specific terpenes. Each of these terpenes is not equally important to the plant, nor equally potent on our nose; therefore, the plant is always going to need more of some specific compounds and it may require less of more specialized terpenes. The most common terpenes that you will encounter on the legal market are β-caryophyllene, β-myrcene with others like pinene, α-humulene, and limonene coming in next.

You'll also start to see repeating patterns of specific terpenes showing up together. For example, one study that analyzed the chemistry from 90,000 cannabis samples found there were three distinct groupings of dominant terpenes[37]. The first cluster was dominant in caryophyllene and myrcene, the second was dominant in myrcene and pinene, and the third in caryophyllene and limonene. This pairing and similar expression is likely because when a specific defense pathway is activated in the plant, it initiates multiple compounds being produced at similar rates through similar pathways. These distinct clusters may also represent distinct effects such as uplifting, sedating, creative, etc.,

THE EFFECT OF SMELL

Not only do terpenes smell, but many of them also have activity on receptors in the body and change the way that cannabis makes us feel. They are also part of why different strains make us feel differently and why some people react positively or negatively to a specific variety.

A common saying in the cannabis world is **"The Nose Knows."** When you try a cannabis strain that really meshes well with your body, whether that means it doesn't make you feel anxious, takes away your pain, wakes you up, makes you giggle, etc., it is important to take note of the terpene profile as well as the cannabinoid profile. Looking at the dominant terpenes or even noting if there are any unique terpenes in your flower or concentrate will help guide you toward other products that you may also react well to in the future. This is less important with edible products because we are still unsure what happens to terpenes once we eat them.

One major factor when choosing a cannabis product is if it's going to keep you awake or put you to sleep. Personally, I like to keep different types of cannabis around for this reason. This way I have daytime cannabis products that are stimulating, creative, and energetic and, when I'm winding down and getting ready for bed, I have something that shuts off my brain and allows my bed to swallow me whole.

If you're looking for the more classic sativa feel, lean towards products that smell gassy, astringent, sour, and tangy that almost make your nose tickle. You'll feel the aroma throughout your entire nose. On the Certificate of Analysis (COA) look for dominant terpenes like terpinolene, limonene, ocimene, and pinene. A lower dose of THC is more stimulating than a high dose for most people, and CBG is a great cannabinoid to explore for daytime stimulating effects without the intoxicating high.

For nighttime use, sedating cannabis varieties usually smell very different from uplifting varieties. The smells are typically spicier, more clove-like, earthy, rich, and often floral. The smell has more depth, both in flavor and in location of the nose. I've also found that the flower is often darker in color, and purple varieties are usually a safe bet for a PM routine.

Below is a diagram illustrating how I would rank the most sedating to most stimulating terpenes based on science and personal experience. Note, this scale is not scientifically proven, although it is heavily based in science. I have categorized the terpenes based on the literature available, my experience, and the shared experience of other consumers.

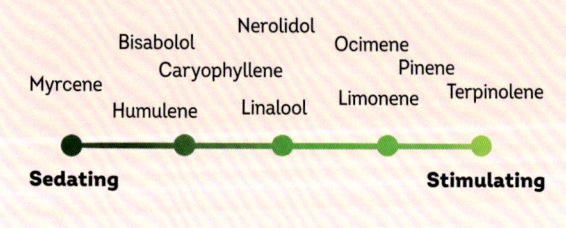

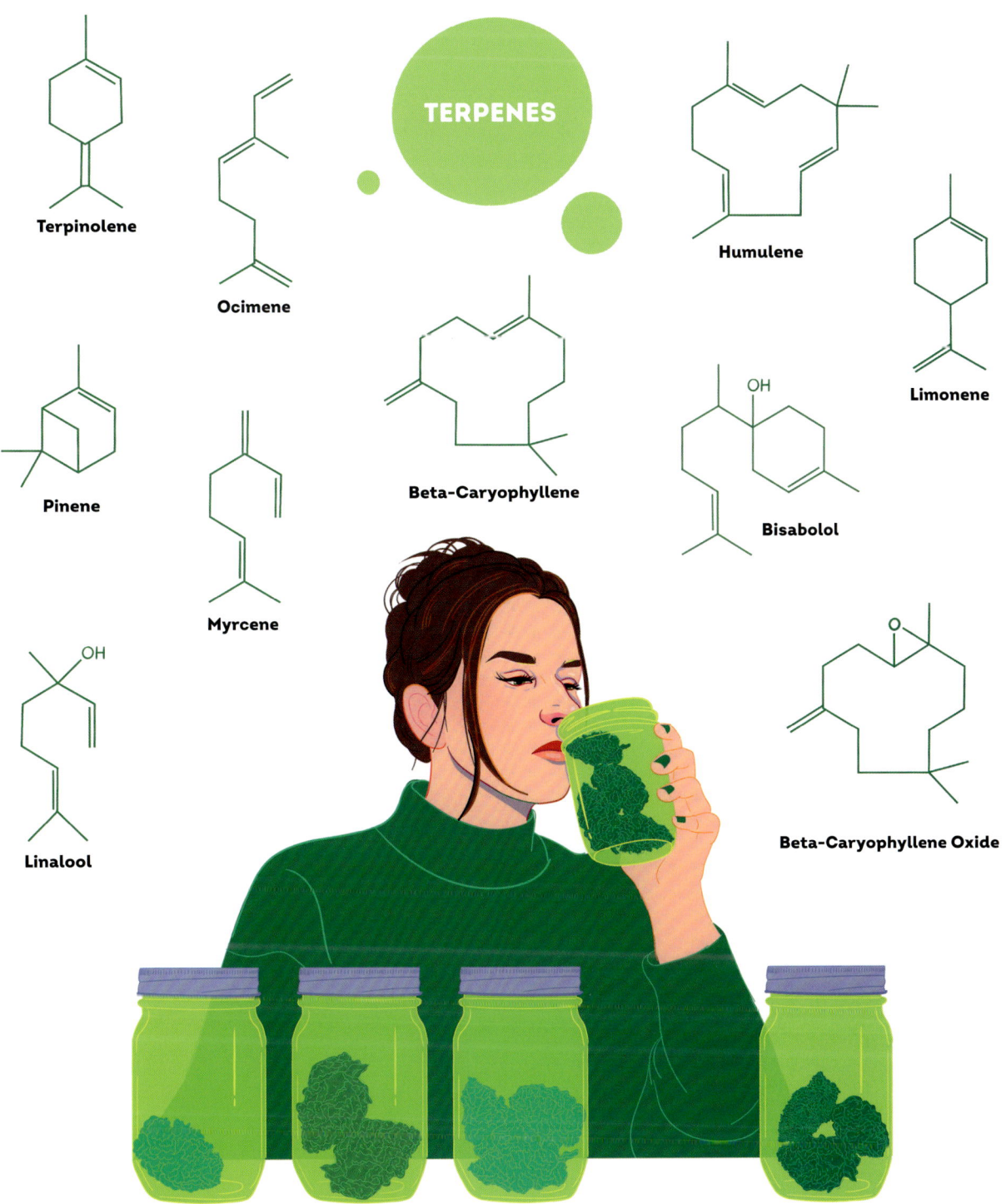

TERPENES

Terpinolene

Ocimene

Humulene

Limonene

Pinene

Myrcene

Beta-Caryophyllene

Bisabolol

Linalool

Beta-Caryophyllene Oxide

KEY TERPENES

Specific terpenes enhance the entourage effect of the cannabis product. Not only are CBD, THC, and other cannabinoids acting on our bodies, now a cocktail of these small scent compounds are added to the mix, allowing us to further personalize our cannabis medicine.

Scientists can engineer plants to produce more of a specific compound or ratios of compounds to meet patients' diverse needs, and this is part of the reason why homegrow of cannabis should be a fundamental right especially for medical patients. If people are able to purchase quality genetics and grow their own plants, they can have affordable, accessible, personalized medicine.

For example, the cannabis plant produces the terpene eudesmol also commonly found in the eucalyptus tree, which has great anticancer benefits by reducing blood flow to tumors but is difficult to find in commercially available strains[38].

Myrcene

Even though myrcene is the terpene best associated with sleep or sedation, when you see myrcene on a COA, note that it is almost ubiquitous in cannabis, so it may not be helpful to ask for a myrcene rich variety at your dispensary. It is likely that myrcene does contribute to the sedating couchlock feel of cannabis, but the amount matters significantly. One study claims that this threshold is 0.5%—meaning that if a cannabis variety has more than 0.5% myrcene it has a couchlock effect, and less than 0.5% has a more stimulating effect[39], but the exact mechanism is still up for debate.

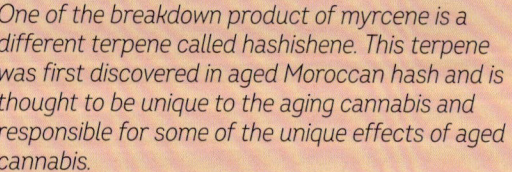

NUGS OF KNOWLEDGE

One of the breakdown product of myrcene is a different terpene called hashishene. This terpene was first discovered in aged Moroccan hash and is thought to be unique to the aging cannabis and responsible for some of the unique effects of aged cannabis.

Bisabolol

The smell of bisabolol is one of rich, sweet, floral honey—it is delicious. If you're familiar with chamomile flowers, much of the aroma comes from this sesquiterpene. Bisabolol is an amazing sedating, calming, and antianxiety terpene. It works to help relax and sleep by acting on the $GABA_A$ receptors[40], and likely at the same receptor subtype that mediates the effects of benzodiazepine drugs. Similar to lavender, bisabolol even smells relaxing.

If you're worried about finding a variety of cannabis that is high in bisabolol near you, worry not. The most enjoyable way to get high levels of bisabolol into your cannabis is to add it in. By either growing or purchasing organic chamomile, which is readily available as a common tea, you can add chamomile flower directly into your bowl or vape. I personally prefer it in a dry herb vape—it creates the most sweet, delicious flavor.

NUGS OF KNOWLEDGE

You can also do this with other herbs, such as adding small amounts of lavender to increase the levels of the calming terpene linalool in your dose. However, it is important to check the source of any herb to ensure it was grown organically and doesn't contain pesticides or heavy metals.

Beta-Caryophyllene

Beta-caryophyllene is a terpene that is also present in black pepper and cloves and has a warm, spicy smell. Beta caryophyllene has shown antibacterial, anticancer (breast, colon, melanoma, glioma, pancreatic, lymphoma,) and anti-seizure activity[41].

Not only is beta-caryophyllene a terpene because it is built of isoprene units, but it is also a cannabinoid because it has activity on the Cannabinoid 2 receptor as a selective full agonist.

As a CB2 selective agonist, this has implications for inflammatory and immune conditions including nervous system illness like Parkinson's disease, Alzheimer's disease, and multiple sclerosis as well as chronic inflammatory conditions like arthritis and inflammatory gut conditions like Crohn's disease and ulcerative colitis[42].

CB2 agonists like beta-caryophyllene or cannabichromene (CBC) can be taken in a variety of ways, including the most popular: smoking and vaping. There are also consumption methods that cater more to the CB2 receptors on the gut, like edibles, and skin-like topicals—as the skin has a multitude of receptors including CB1, CB2, TRPV1, etc.

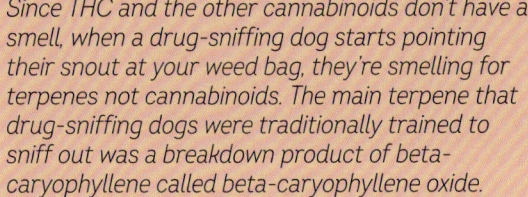

NUGS OF KNOWLEDGE

Since THC and the other cannabinoids don't have a smell, when a drug-sniffing dog starts pointing their snout at your weed bag, they're smelling for terpenes not cannabinoids. The main terpene that drug-sniffing dogs were traditionally trained to sniff out was a breakdown product of beta-caryophyllene called beta-caryophyllene oxide.

Humulene

Alpha-caryophyllene, also known as humulene, is another sweet smelling sesquiterpene. Humulene is best known for the aroma of hops or dank IPAs. Similar to beta-caryophyllene, humulene is a great anti-inflammatory compound, and may be further studied for cases of allergic inflammation, as humulene prevents histamine release and promotes healthy mucosa[43]. It has also been studied for alcoholic gastritis.

Limonene

Limonene is a terpene commonly found in cannabis, as well as in citrus fruits like oranges and lemons. It contributes a characteristic citrus aroma to strains and has gained attention for its potential therapeutic effects. Research shows that limonene has anti-inflammatory, antioxidant, and antimicrobial properties, which could be beneficial for users seeking relief from inflammation and stress[44]. Limonene is believed to contribute to mood elevation and anxiety relief, making it a popular choice for consumers looking for an uplifting experience with reduced anxiety. Some strains high in limonene include Super Lemon Haze, Do-Si-Dos, and Lemon Skunk.

Limonene's potential benefits go beyond mood enhancement. Studies have indicated that it may have anticancer properties by reducing tumor growth through pathways like apoptosis (cell death) and preventing metastasis[45]. Additionally, it has been explored for its digestive health benefits, acting as an antiacid and reducing gastric reflux.

Linalool

The signature scent of lavender is mainly due to the the terpene linalool. Studies have shown that inhaling or simpling smelling linalool has sedating and antianxiety effects[46]. Which is another reason why you should always stop and take a second to smell your weed before medicating,

Not only is linalool a great terpene to target for nighttime use because it is relaxing and sedating, but evidence also shows it may be helpful in **canceling some of the memory impairing effects of THC in the brain through serotonergic pathways**[47]. Another terpene that may help with short-term memory is pinene, but pinene tends to be more stimulating than linalool-rich varieties.

If you are someone who suffers from anxiety, consider trying a cannabis strain that contains linalool and CBD. If you can't find a variety with both, try mixing in a hemp variety with one or both other components to ensure the THC is balanced.

The sesquiterpene **nerolidol**, which has smells of rich orange peels, has shown similar benefits and effects as linalool. It is sedating, anti-seizure, and reduces anxiety.

Pinene

Pinene is the most widely distributed terpene in nature—you can thank softwood trees like the white pine for it. Pinene has a distinct sharp aroma that smells like a cleaning agent. In the plant, pinene likely functions as an insect repellent. It has antimicrobial effects due to its toxic effect on some membranes and has been used as a topical antiseptic[48]. It may even help naturally extend the shelf life of your topical cannabis products.

At low levels, pinene can be beneficial in opening the lungs and airways, acting as a bronchodilator as well as providing anti-inflammatory effects[49]. However, at high levels, it can be irritating. Some varieties that you smoke or vape may make you cough WAY more than others. Although this sometimes has to do with how the product was processed, dried, and cured, it could also have to do with the terpene profile. And yes, it is possible to be allergic to or intolerant of specific terpenes.

The terpene **ocimene**—with complex floral, woody notes—has been studied in combination with pinene and is thought to have synergistic effects. Ocimene has been described as more stimulating than pinene and is also found in high levels in basil.

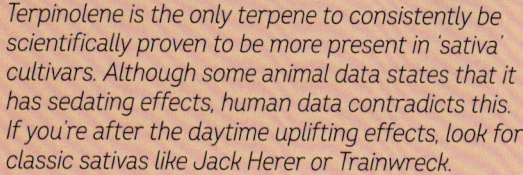

NUGS OF KNOWLEDGE

Terpinolene is the only terpene to consistently be scientifically proven to be more present in 'sativa' cultivars. Although some animal data states that it has sedating effects, human data contradicts this. If you're after the daytime uplifting effects, look for classic sativas like Jack Herer or Trainwreck.

Terpinolene

The aroma of terpinolene is very complex. There is a distinct pine odor similar to pinene, but it is more woody, floral, and citrusy and generally complex. Terpinolene is also found in other botanicals like rosemary and lilacs. Interestingly, mouse studies have shown terpinolene to have a sedating effect[50], but human experience says the opposite, noting it as a powerful stimulating compound in popular sativa-type varieties like Jack Herer and Durban Poison.

Chemical data supports that terpinolene is often found alongside another terpene called **alpha-phellandrene**, with a refreshing minty pepper aroma, in sativa-type varieties, adding to the stimulatory effects. They are likely produced through the same biochemical pathway in the plant, allowing them to be co-expressed. Research also indicates that these compounds may be used in synergy to enhance wound healing for topical purposes.

Note there are dozens of other terpenes that exist in the cannabis plant, oftentimes produced in very low quantities, that are not discussed in detail in this section but may play an impactful role on how a strain feels and smells.

VAPE TEMPERATURES FOR TERPENES

If you are someone who likes to vape at low temperatures, and you are using a specific variety of cannabis for its therapeutic effects, check to make sure that your temperature is set high enough to vaporize the compound. Some terpenes like bisabolol, eudesmol, humulene, and caryophyllene have higher vaporization temperatures because they are larger molecules.

Personally speaking, I love dry herb vaping cannabis flower, but I'm always a little torn as to what to set my vape temperature at. On one hand, when the temperature is on the lower side, around 356 to 392°F (180 to 200°C), the flavor of the flower shines through and you can literally taste the complexity of the flower on your tongue. However, at these lower temperatures there are some compounds like heavier sesquiterpenes, cannabinoids, and flavonoids that are not being vaporized. At higher temperatures, you are able to vaporize more compounds but lose some flavor because the aroma compounds are now paired with the non-aromatic components that drown out the flavor.

What I've landed on is: when I get new flower or when I'm looking for more uplifting effects during the day, I keep the temperature lower. When I want to feel more sedated, couchlocked and really feel the full potential of the vape, I crank the temp up to its max, which on my device is 446°F (230°C).

Flavorants

Terpenes are undeniably important to the aroma of a plant, our preference towards products, and for biological and medicinal effects. However, there are other molecules present that may alter the effects or aroma of a given strain as well and greatly contribute to the exotic flavors of modern cannabis.

Beyond terpenes, another class of compounds that contribute to the distinct aroma of cannabis are the flavorant compounds. Note that flavorants are different from flavonoids, which we discuss below. Rather than terpenes, which are characterized by isoprene units, flavorants are a conglomerate of other types of molecules including alcohols, esters, fatty acids, indoles, aldehydes and sulfur-containing compounds called volatile sulfur compounds (VSCs[51]). These represent the extreme smells of exotic cannabis from sweet and fruity to savory notes of garlic, onion, and skunk.

Indole and skatole

Skatole is the molecule partially responsible for the offensive smell of poop and can be found at very low levels in some very savory varieties of cannabis. The cannabis community has known there is a poopy smelling compound in cannabis for decades, even establishing the name poopenes somewhere along the way.

Interestingly, the chemical structures of skatole and another flavorant in cannabis named indole are similar to compounds known to have psychedelic activity on the brain and enhance perception like DMT and serotonin—which is why some people hypothesize certain varieties of cannabis have enhanced spiritual effects.

Other flavorants are responsible for the classic skunk smell of some varieties. The scent is from a series of small, sulfur-containing compounds; although one compound (3-methyl-2-butene-1-thiol) is most responsible for the signature eggy aroma, six other sulfur-containing compounds contribute to the unique smell.

FLAVONOIDS

You encounter flavonoids all the time in nature and in your everyday lives. Many of the natural blue, purple, red, yellow, and orange pigments are from flavonoids. In the fall, in the northeast portion of the United States, just before leaves drop from trees, they turn a variety of beautiful colors, displaying their flavonoid rich pigments. Areas like the White Mountains of New Hampshire have such beautiful colors on display because, in regions where the temperature has massive fluctuations, the trees need to protect themselves from the intense conditions and freeze-thaws.

They do this by producing more flavonoids acting as antifreeze protection compounds; during most of the year, the high levels of colorful protective pigments are hidden behind the powerful green color of chlorophyll. However, in the fall when temperatures drop, the chlorophyll dies off, leaving the flavonoids on full display. When you see a beautiful purple variety of cannabis, that is also the flavonoid colors showing through the chlorophyll. If you are growing cannabis in certain regions, you will likely notice your plant gets darker in color as the season crawls to an end and the weather gets colder.

Biological Effects

Flavonoids are best known for providing the beautiful colors of nature. However, these colors also have potent biological activity in the body.

The cannabis plant produces about 30 different flavonoid compounds—some that are common in many other plants, and some that are unique to cannabis[52]. Quercitin and apigenin are common flavonoids and powerful antioxidants. Flavonoids in general are typically good antioxidants because they are electron-rich compounds that can donate an electron to neutralize dangerous free radicals in the body. The electron-rich nature of the molecules is also why they are so highly pigmented. These molecules contain strings of double bonds that can absorb and reflect light in unique ways, portraying different colors of the rainbow.

The flavonoids that are thought to be unique to cannabis are Cannflavin A, B, and C. Cannflavin A has shown potent bioactivity as an anti-inflammatory agent, showing 30 times more potent activity compared to aspirin in inhibiting the inflammatory signal with fewer side effects[53]. Cannflavin A and Cannflavin B inhibit two enzymes essential for inflammation (prostaglandin E synthase-1 and 5-lipoxygenase). Beyond inflammation, the cannflavins are neuroprotective, anticancer, antiviral, and antiparasitic[54]. Because of the limited capabilities of the plant to produce the cannflavins, researchers have found ways to either synthetically produce the compounds or produce them by inserting the cannflavin gene into yeast.

CURATING YOUR CANNABIS EXPERIENCE

In many cases it is possible to purchase isolated cannabinoids or terpenes to formulate into your own products or add in additional botanicals to supplement your needs. This is helpful if you are someone who likes to extract and formulate your own products, if you can't find what you're looking for at a dispensary near you, or if you're on a tight budget.

When I make tinctures at home, I purchase CBN isolate to add into my nighttime formulations. CBN, CBG, CBC, CBD, and many other compounds can be purchased online in isolated form, essentially as ingredients for dietary supplements. If you are purchasing isolate online or any readily available cannabis product, remember to check:

> 1. The product is from a reputable company with a certificate of analysis (COA), showing that it is a pure compound, the date it was tested, and which lab tested it.

> 2. The dosing on the specific cannabinoid to make sure you're within the safety parameters. This is an easy way to personalize your extracts for specific needs.

THE ENTOURAGE EXPANDED

Beyond the chemistry of a strain or product, there are other aspects that can alter the quality of the overall cannabis experience. The overall quality of a product, whether that be flower, rosin, edibles, etc., will shine through based on how the product was grown, dried and cured, stored, processed or extracted, packaged etc. Depending on how it was produced, there could be varying levels of material, chemicals or moisture that alters how the product feels. Other contributing factors to the overall experience include the consumption method, other products/drugs/food in your body, your environment, age and metabolism, genetics, and so on. In the following chapters we will specifically discuss how the 'entourage of chemistry' changes depending on how you consume cannabis.

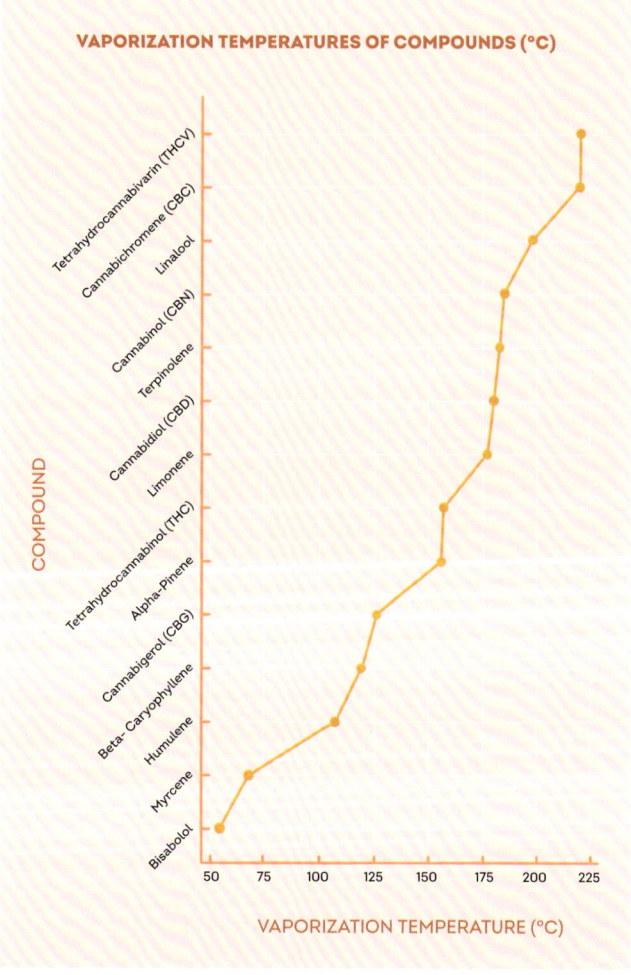

VAPORIZATION TEMPERATURES OF COMPOUNDS (°C)

COMPOUND

Tetrahydrocannabivarin (THCV)
Cannabichromene (CBC)
Linalool
Cannabinol (CBN)
Terpinolene
Cannabidiol (CBD)
Limonene
Tetrahydrocannabinol (THC)
Alpha-Pinene
Cannabigerol (CBG)
Beta-Caryophyllene
Humulene
Myrcene
Bisabolol

50   75   100   125   150   175   200   225

VAPORIZATION TEMPERATURE (°C)

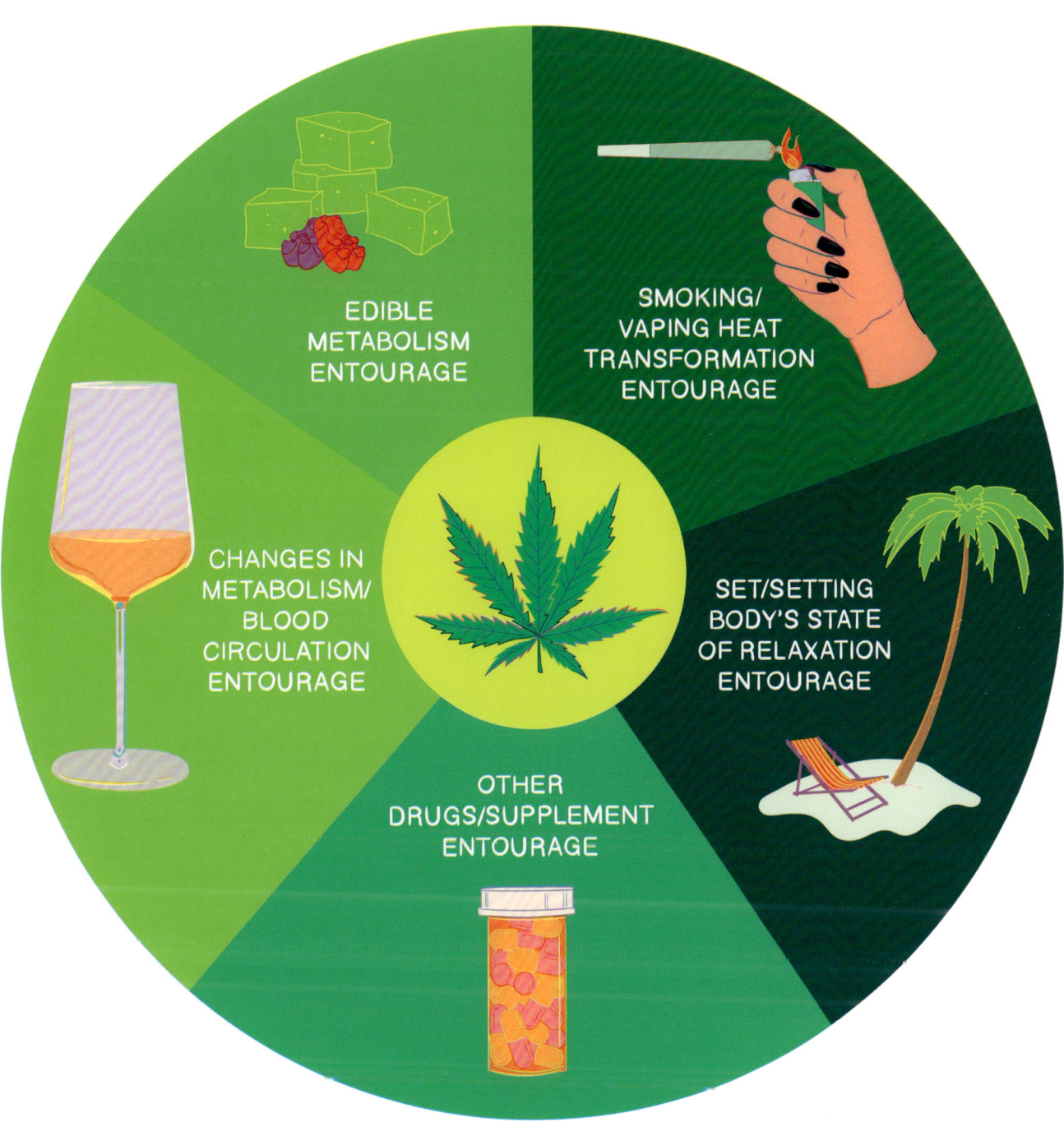

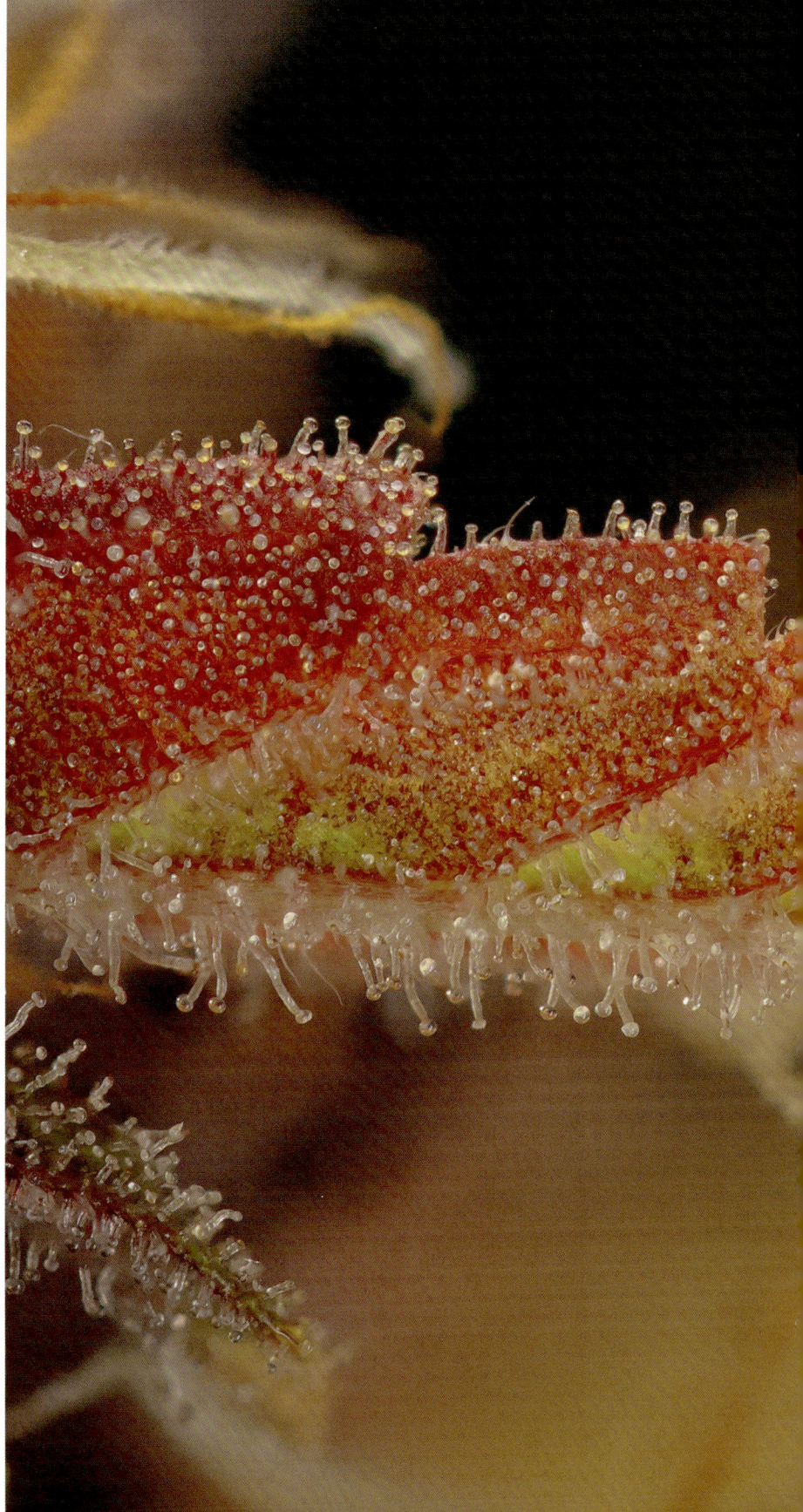

SMOKE BREAK

LET'S RECAP WHAT WE LEARNED:

⇒ Cannabis interacts with the Endocannabinoid System (ECS), which is found throughout the body and helps regulate functions like pain, mood, and inflammation.

⇒ The ECS consists of endocannabinoids, cannabinoid receptors (CB1 and CB2), and enzymes that synthesize and break down these molecules.

⇒ Receptors in the body act like locks, and cannabis molecules like THC and CBD are the keys that either activate or inhibit these receptors, leading to various effects. Different cannabinoids can affect different receptors, leading to a wide range of medicinal outcomes.

⇒ Cannabinoids like THC and CBD mimic endocannabinoids naturally produced by the body. THC is a partial agonist at the CB1 receptor and responsible for the psychoactive effects, while CBD works on multiple receptors and is non-intoxicating, helping with inflammation, anxiety, and pain.

⇒ Smell plays a critical role in the cannabis experience due to the terpenes, aromatic compounds produced by the plant. Terpenes not only give cannabis its distinctive scent but also have therapeutic effects, influencing how the strain makes you feel— whether relaxing, energizing, or mood-lifting. Your nose can often guide you toward the best strain for your body's needs.

⇒ The entourage effect describes how cannabinoids, terpenes, and flavonoids work together to enhance cannabis's therapeutic effects. Each compound interacts in a unique way, and the consumption method influences how the body experiences the entourage effect.

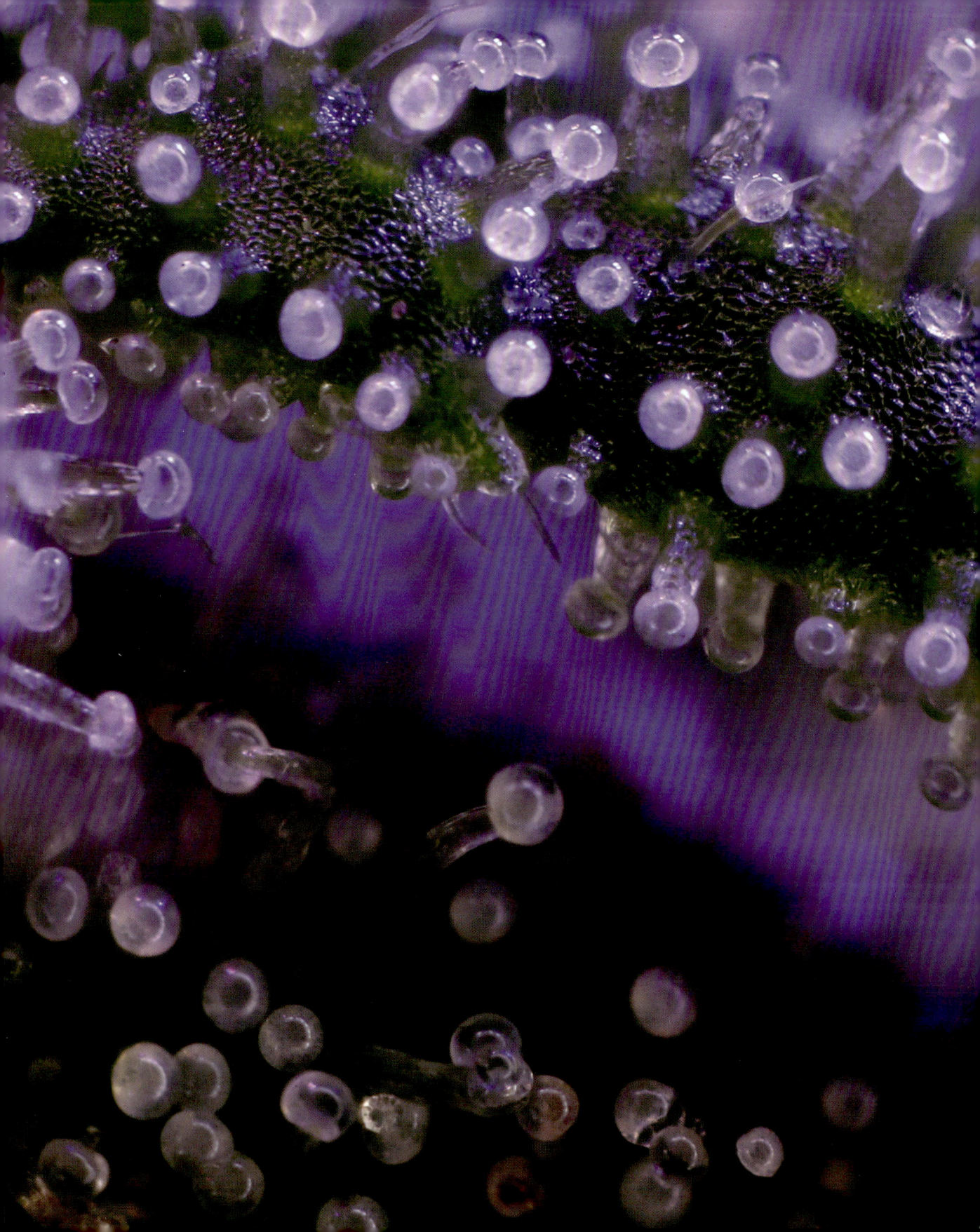

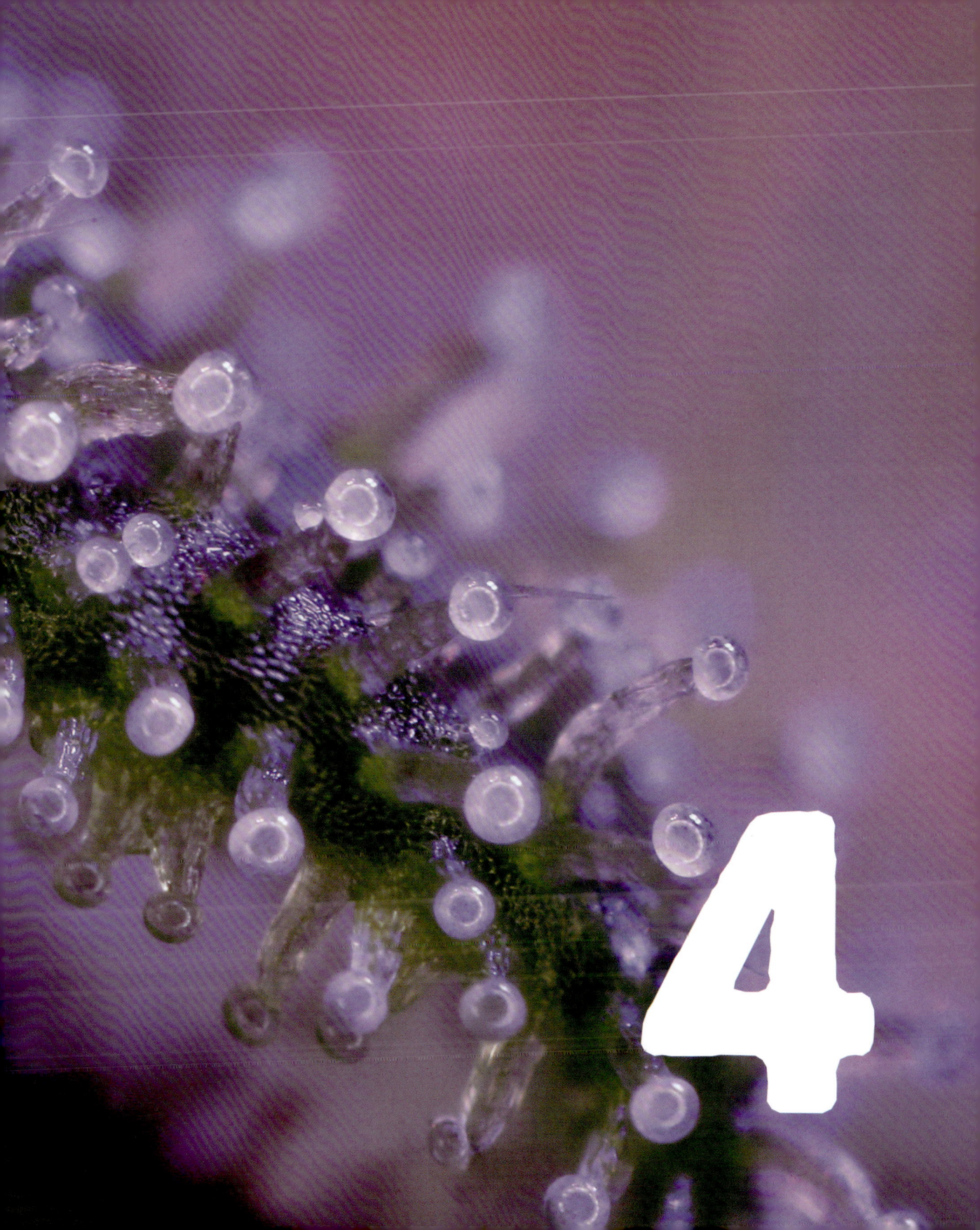

4

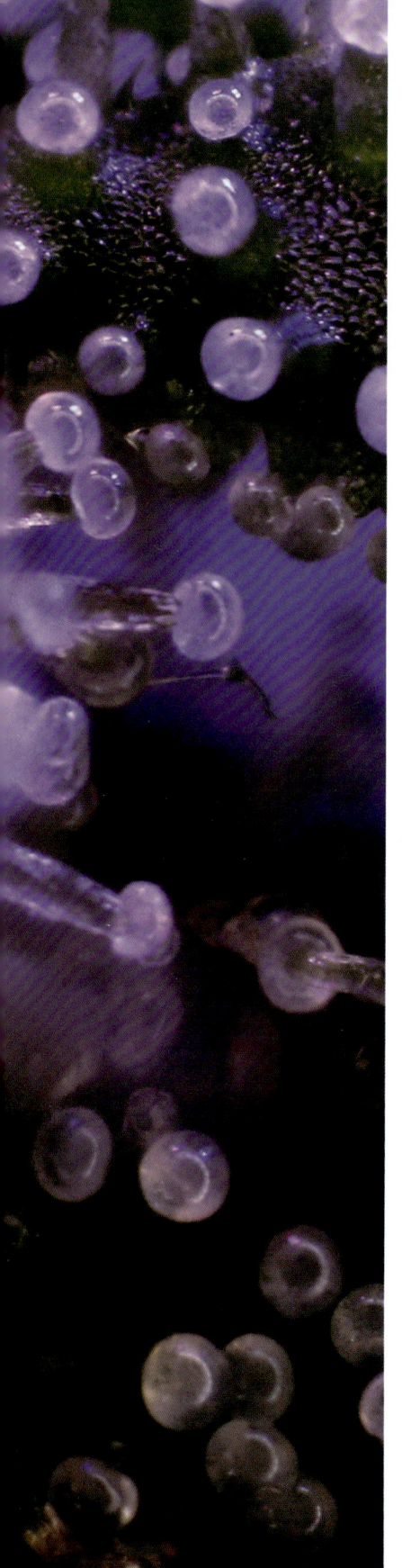

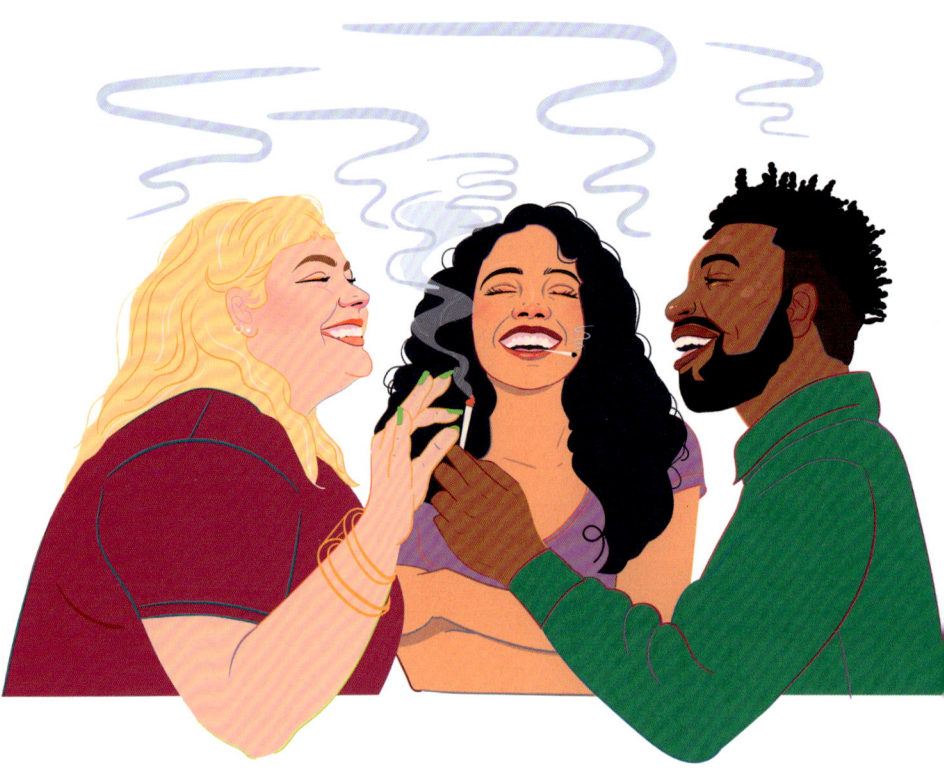

HOW TO CONSUME CANNABIS: METHODS AND DOSING

Our bodies are unique and change throughout our lives—especially our endocannabinoid system. Because our endocannabinoid system is dynamic and fluctuates by age and even time of the day, our own consumption should be thought of as dynamic as well. There are a variety of ways you can consume the plant, and you will find your preference for products and dosages will change based on your age, hormone levels, menstrual phase, level of activity, time of year, and many other factors. The most valuable tool that you learn is how to listen to your body and gauge your dose accordingly.

Using cannabis does not just mean smoking weed anymore. Some of the different factors to consider when you're choosing which method to use are:

1. Availability and cost of products

2. Duration of effects

3. Localized effects or systemic

4. General health impacts

5. Indoor vs. outdoor use

6. Group settings or alone

7. Discreteness (cannabis is SMELLY and that isn't always safe)

8. Personal reactions to products based on genetics and metabolism.

When starting with cannabis or trying a new consumption method the general rule is **"start low and go slow"**—taking a small dose and waiting it out to see what the effects are. If you were trying a new IPA for the first time, you would probably start by taking a sip, not shotgunning the entire can. Take notes on your experience, observing which brand of products you use, what dose you took, how long until you felt the effects and if you enjoyed the experience or not. Although this exercise is especially important to new users, it can be practiced by frequent users as well to track favorite products or help with consuming intentionally.

It is important to remember that the consumption that you choose will impact how you feel and what chemistry is entering your body. **The entourage effect of cannabis is dependent on the consumption method.** Smoking will provide unique chemistry of transformed and degraded molecules while edible consumption will result in various metabolites from cannabis interacting with the body. I pay as much attention to HOW I'm consuming as to WHAT I'm consuming because the difference in effects are like night and day.

A common mistake for new cannabis users is thinking that a product didn't work or isn't making you feel elevated enough, so you take another dose and end up overdoing it. Although you can't die from taking too much cannabis alone, you can overdo it, and it can be a scary and uncomfortable feeling. This feeling of mega dosing yourself on THC is often called **"greening out"** and some symptoms are nausea, dizziness, and confusion. If you or someone else is experiencing this you should sit down, get some water, and find anything else that can increase your comfort or distract you for the next few hours. Personally, I have only greened out one time and it was from taking too much cannabutter on pierogies; I knew pretty quickly I took too much THC, laid on the couch with water and a weighted blanket, and slept for the foreseeable future. Some evidence suggests that chewing on peppercorns may also help with grounding yourself as they contain the terpene beta-caryophyllene, but time is the best way to get through it. Make sure, if you do overdo it on cannabis, you use your cannabis journal and write what you did wrong to make sure you don't do the same thing again in the future.

Dosing can be easier with faster acting methods like smoking or vaping compared to slower methods like edibles. These inhalation methods make it easier to **"titrate"** your dose—meaning slowly increasing your dose until you feel like you're at a comfortable level. Methods that require your body to metabolize the product, like edibles, can be much more variable and it could take a lot longer for you to feel the effects.

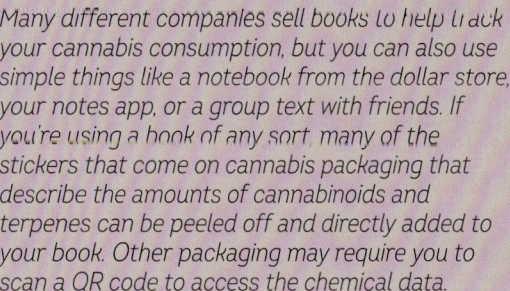

NUGS OF KNOWLEDGE

Many different companies sell books to help track your cannabis consumption, but you can also use simple things like a notebook from the dollar store, your notes app, or a group text with friends. If you're using a book of any sort, many of the stickers that come on cannabis packaging that describe the amounts of cannabinoids and terpenes can be peeled off and directly added to your book. Other packaging may require you to scan a QR code to access the chemical data.

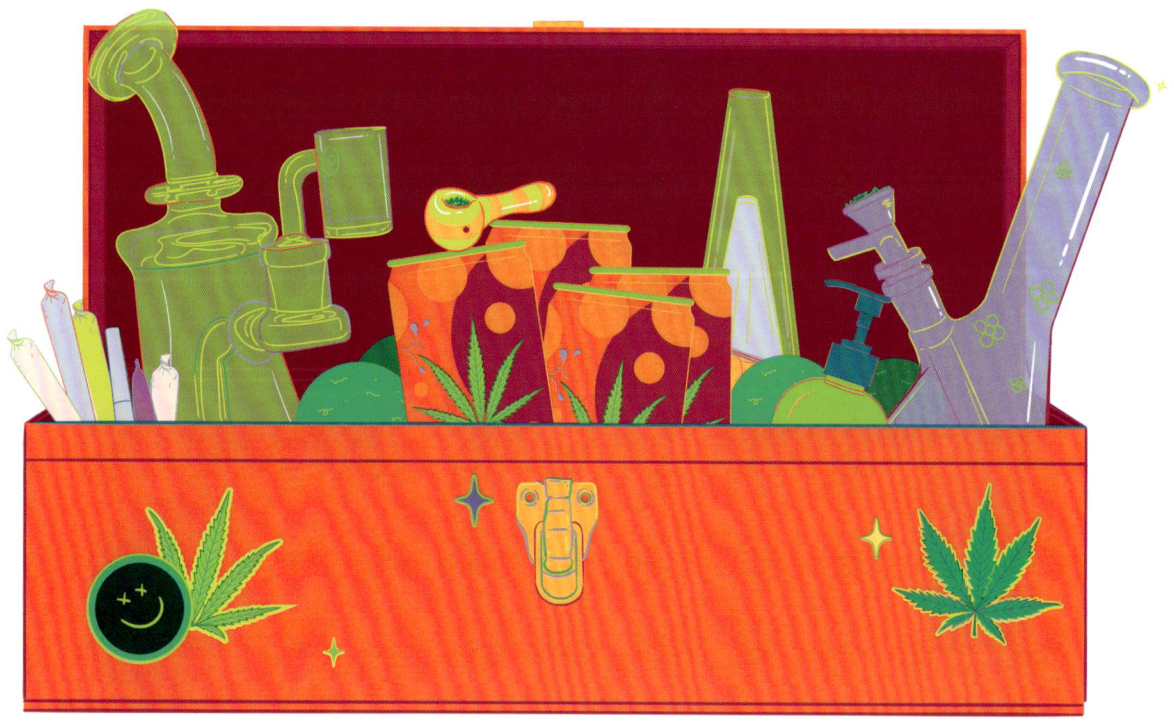

Every consumption method is a tool in the toolbox. Each one has its pros and cons from a chemical, health, societal, or genetic or a combination of these. It is up to you as a sentient and educated consumer to make the decision of what is best for you and your body. And remember, if you have a bad experience with cannabis, it isn't the fault of cannabis; it's something for us to take as a learning experience. With each of the consumption methods, consider what the net benefit is. Knowing what your choices are and trying out the different methods to see how they vibe with your body is a critical part of being an educated consumer.

Almost all products can be made at home if you cannot afford or do not have access to the cannabis products. While I encourage everyone to experiment with making and growing their own medicine at some point in their cannabis journey, if it is your first time using cannabis, I would recommend a low dose of a dispensary product, so you know exactly what you're putting into your body. It is much easier to plan your makeup and predict your experience if you know the exact dose of your product. With homemade products it is more of a guessing game as to what your dose of CBD or THC is. There are calculations that can be made to get a better prediction, but without analytical machinery it won't be precise. Once your body is acclimated with cannabis you will feel more comfortable expanding into new consumption methods and homemade products.

Additionally, if you are a medical cannabis patient or immunocompromised, dispensary products are tested to ensure there aren't any heavy metals, molds, or other inflammatory materials in your cannabis products that could be causing more harm than good.

SMOKING

Smoking is still the preferred consumption method of many cannabis users. The act of smoking has rooted significance in cannabis culture. Joints and blunts are often shared in circles where they are passed from one person to the next. People share stories, experiences, love for the flower, deep thoughts, or lighthearted funny comments inspired by THC. Lighting up a joint is often a beacon of trust and comradery. It is not always safe to consume cannabis and finding community almost anywhere in the world with the familiar skunky smell holds significant meaning to many. The act of sharing medicine while coming together and getting to know other people who also gravitate towards this plant is an undeniably important factor in the therapeutic nature of cannabis smoking. **When you get together to share a joint, you already have one thing in common: you love weed.**

Cannabis can be smoked many ways, but it typically includes grinding up the nugs of weed so it is a fluffy pile of ground herb with no stems or seeds, then either placing the ground herb in a smoking device like a bong or a bowl and lighting it on fire or rolling up the ground weed using rolling papers to smoke.

PROS AND CONS

Smoking cannabis does not have the same harmful impact on the lungs as nicotine products, as combusting nicotine produces hundreds of carcinogenic compounds. However, cannabis smoke has been shown to produce some carcinogens and toxicants[1] that could impact human health and, at the end of the day, smoking anything exposes your delicate lung tissues to heat, particulates, and gasses that could impact your health from constant exposure[2].

Smoking produces carbon monoxide[3], a gas that can have a negative impact on heart health by preventing oxygen from binding to blood cell[4]. Cannabis smokers are exposed to more carbon monoxide than cigarette smokers, which is partially because cannabis smokers hold the smoke in their body longer and take deeper inhales compared to tobacco smokers. Cannabis smoke is rich in cannabinoids, which are sticky, resinous molecules, and by definition, cannabinoids would essentially be considered "tar". Smoking cannabis produces more

tar in the lungs than tobacco smoke does, but again, produces far less cancer-causing compounds.

There are many physicians who believe that nobody should be smoking, period; but that's not the reality of the world. There are benefits to this consumption method chemically, spiritually, and socially. When cannabis is lit on fire (smoked) the heat acts as a catalyst to change some of the chemistry, creating new compounds and changing the ratios of active compounds. **The compounds that are present in the bud before it is smoked are not the same as the molecules entering your body after lighting it on fire.** The smoke will still mainly contain high amounts of major compounds like THC, CBD, or CBG, but now there are also higher levels of rare and minor cannabinoids like CBE (Cannabeilsoin), CBT (Cannabitriol), CBL (Cannabicyclol), and CBND (Cannabinodiol) that were not present in the starting material but are now going into your body. These cannabinoids add to cannabis's therapeutic potential, and may be part of the reason so many people prefer this consumption method. However, we need more research on the minor and rare cannabinoids before we can fully understand this potential.

Choosing to smoke is a decision you can make based on the net benefit that you receive from smoking. If you already have compromised lungs, it is generally recommended to choose a different consumption method.

Grinding Cannabis

Grinders are not necessary for cannabis consumption—you can absolutely break up the cannabis nugs with your fingers—but grinders make it a whole lot easier and save time! They also increase accessibility if you or someone you know does not have good dexterity.

Grinders typically have more than one chamber, but not all are the same. Often there is a top piece where you add in your nugs, then there is a middle section where the ground herb is collected, and a final lower compartment that collects the very fine, and precious) grind, called **kief**.

Kief is the trichomes of the cannabis plant, which have broken off the flower and fallen to the bottom. Kief is what hash is made from because it is a concentration of the trichomes of the cannabis plant, which are smaller than the ground up plant parts. Kief is often collected over time and eventually added to the top of a special bowl or joint or used to make specialty concentrated products at home. But don't worry, if your grinder doesn't have a kief collector, it simply means the kief is still with your flower!

To grind up your cannabis for smoking or rolling, first hold the nug by the stem. Start to separate the sections of the nug from the main stem by pulling it apart. The goal here is to remove the main stem of the flower and any seeds that may be present.

Place the nug pieces in a grinder (make sure not to overfill it), put the top of the grinder on, and turn it ½ a turn to the right, then to the left a few times—you will be able to tell when the grinder turns easily, noting that the cannabis is ground. Open the main chamber of the grinder and you should see your ground cannabis. Grinders can be found in any smoke shop, or are available from online stores. There are often different sizes, and some grinders can have filters for different preferences of grind, similar to coffee. Some people still prefer to use their hands to break up the nugs to be gentler on the flower—I encourage you to do whatever works best for you!

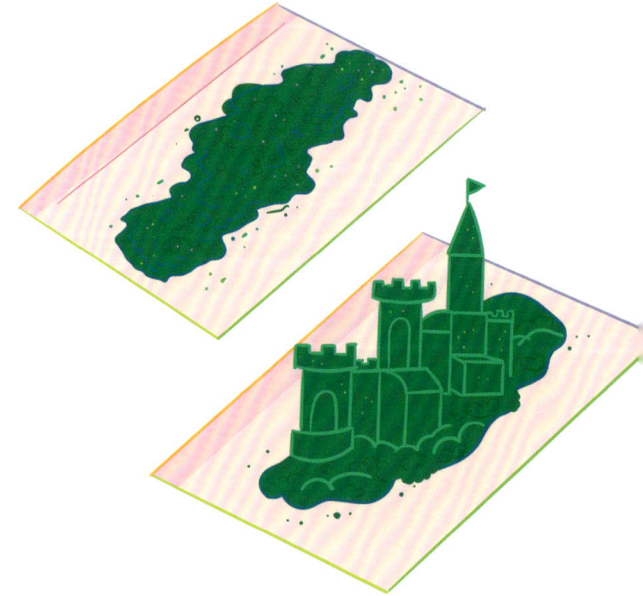

NUGS OF KNOWLEDGE

You may have noticed that the weed you got decades ago had a lot more seeds in it compared to the cannabis available now. This is because seeds will develop if the female plant is exposed to pollen from a male plant, but since growing has become much more controlled with the emergence of a legal market, seeds are far less common!

Rolling up

The classic way to consume cannabis, and still a favorite of many (including myself) is rolling up the ground flower into a small, smokeable cylinder using paper made typically of hemp paper or rice paper; this is called rolling a joint. You can find other natural rolling papers like rose petals or palm leaves, but when cannabis is rolled in a tobacco leaf, it is called a blunt. There are MANY different techniques to rolling joints, and everyone has their own tips and tricks. There are even rolling competitions where people create works of art like dragons, crosses, or skulls that are all smokeable!

My best advice for people new to rolling is to first **use quality cannabis.** Cannabis with sticky trichomes that has been dried and cured to a proper moisture level allowing it to stick together, is much easier to roll, than crusty, dry weed. **Think of it like making a sandcastle with wet sand vs. dry sand—the wet sand holds its shape and is easily manipulated whereas the dry sand wants to crumble and is difficult to control.** The second tip is to practice, practice, practice. It may seem difficult at first, but as your hands get used to the motion it will become progressively easier until you barely need to think about it anymore. The tools I have on hand when rolling are a rolling tray, rolling papers, scissors, a grinder or mill, tips or crutches, and a chopstick. Here is a quick guide to how I roll a joint:

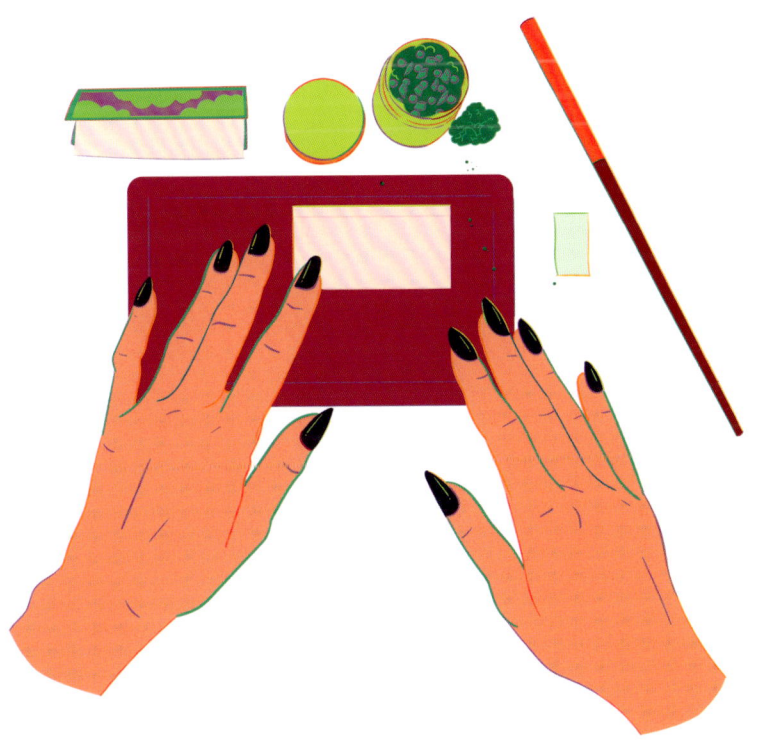

1. Take a piece of rolling paper and lay it down on the table or rolling tray with the sticky gum on the very top, facing you.

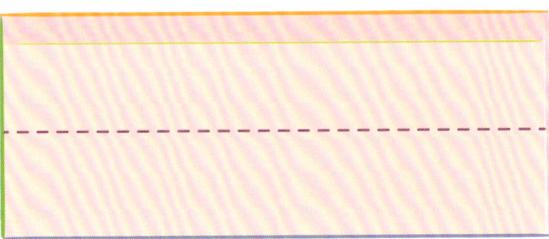

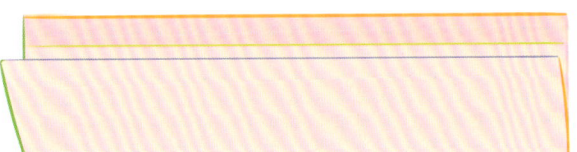

2. Fold the bottom half once more lengthwise, creating an additional crease on the bottom half. This makes a little boat that you will fill with ground flower.

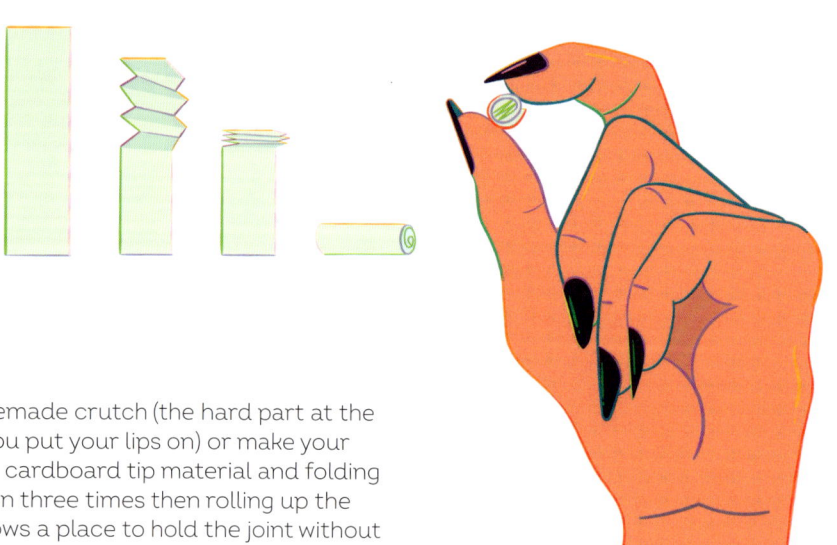

3. Use either a premade crutch (the hard part at the end of the joint you put your lips on) or make your own by taking the cardboard tip material and folding it like an accordion three times then rolling up the rest. A crutch allows a place to hold the joint without compressing it, but they are not necessary, and many people roll without them.

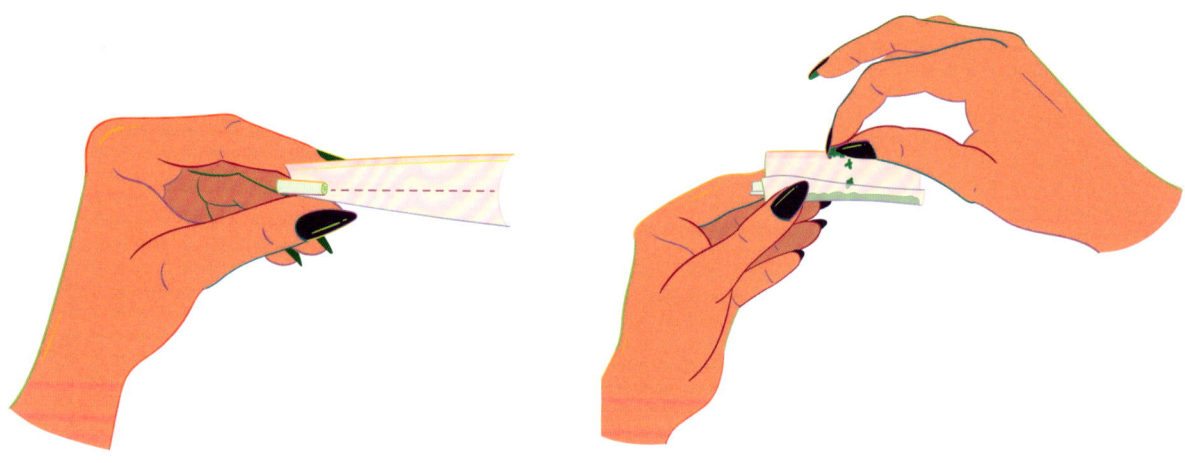

4. Place the tip (crutch) that you just folded onto one of the sides of your paper; I like to place it on the right side with about ¼ – ½ sticking out of the paper.

5. Add your ground flower onto the paper, spreading evenly. Make sure to add enough flower so when you compact it, it's roughly the diameter of a cigarette. Having too much or too little flower will make it more difficult to roll.

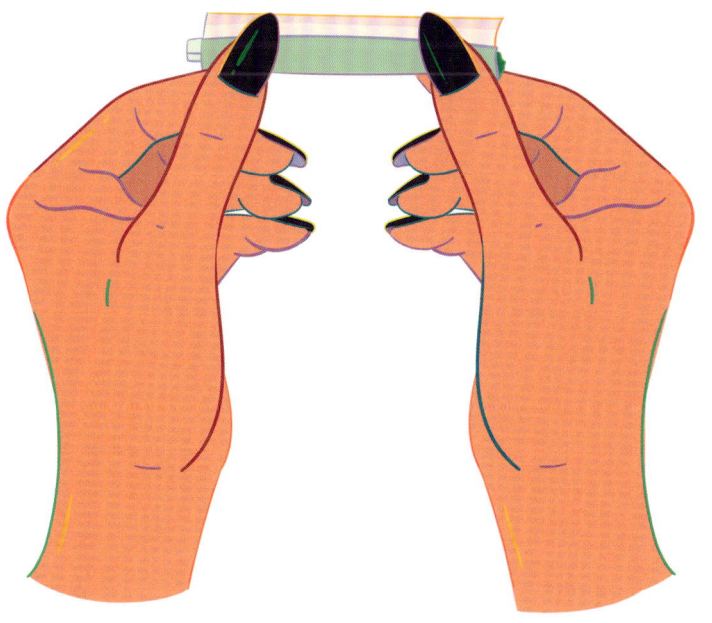

6. Hold the paper in your hands and, using your pointer fingers and thumbs, gently begin massaging the flower into a cylinder by bringing the ends of the paper together and moving your thumbs up and down. The pressure from your hands should be on THE PAPER not on the weed, using the pressure from the base of your fingers to push the flower into a cylinder. If you mess up and don't like the way it's turning out, feel free to pour out the flower, fluff it up, and restart with new paper.

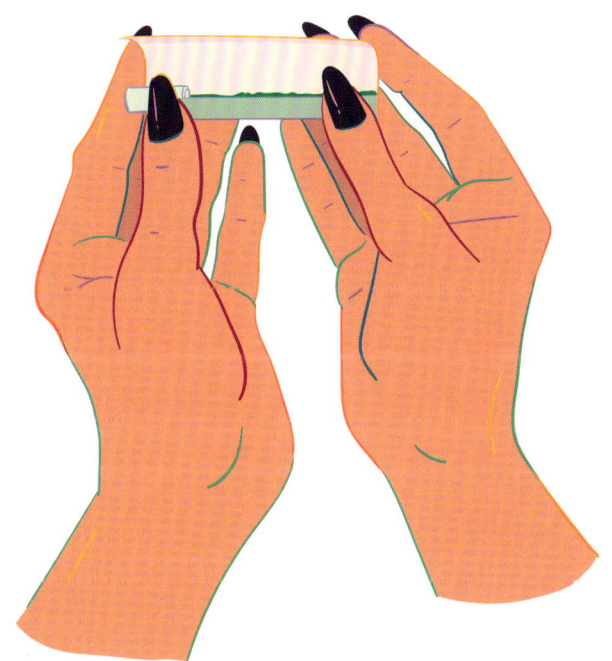

7. Once you can feel that the flower has been shaped into a cylinder, roll the paper all the way down so the flower is visible and the most paper is on the back side. Using the crutch (tip), pinch the paper with your right hand and use your left hand to hold the joint and to slide your thumb slowly across the cylinder as it's being rolled to help guide the paper.

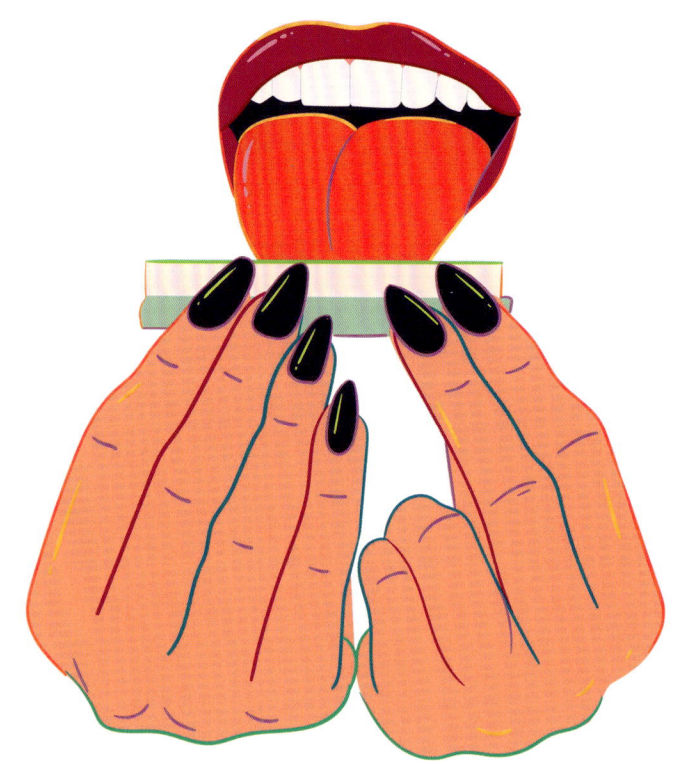

8. Lick the gum (sticky part) when it is the only part of the paper remaining and continue rolling until all the paper is in the cylinder.

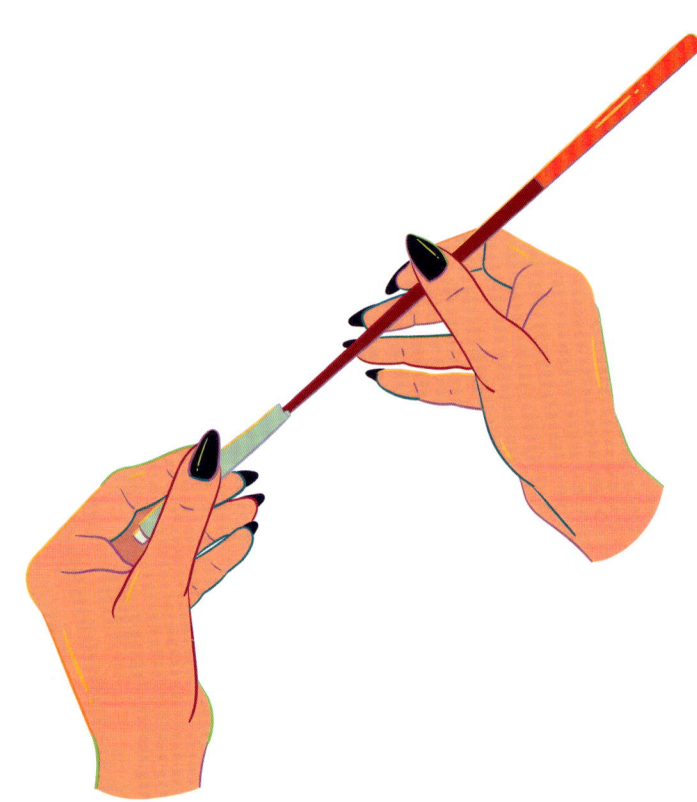

9. Using a chopstick or other pointy object, push the flower down to compact it from the open side that is not the tip. Once compressed, twist the top to close it.

10. Light the joint from the twisted side, first giving it an even burn all around the top then taking small puffs to get it ignited. Don't take long pulls right at the start—this can cause uneven burning called canoeing that isn't ideal.

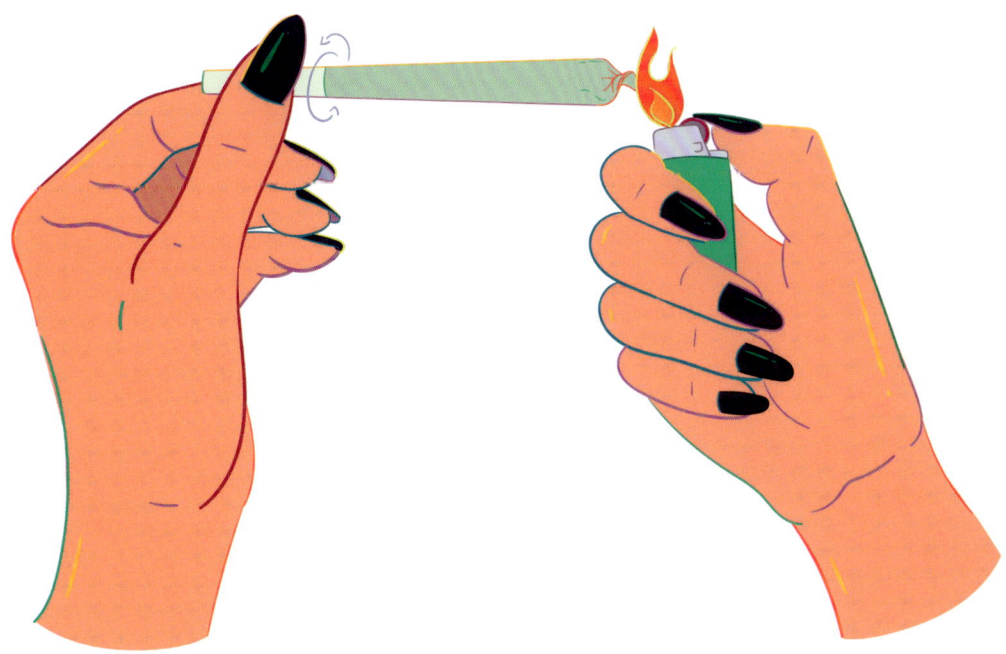

This ten step process to rolling a joint is one reason why smoking is one of my favorite consumption methods—the intention, the time, and the spiritual nature of smoking. There is a component of forced intention associated with smoking because of the time it takes, and because it often involves going outside to consume. Going outside and walking or just simply taking in the sunlight and fresh air can boost serotonin production and add to the therapeutic potential of cannabis. For me, this is why smoking maintains the top spot as a preferred consumption method. Additionally, during the actual act of smoking, we take the practice of long deep breaths, similar to meditation, that can continue to activate the parasympathetic nervous system and add to the relaxation of the overall experience.

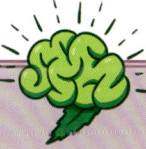

NUGS OF KNOWLEDGE

One way to try out the flavor of a joint before you smoke it is to take a "dry hit". Just after you roll a joint, untwist the very top and inhale air through the joint as if it were lit. This allows you to taste the flavor on your tongue before it is ignited.

SMOKING A JOINT

There are some tricks to smoking to ensure you get an even burn. Starting with quick, small puffs rather than long drags allows the joint to light and start burning evenly. The length of the pull can increase once the ember has been created and starts on an even burning journey; however, if you take those long, hard pulls early on it may cause canoeing, or uneven burning, which you will want to avoid. When you inhale the smoke, you do not need to hold it in for longer than a couple of seconds. What can be absorbed from the cannabis will be almost immediately, and after that you typically want to limit the amount of time that the nontherapeutic compounds in the smoke and the hot air interact with the sensitive tissues of the lungs. If you ever feel that your lungs are inflamed, irritated, or just don't feel good, consider switching to one of the non-inhalation techniques below at least temporarily to allow your lungs to recover.

As you smoke a joint you will need to ash it. Ash is the organic material left over after the cannabis is smoked. There is a wives' tale in the cannabis community that black ash means poor quality flower that has not been flushed of the excess nutrients from growing and white ash means good quality flower—this theory is greatly lacking scientific data, although I do believe there is some rationale behind it. One project I'm currently working on called the Science of Smokeability aims to figure this out.

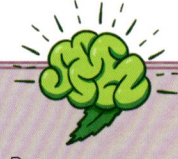

NUGS OF KNOWLEDGE

A friend and colleague, Dr. Markus Roggen, notes that when you smoke a joint, you are engaging in three different consumption methods: smoking, dry herb vaping, and using a concentrate. The smoking is obvious, but as you pull hot air through the joint it vaporizes some of the compounds as the warm air passes over the flower, and as the flower heats up the resin builds and begins to accumulate towards the bottom of the joint—effectively making a concentrate. This is why smoking the second half of the joint can feel different than the first half.

OTHER SMOKING METHODS

Although we often attribute smoking cannabis to smoking joints, there are a variety of other ways to smoke weed. Some examples include bongs, bowls, bubblers, chillum, spliffs, and blunts. In general, these are all very similar techniques, except blunts and spliffs, which contain tobacco. But there are some things to consider when purchasing a new piece or trying a new method of consumption. First, quality pieces are typically made from glass or ceramic material, and occasionally metal. I would recommend staying away from silicone pieces as they are almost always harsh, present a very unpleasant smoking experience and cannot be recycled like the alternatives.

When considering glass pieces like bongs, bowls, and bubblers, the size of the glass matters as well as if it contains water or not. The larger the piece, the more smoke it will hold, and the larger the hit is going to be. However, larger pieces also allow more time and space for the smoke to cool off before reaching your lungs and can often be less irritating. Really small bongs can be difficult because you light them so close to your face it almost feels like you're going to light your eyebrows on fire.

Bowls do not have any water filtration and are often especially harsh because they are small and there is limited space for the smoke to cool before entering your lungs. However, bowls are more portable and discreet compared to something like a 3-foot (91-cm) bong. When lighting up a fresh bowl with a group of other people, if you're planning on sharing people will typically "corner the bowl" meaning only light a

NUGS OF KNOWLEDGE

Some herbal teas are used to reduce inflammation and clear excessive phlegm from the lungs. The best known herb for this is mullein, which is a common wild plant found across the U.S. and other parts of the world. Dried mullein can be added to a mason jar and filled with hot water to extract the active compounds. After extracting for 1 to 2 hours, drink the tea a few times a day until the lungs feels better.

portion of the fresh greenery on fire—not the entire thing. This way when you hand the bowl to the next person, they get to enjoy some fresh flower too.

Some pieces like bongs and bubblers use water filtration. The water inside the piece not only cools the smoke but also filters out particulates and water-soluble compounds that may be irritating or inflammatory to the throat. This filtration step can contribute to a more enjoyable experience and cleaner taste. You can control the temperature of the air hitting your lungs by either adding ice, allowing a very cool, almost menthol, feeling or using warm water in your piece which often feels much smoother because the warmth relaxes the tissues in the throat.

If you choose water filtration, make sure to change the water every single day, and clean your piece regularly. Bacteria and mold can grow on stagnant water in a single day, and you absolutely do not want to be smoking and inhaling the microbial contamination when you're trying to medicate. Additionally, the stagnant smoke flavor in the water will accumulate over time and begin to present itself when you inhale. You are compromising the value of cannabis if you are subjecting yourself to inhaling moldy water, and if you can't stay on top of cleaning your piece, I would recommend choosing a method without water.

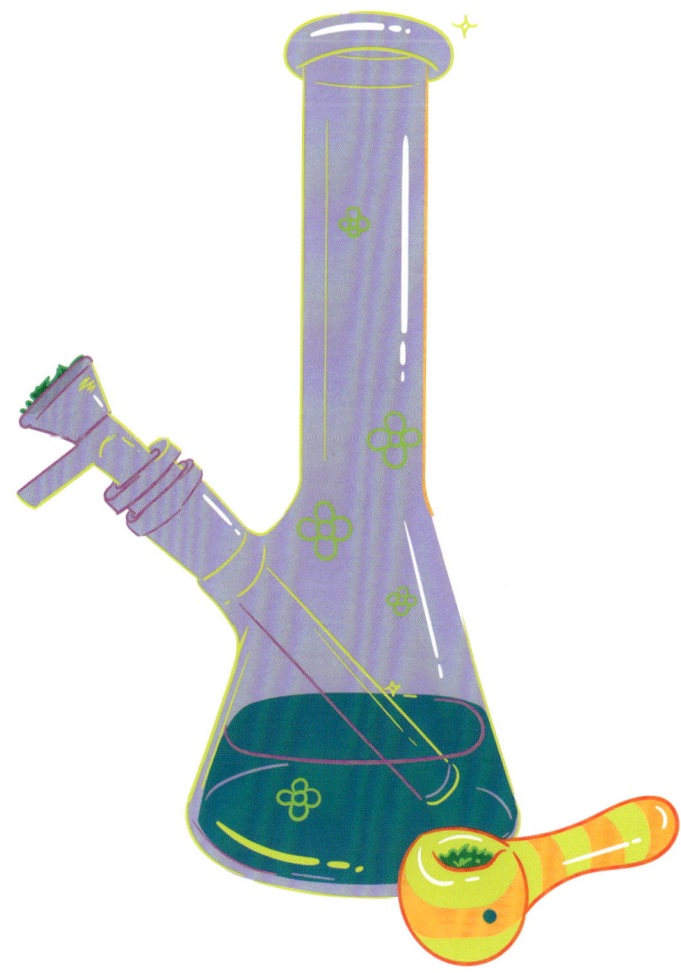

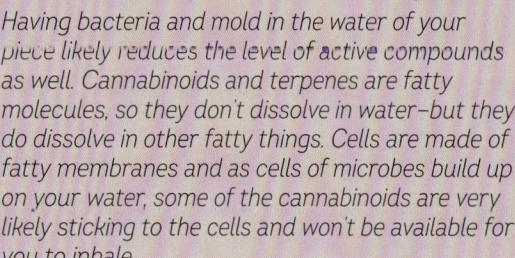

NUGS OF KNOWLEDGE

Having bacteria and mold in the water of your piece likely reduces the level of active compounds as well. Cannabinoids and terpenes are fatty molecules, so they don't dissolve in water—but they do dissolve in other fatty things. Cells are made of fatty membranes and as cells of microbes build up on your water, some of the cannabinoids are very likely sticking to the cells and won't be available for you to inhale.

TOBACCO MIXES

Blunts, spliffs, and chillum are very common ways to consume cannabis with tobacco. These consumption methods have deep-rooted cultural significance, especially in Black and brown communities. Blunts are made from rolling cannabis flower in tobacco leaves, and spliffs typically consist of cannabis flower mixed with tobacco leaves, rolled into a joint using hemp or rice papers. Additionally, cannabis hash has long been consumed with tobacco rolled up, similar to spliffs. A chillum is a traditional smoking device that is a straight, conical pipe usually made from clay or stone, and it is typically used for smoking cannabis and tobacco. The traditional method is hand mixing tobacco and aged hashish. However, chillums now come in all shapes and sizes– even the classic "one hitter", which is the size of a cigarette, is a chillum. This combination of cannabis and nicotine offers unique therapeutic benefits, provides a more stimulating feeling for daytime use, decreases the relative ratio of intoxicating cannabinoids, and increases the chemical diversity in the inhalation product.

No products or molecules are inherently bad, but it is important to understand the pros and cons of consuming tobacco products as an educated smoker. Nicotine has proven to be very beneficial for people who suffer from chronic inflammatory and autoimmune conditions like ulcerative colitis (UC) and sarcoidosis. Nicotine lessens the body's secretion of antibodies, which are often elevated in patients with autoimmune conditions. Reducing anitbody secretion results in an anti-inflammatory response and ultimately immunosuppression, which can be beneficial for those with overactive immune systems[5]. **Some research has also noted that adding tobacco in with cannabis increases the vaporization efficiency of THC by as much as 45%, so you get more THC per puff if tobacco is mixed in with cannabis**[6].

But there are clear downsides to nicotine as well. Globally in 2019, there were approximately 1.14 billion people who smoked tobacco products, accounting for 7.7 million tobacco, related deaths[7]. When tobacco leaves are smoked, it produces different chemistry compared to smoked cannabis and has significant implications on our health. Nicotine itself doesn't cause much harm. However, when the molecules in tobacco including nicotine are smoked, they break down into well-known cancer-causing compounds called **nitrosamines**. Additionally, burning tobacco produces a more acidic environment in the joint[8] and burns hotter than cannabis, producing additional chemical changes that can result in more carcinogens produced.

TRADITIONAL HASH

Traditional hashish deserves its own category in this book; it is a traditional art form that is still practiced in the cannabis industry and has a long cultural history across the world. Different parts of the world are renowned for their unique techniques of making hash, leading to signature colors, textures, or methods of preparation. Traditional Moroccan hash will be different from Afghan hash. However, there are similarities between what goes into making hash across the world.

Hash is the art of removing the cannabinoid-rich trichomes from the plant material (which can be frozen or dried/cured). The trichomes can be removed a few different ways, including using ice water to chill the flower so the delicate trichomes break off the flower and sink to the bottom of the vessel, or by spreading dried cannabis flower on a sheet or sieve so the small trichomes are separated from the larger plant material. **In general, making hash involves using sieves to separate the trichomes from the rest of the plant.** Then the trichomes are either pressed by hand (this method is called charas) or can be pressed by warm bottles to release the oils and stick together in a ball or a brick. When rolled into a ball, it is called a Temple Ball–a method popularized by the late cannabis enthusiast and hash expert, Frenchy Cannoli. Hash is technically a cannabis concentrate but does not use any solvents.

Hash is traditionally smoked with tobacco flower, by itself, or with cannabis flower. Traditionally, hash is aged a minimum of three months before consuming, and the aging changes the chemistry substantially. Additionally, the process produces new compounds, one of which is **hashishene**–a terpene first isolated from aged hash.

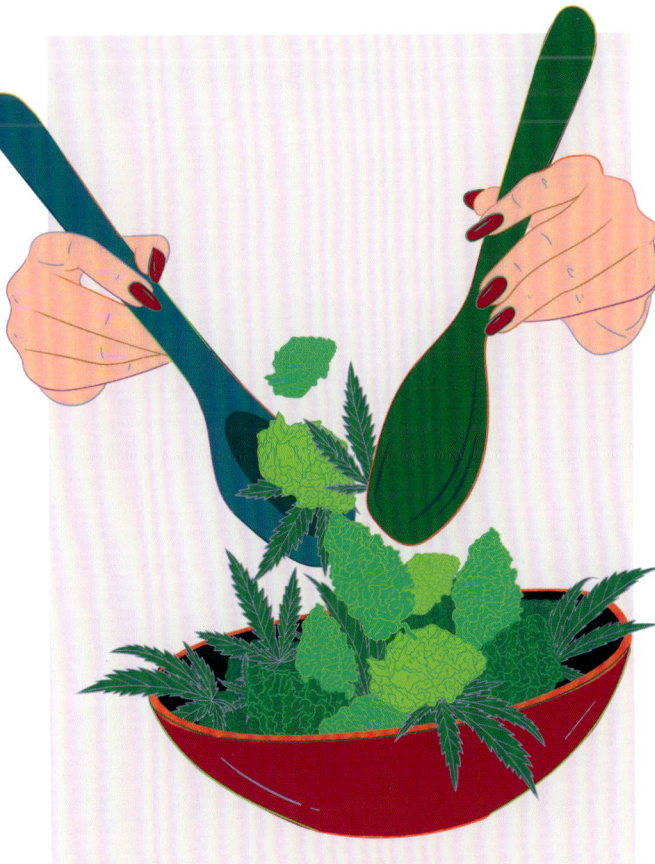

VAPING

Vaping is an umbrella term; it does not mean one thing. Vaporization is the process of heating up a cannabis product BELOW the point of combustion—aka smoking which occurs around 480°F (250°C). The point of vaping is to vaporize or inhale the active compounds such as cannabinoids and terpenes and to avoid the other non-active byproducts produced in the smoking process. Because vaping is an inhalation method, it is fast-acting like smoking—this can be especially important for people with flare conditions like migraines and inflammatory gut conditions because you need relief FAST.

Most vapes allow you to control the vape temperature, so there is some control over which compounds you're inhaling and which you are leaving behind. Vaping can often make you feel really high, especially if you are used to smoking. This is because the relative amount of THC and CBD per puff is greater compared to smoking. Not only are you only vaporizing the active compounds of interest and no others, but THC, CBD, and other active compounds aren't being degraded or transformed as much as they are during the combustion process, so you are inhaling more of the actual THC and CBD and not the by-products created via combustion.

DRY HERB VAPING

I believe this is one of the "healthiest" consumption methods, alongside edibles, and it is one of my favorites. Dry herb vaping is when you take cannabis flower and heat it up to vaporize the active compounds. One of the benefits of dry herb vaping is that it uses flower, unlike the other vaping methods which use extracts. If you grow your own flower or have access to quality cannabis, this is a great method to use the flower without smoking it. Using flower allows you the flexibility to still create the "salads" with different types of cannabis flower containing either mainly THC, CBD, THCV, or CBG.

Like smoking, the process starts with first grinding the flower. Once the flower is ground it is a simple process of putting it in the chamber of the vaporizer, then setting the temperature and inhaling the vapor.

The temperature that you vaporize at will also impact your experience. At lower temperatures you will get the most flavor from your cannabis. When I get a new strain or variety, I always try it first on my dry herb vaporizer at a low temperature, allowing me to fully taste the flavor profile. Low temperature vaping

Whether you're interested in smoking, vaping, topicals, suppositories, or tinctures, keep in mind that you do not need to restrict yourself to THC products or to THC flower. With each consumption method other active compounds like CBD, CBG, CBN, THCV, CBC, etc., can be used for a less intoxicating, but still medicinal, effect.

If you are very sensitive to THC, or simply do not want to feel the high effects from cannabis, I strongly encourage you to experiment with using different types of cannabis flower. For instance, hemp varieties can be bred to produce majority cannabinoids other than THC, such as CBD-dominant hemp, CBG-dominant hemp, and THCV-dominant hemp.

As a consumer, you can use these different varieties of cannabis to produce "salads" where you mix the different types of flower together to find your personalized ratio for how you are feeling at that moment. Depending on where you live, you may be able to purchase these other non-THC varieties of cannabis online. In the United States, due to the 2018 Farm Bill, products that contain less than 0.3% THC can be purchased from online retailers.

also allows for the small monoterpenes to be vaporized, often providing uplifting effects, great for daytime use. When I'm looking for more sedating effects; I turn the vaporizer up to typically around 428°F (220°C), at higher temperatures the flavor gets drowned out by the other particles in the smoke, but the feeling is much more heavy hitting.

You will notice a difference in the end product of flower that has been dry herb vaped compared to combusted. Vaped flower is brown but still contains the structure and integrity of the flower. Combusted flower turns into ash and lacks structure as all the organic material has been burned compared to vaporizing that selectively vaporizes the active compounds.

NUGS OF KNOWLEDGE

One-hitters: one-hitters are small cannabis devices that are meant to be discreet and offer one hit of weed. These are great for people on the go, or people who want to keep their tolerance low by only using the smallest amount needed or the therapeutic minimum. Both smoking and dry herb vaping one-hitters exist, some even are disguised to look like a cigarette for maximum discreteness.

DABBING

Dabbing is a form of vaporization where cannabis concentrates, which come in a variety of textures, are heated up in either a dab rig that looks similar to a small bong, or an electronic device that is typically a handheld, water-filtered device.

When using a dab rig, the rig is heated with a blowtorch, then allowed to cool to the desired temperature (typically ranging from 400 to 600°F [204 to 315°C]), the extract is then added into the chamber for inhalation. Many people use either temperature guns or other specialized devices to measure the temperature of the rig before hitting the dab, so it doesn't create an excess of carcinogens like benzene and doesn't burn your throat from the heat[9]. Electronic devices usually have a variety of settings for different dab temperatures, and you simply hit a button, and it automatically heats to the right temperature.

Electronic devices are great for beginners because you don't need to worry about temperature settings being too high or accidentally burning your house down with the torch.

Concentrated cannabis oils and hash which come in a wide variety of textures, colors, and aromas, are used for dabbing. Because the products are concentrated, dabbers typically use a lot less product at a time compared to smokers, so only small amounts of product are needed. If you are used to smoking a one-gram joint, you may only need a pea-size dab in order to feel similar effects. This way, if you are a low-responding person and need higher doses, you can get a higher-potency product like a dab and save your lungs some smoke exposure.

The effects you feel from dabbing are going to vary based on the type of extract you use and the type of plant it was extracted from. For example, there are "live" extracts and cured extracts. Live extracts like live resin and live rosin are made from freshly harvested cannabis buds, and are unlike other forms of extracts that utilize cannabis that has been dried and cured. During the dry and cure process, some of the chemistry changes in the plant. Many of the terpenes that provide the uplifting effects and some of the potent aromatic compounds are lost to the environment, leaving behind the heavier, more sedating compounds which have been attributed to reduced anxiety.

One popular type of solvent-based extract for dabbing is butane hash oil (BHO), which is made by extracting cannabis with butane as a solvent. Once it is extracted, the oil can be manipulated to have many different textures—that's where the terms shatter, butter and wax originate.

Dabbing is a great therapeutic method of consumption for people who require higher doses of cannabinoids, but is often not the first consumption method that people try because cannabis concentrates can hit really hard for new users who have not built a tolerance to THC.

Ice hash rosin and full melt hash are regarded as premium cannabis products due to their purity, potency, and solventless extraction methods. Ice hash rosin is made by collecting trichomes from cannabis using ice water and agitation, followed by pressing the hash under heat and pressure to create a concentrated, terpene-rich extract. This process preserves the plant's natural cannabinoids and terpenes without the use of solvents, offering a clean and flavorful experience. Full melt hash, on the other hand, refers to a form of hash that completely melts when vaporized, leaving no residue, indicating its high purity and minimal plant matter. Both products are valued for their potency, flavor, and craftsmanship, making them sought after by connoisseurs. Hash can also be smoked as a "hash hole" where a line of quality hash is added on top of cannabis flower and rolled up in a large joint. When smoked there is a clear "hole" in the center where the line of hash was. It presents a flavorful, strong smoking experience that is great for sharing among groups of people.

After you take a dab, immediately clean your piece. This is the easiest time to clean because the wax and glass (or ceramic) are already hot. To clean, take a cotton swab and rub it along the bottom and sides of the area where you put your wax. If it isn't easy to clean up, simply add some isopropyl alcohol to the cottom swap then try again. This will make the flavor come through on your next hit just as strongly and allow you to make friends easier because you don't have a gross piece.

VAPE CARTRIDGES

Vape cartridges or vape pens are a very discreet way to use cannabis and can be a great consumption method for medicating on the go. Vape cartridges come in a variety of shapes and sizes, but all contain a cannabis oil that is heated to the point of vaporization. There are different types of heating elements used to make the pens, including ceramic and metal. Recent scientific studies have indicated that metals from the heating elements inside the vape cartridges can leach into the oil over time and can be vaporized by the consumer[10]. This is of most concern if you are keeping your vape in an area like a hot car that has extreme heat and temperature fluctuations, or if you're using an old vape cart, that you found while cleaning out your room.

The important thing to know about vapes that is not all oils are the same; some vape oils are extracted from the plant using no solvents, other types of vapes are highly processed and may **only** contain THC that has been stripped from the rest of the plant. The three types of vape cartridges you will typically find are:

1. Rosin: Rosin is typically the premiere quality of cannabis oil because it is made without using

solvents. Therefore, there is no risk of residual solvent, and you know that the oil contains a large diversity of medicinal compounds in the natural ratio that the plant makes them in.

2. Live resin and live rosin: When you see the word live in front of a cannabis product, it means that the oil was extracted from a cannabis plant that was frozen right after harvest to preserve the entire chemical profile within the plant. Usually some of these compounds are lost during the dry and cure process. Live resin is a cannabis oil that is made from extracting the plants after they have been frozen with solvents to get the full profile of the living plant in the final oil. Live Rosin also captures the full profile from the freshly harvested and immediately frozen plant, but this method does not use solvents to produce the final product. Rather, the flower is pressed using pressure and heat to remove the oils.

3. Distillate: There are a LOT of products in the legal cannabis market made from THC distillate. Distillate is made by distilling or purifying out the THC from the rest of the plant material. Because distillate cartridges are mainly THC, they lack the chemical diversity found in other products like rosin or live resin and often result in a more hollow feeling compared to these other oils that present a robust liveliness. However, one advantage of distillate is that it is extremely reproducible and will provide consistent effects. Additionally, pure distillate does not smell and may be a good option for travel. Other products similar to distillate are liquid diamonds or liquid shatter that is purified THC with some added terpenes to provide more flavor, but it is still lacking the complexity of other extracts like rosin and live resin.

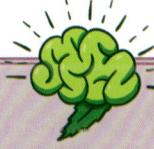

NUGS OF KNOWLEDGE

Botanically derived terpenes vs. cannabis derived terpenes: Some cannabis products contain added terpenes. If the terpenes were extracted from the cannabis plant then added back into the final product, this, is a cannabis-derived terpene. If the THC was distilled out and then terpenes from other sources like the lavender plant or hops are added back, in these are called botanically derived terpenes.

We are still learning about the overall safety of vape pens. In general, I advise against this method unless you are someone who suffers from a chronic condition and need a discreet and safe way to medicate regularly like many parents experience, or it is the only option available to you in your area. Vape cartridges are very easy to use, and many people develop a poor relationship with their vape because they start using it all the time without any intention or purpose to their consumption.

Because many cannabis oils are too thick to be vaporized, manufacturers use additives, like high terpene amounts to combat this. Although terpenes do have medicinal value, artificially high terpene content is potentially harmful to vape and can cause throat irritation. This is one of the reasons I like to emphasize the **natural ratio** of compounds produced by the cannabis plant. The plant is producing molecules at levels that have traditionally been compatible with our bodies. As we refine, manipulate, and manufacture cannabis products we are often changing this ratio and no longer have thousands of years of safety data like we do with flower; more is not always better.

EDIBLES

Edibles are a broad category that include gummies, caramels, chocolates, and even drinks—but you can think of it as essentially anything that you are ingesting that must pass through your gut. One of the massive benefits to edibles is how discreet they are, unlike smoking or vaping which you can smell from a mile away, edibles can be taken without anyone knowing and brought with you pretty much anywhere. Edibles often offer a feeling of a "body high" or complete relaxation all over, as opposed to the brain-focused "head high" that is often associated with inhalation methods.

If you are just starting with your edible journey and you are unsure if you are going to be a low-responder or high-responder, I would suggest starting with 2.5 mg of THC. This may require you cutting a gummy in half or even a quarter. It can be helpful to eat something fatty before taking the edible, which allows for greater absorption and more consistent results. After taking the edible, wait it out and keep track of when you took it and what effects you feel. At the end of the night, take notes for next time—whether you would stay at the same dose, or increase your dose. The following day, eat something fatty before taking the edible, and try the next dose. Once you've homed in on your dose, you can try different products and start to understand how your body reacts.

WAITING PERIOD

Edibles also last much longer compared to inhalable methods, which you feel the peak effects of within 10 minutes. Depending on your metabolism and the type of product you're using, it could take upward of two hours to feel the full effects from an edible. This is why we need to be very careful when dosing edibles because a common mistake people make is taking a second dose because they don't feel the effects from the first dose, leading up to the classic story of both edibles hitting at the same time.

Our body needs to process the THC (& other compounds) before we feel

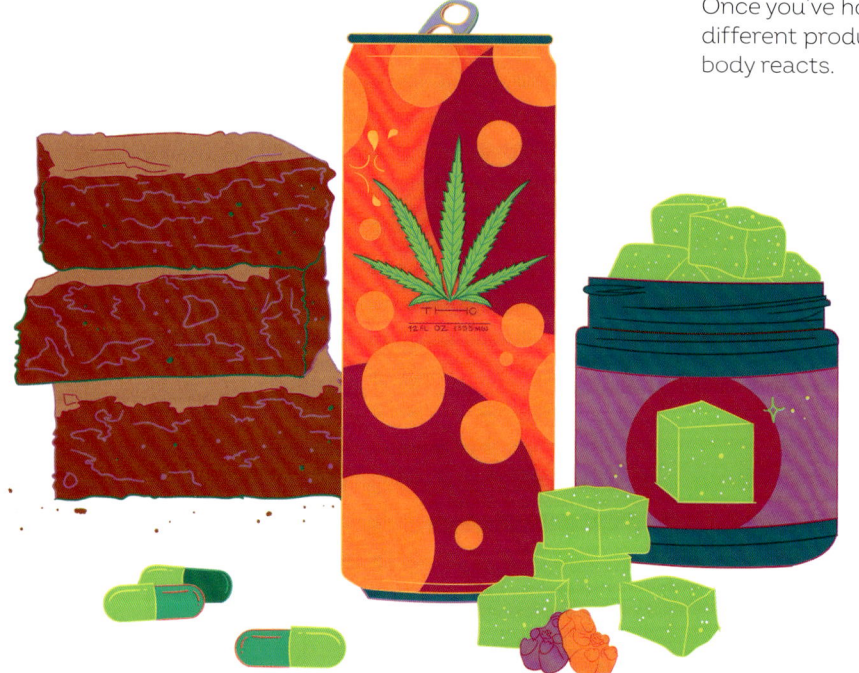

the effects. When we swallow THC-containing products, it eventually makes it to the liver where everything we ingest is processed and prepared for its exit from the body (pooping and peeing). The liver has special enzymes that process all drugs and substances in the body, and it 'processes' them by literally changing the chemistry of active molecules. For THC, as it passes the liver, it is changed into a different molecule called 11-hydroxy-THC, often abbreviated as 11-OH-THC because there is a hydroxyl chemical group (-OH) on the 11th carbon of the molecule. This metabolite still makes us feel high and is very active in our body, potentially even more active than THC on the CB1 receptor; some evidence suggests it can pass our blood brain barriers and more easily penetrate our brain compared to the un-metabolized THC.

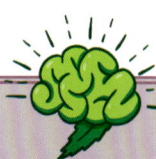

There are a variety of edible products that are made to be 'strain specific' or contain added terpenes to provide a similar strain-specific effect as smoking flower would provide. However, many of the terpenes are lost or changed during the cooking process, and it is still mainly a mystery as to what happens to these compounds during metabolism.

THC → 11-OH-THC → THC-COOH

Newer technology is allowing edibles to act faster than ever; this is called nano-emulsion technology. This technology breaks the cannabinoids up into very tiny particles rather than large ones that normally would enter your body and allows the fatty compounds to mix with water—allowing you to feel an edible or drink in as little as 15 minutes. Your body is mostly water, and incorporating nanoemulsions allows the active compounds to mix and enhances the bioavailability and absorption of the active molecules like THC and CBD. Additionally, nano-emulsion technology contains other digestive components that your body would typically add to process and absorb the edible.

The Entourage of Edibles

When the liver processes THC it is using enzymes to transform THC into an easier form to process and excrete. However, it's not just THC that is being metabolized, it is also all the other compounds in cannabis which are sometimes being processed by the same enzyme as THC and sometimes by other enzymes. This leads to a whole new swath of chemistry circulating in the body, now containing the metabolites of cannabis.

Some people can't feel edibles at all. No matter what the dose is, some people are unable to process edibles, and this is currently not a viable consumption method for many. For some, it may take upwards of 50-100 mg to feel any effects, and for others 5 mg may make you feel incredibly high. This variability in how cannabis consumers feel the effects from edibles comes down to our body's ability to process the THC. Evidence collected from the nonprofit organization I co-founded, the Network of Applied Pharmacognosy, suggests that up to 16% of cannabis consumers can't feel the effects from edibles, but hopefully we will be able to find a way to formulate around this because that is a substantial portion of the population who can't use this valuable consumption method.

Making Edibles at Home

Edibles can easily be made at home but remember you won't have the precision and comfortability of knowing your dose like you do with dispensary products—so continue with caution.

If you want to make edibles at home, you have to **decarboxylate** your flower first. This is a big word that essentially means heating up your flower in an oven to activate it. We don't need to worry about this with other consumption methods because we are already heating up the material via smoking or vaping. But with edibles, we need to heat up the flower first, then extract it, then ingest it.

Heating up the flower converts the active compounds from the acidic versions that are made in the plant to the non-acidic version that is active in our body. Every cannabinoid is produced in the acidic version in the plant, because it helps protect the plant from the sun and other environmental stressors, but that acidic version will not make us feel high and has limited medicinal value. This activation process is called decarboxy-lation because when we heat up the flower in the oven, it removes a group on the molecule called a carboxylic acid, or simply put, a CO_2 group.

Here are four simple steps to making your own cannabis butter or oil to cook with:

1) Put your bud on a tray and preheat your oven to 230 to 265°F (110 to 129°C) depending on the type of cannabis you have. Roast in the oven 30 to 40 minutes.

2) Once it is out of the oven, place it in a double boiler then add your fat product (clarified butter or oil such as MCT coconut oil, olive oil, or avocado oil) over the flower.

3) Allow the cannabinoids to infuse into the oil for about 1 hour on low to medium heat. I like to use a muddler or other kitchen tool to break up the nugs for maximum extraction.

4) Strain out the flower and use in any recipe by substituting oil or butter with your infused product.

There are also a variety of cookbooks, YouTube videos, and online recipes to follow to make homemade edibles. Additionally, modern devices exist that will decarb your flower with the touch of a button, then all you need to do is add your oil of choice and hit another button to infuse—it's foolproof but can be a bit pricey.

New tools allow you to measure the concentration of your edibles at home, but again they are typically not in the budget of a regular consumer, so if you know the amount of THC and CBD in your starting material, you can easily calculate the amount in your final product or simply look up 'edible dosage calculator' and a website will do it for you!

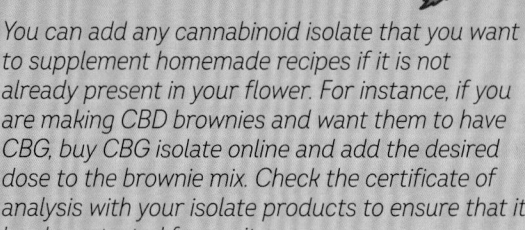

NUGS OF KNOWLEDGE

You can add any cannabinoid isolate that you want to supplement homemade recipes if it is not already present in your flower. For instance, if you are making CBD brownies and want them to have CBG, buy CBG isolate online and add the desired dose to the brownie mix. Check the certificate of analysis with your isolate products to ensure that it has been tested for purity.

TINCTURES

Technically speaking, tinctures are alcohol extracts, but cannabis products made from oils are commonly referred to as tinctures. Tinctures may be the **most versatile consumption method** for cannabis as they can be added into food, lotions, bandages, or taken sublingually.

Don't have any edibles on hand? Don't worry about it—just add a few drops of your tincture to a gummy that you already have and BOOM. Need a THC infused lotion for a sore spot on your back? Not a problem—add some of your tincture into your favorite lotion and voilà. When making 'tinctures' at home, I like to use coconut MCT oil. MCT means medium chain triglycerides—this is a refined version of coconut oil that is liquid at room temperature and is very effective at extracting cannabinoids. If you prefer, you can also make a traditional alcohol-based tincture at home using a high-proof neutral alcohol like vodka. When making tinctures, you also need to decarboxylate the flower to activate the cannabinoids, similar to making edibles unless of course you are aiming to extract the acidic cannabinoids which do have medicinal benefits.

Sublingual Consumption

Tinctures can be taken sublingually (under the tongue), as the product can be absorbed via the tongue's mucous membranes. This allows the active compounds to be absorbed directly into the bloodstream, so you feel the effects much quicker compared to eating an infused product. There are other non-tincture-based sublingual methods of administration available on some legal markets including: sprays, tablets, and strips. Sublingual methods are also easy to dose using the measurements on a tincture bottle.

RSO

Rick Simpson Oil (RSO), also called **full extract cannabis oil (FECO)**, is a concentrated cannabis alcohol extract that differs from traditional alcohol-based tinctures. RSO is made by extracting cannabis in alcohol, then evaporating off the alcohol so it is only the concentrated black oil. This oil is typically used by medical patients and administered via syringe (not injected into the body, rather used for precise measurement of dose) because dosing is critical, as it is a very concentrated product. RSO was named after a Canadian cannabis activist who used the concentrated oil to treat cancer and other chronic conditions.

TOPICALS

Topicals are products that you put on top of your skin which include common products like creams, lotions, gels, and salves. These products are great for relieving localized pain and inflammation and are one of the best ways to introduce people to cannabis, because they work extremely effectively and do not get you high. When my grandma wanted to use a cannabis product for the first time, topicals were all she was comfortable with, and they worked extremely well for her arthritis and knee pain.

Topicals can be formulated to contain THC, CBD, CBG and many active compounds in the plant. There are often options for whole plant formulations or products made with isolated compounds—such as terpenes. Terpenes like limonene and pinene have even been shown to help enhance the permeability of cannabinoids in the skin and make a more effective topical[11] product[12].

How Do Topicals Work?

The skin has cannabinoid receptors all over it, including on the hair follicles and sweat glands. When the topical product is applied to the skin, these receptors are locally activated. However, the active compounds are unable to fully penetrate through the skin and reach the bloodstream which is why you won't feel the psychoactive effects from using topical products. You also will not test positive on a drug test for using topical products for the same reason, as it will not reach your bloodstream.

Cannabinoids can have medicinal effects on the skin outside from direct interactions with the cannabinoid receptors. Studies have identified cannabinoids to be effective for reducing inflammation, oxidative damage, reducing damage from UVA/UVB radiation, anti-aging, and well as anti-acne properties. For instance, CBD inhibits the genes involved in the pro-inflammatory response and can help lower localized inflammation. Additionally, cannabinoids like CBD and CBG have shown to be antimicrobial, meaning they kill bacteria and fungi on the skin and don't negatively impact the skin's natural ecosystem[13].

Applying Topicals

Topicals need to be applied REGULARLY, not just once per day. Bring the product around with you if you're leaving the house and apply whenever it is convenient. However, if you're using topicals regularly for long periods of time, your skin receptors can also develop a tolerance, and you may need to occasionally use less product or change products to allow your skin's ECS to recover or change up the products you are using to introduce new active ingredients or a different dose.

Transdermals

Transdermal patches are different from topicals as they deliver cannabinoids directly to your bloodstream, ensuring you feel the psychoactive effects from these patches. Transdermal patches are specially made to adhere to the skin and allow the active compounds to pass through the skin's protective barrier; this can be done using electric pulses, microneedles or special penetration-enhancing compounds. The patch is placed on the skin and a specific dose is administered. Some cannabis transdermal products are formed for specific conditions, and many can be found via online retailers. Many drugs are administered via transdermal patch as it is a safe and non-invasive way of administering medicine.

SUPPOSITORIES

A valuable option for medical cannabis patients who can't swallow, have trouble swallowing, have pain below the waist, or simply need a long-lasting and effective method of administration are suppositories. People with Crohn's disease, ulcerative colitis, endometriosis, pelvic floor dysfunction, painful periods, ovarian cysts, chemotherapy-induced nausea and vomiting, and other localized pain and inflammatory conditions benefit immensely from this method of administration. Patients with gut conditions often gravitate towards this method because it does not require passing through the GI tract to benefit from this medicine.

Although a patient will still feel the intoxicating effects of THC administered rectally, it often leads to less intoxication compared to the same dose taken orally and has a longer release time, which facilitates a gentler experience.

Both vaginal and rectal suppositories are available; some can be used in both areas, while others are specially formulated for either the vagina or the rectum. Suppositories typically contain THC, CBD, or other cannabinoids in varying doses and oil such as coconut or avocado oil to dissolve the active compounds and allow effective absorption.

Because they are simple yet often difficult to find, suppositories can be made at home with minimal ingredients. One of the simplest ways is to add equal parts of infused coconut oil and non-infused cocoa butter, heat them up to mix together, and pour into suppository molds. You may want to line your undergarments with protective barriers to ensure the oil doesn't damage the fabric if it leaks out.

DOSING CONSIDERATIONS

Storage of Cannabis Products

One way to ensure you have a consistent experience with a cannabis product is to make sure it is stored properly. Always store your cannabis products in a closed container and out of the sunlight and extensive heat. Many cannabis connoisseurs who want to maintain the quality of their products have small refrigerators they store their concentrates and edibles in, others simply have a cabinet or drawer.

If products are left in the sun, a hot car, or in an open container, the chemistry will start to change, and compounds will begin to degrade. THC will begin to degrade into CBN and other cannabinoids, and CBD can degrade into another class of compounds called quinones that may not have the same broad safety profile as the parent molecule.

If you see a rapid color change, smell change, or any mold and bacterial growth on your products, stop using them, throw them out, figure out a better storage method, and then find new products.

If you have children around, keep your cannabis products locked and stored away from children. Cannabis companies must follow stringent guidelines to ensure products are not attractive to children and difficult to open. As an adult, it is your job to follow through with these safety measures and keep them out of reach. While children likely won't be rolling up a joint and lighting it on fire, if you have gummies, lozenges, brownies or drinks around keep them under lock and key.

Cleaning Your Pieces

There are a variety of methods and new products to help you clean your glass pieces. You will notice after you have been smoking from your bong, bubbler, or bowl for a few days (or even a few hits) it will start to accumulate a brown sticky substance called **resin**. Resin is the leftover cannabinoids, terpenes, tar, and other sticky molecules from smoking.

If you want to clean off the resin, you need a fat-loving solvent to dissolve the fatty molecules. There's a saying in chemistry "like dissolves like"—if you are trying to get rid of something fatty you need to use something fatty, water will not work. What many people do, including myself, is a simple process of using coarse salt and isopropyl alcohol. Add the isopropyl into the piece where the resin is, then add a generous amount of coarse salt. Cover the holes on the piece and shake the isopropyl around, using the salt as a scrubbing agent. This should work pretty quickly. If you really let the resin build up, allow the alcohol to soak in the piece for a few hours or overnight. For smaller pieces like stems of bongs, bowls, and reusable glass rollings tips, you can add them to a jar with isopropyl alcohol and salt and let them soak. Once they appear to have no resin left on them, give a final wash with soap and water to remove any residual solvent and keep on smoking.

Consent

Even though cannabis is a safe plant for most people, it still does require someone's consent if you are going to give it to others. Never put infused products in people's food or drink without them knowing. If someone chooses to trust you with introducing them to their first cannabis experience, I encourage you to take that very seriously. First impressions are important and can make or break someone's perception of this medicine.

Additionally, never take advantage of someone's physical or mental state when they are under the influence of cannabis or any other substance.

Intention

There is no correct way to consume cannabis and there is no bad or good consumption method. Finding a consumption method that is available to you and fits with your lifestyle is important, but what is also important is your intention when using the medicine.

Intention is having a plan and setting your mind in the right place to get the most out of cannabis. Your intentions with cannabis use don't need to be written down or verbalized, although they can be if that's how you prefer, but thinking about WHY you are using cannabis can help with creating a sustainable relationship with the plant.

Some examples of what your intention could be when consuming are things like being nicer to your partner, being creative for a project, enjoying the nice weather, letting go of small annoyances, cleaning your house, not scrolling on your phone, finding a better mindset for an event, enjoying a friend's company, etc.

Intention helps avoid escapism. Escapism is the act of using a substance to essentially escape your problems and escape reality. Escapism is not always bad, but it is not sustainable for the long run. If you have a very traumatic or difficult time in your life, such as someone close to you passing, a fire, a broken bone, a failed exam, etc., it is okay to use cannabis as a crutch until you are ready to process. In fact, in many cases cannabis can be used alongside therapy or within the community to facilitate these conversations. However, if this turns into your day to day and you're finding that you're unable to do anything without cannabis or you're

constantly over-medicating to avoid feelings, work, or decisions, it is time to reevaluate your relationship with cannabis.

If you and/or your family are prone to addiction, I would highly recommend choosing a consumption method that takes some time to prepare, and perhaps one that you don't feel the effects from immediately. People tend to develop negative relationships with cannabis cartridges or pens because they're so easy to hit anytime, anywhere and you feel the effects instantly. This instant effect is part of the reason why drugs that are injected or snorted are more addictive because the shorter the time for you to feel the effects, the more your brain craves it. Look into methods like edibles that have a lag before you feel anything, or perhaps smoking or dry herb vaping which require you to prepare the flower before consuming.

If you see your friends or family are having a negative relationship with cannabis, reach out to them and see if there are other things happening in their life that they may want to talk about or seek help from a professional to discuss. It is important for other members of the cannabis community to keep each other in check. Although cannabis is safe and not addictive for most, we have a diversity of brains, and our brains may react differently to different substances.

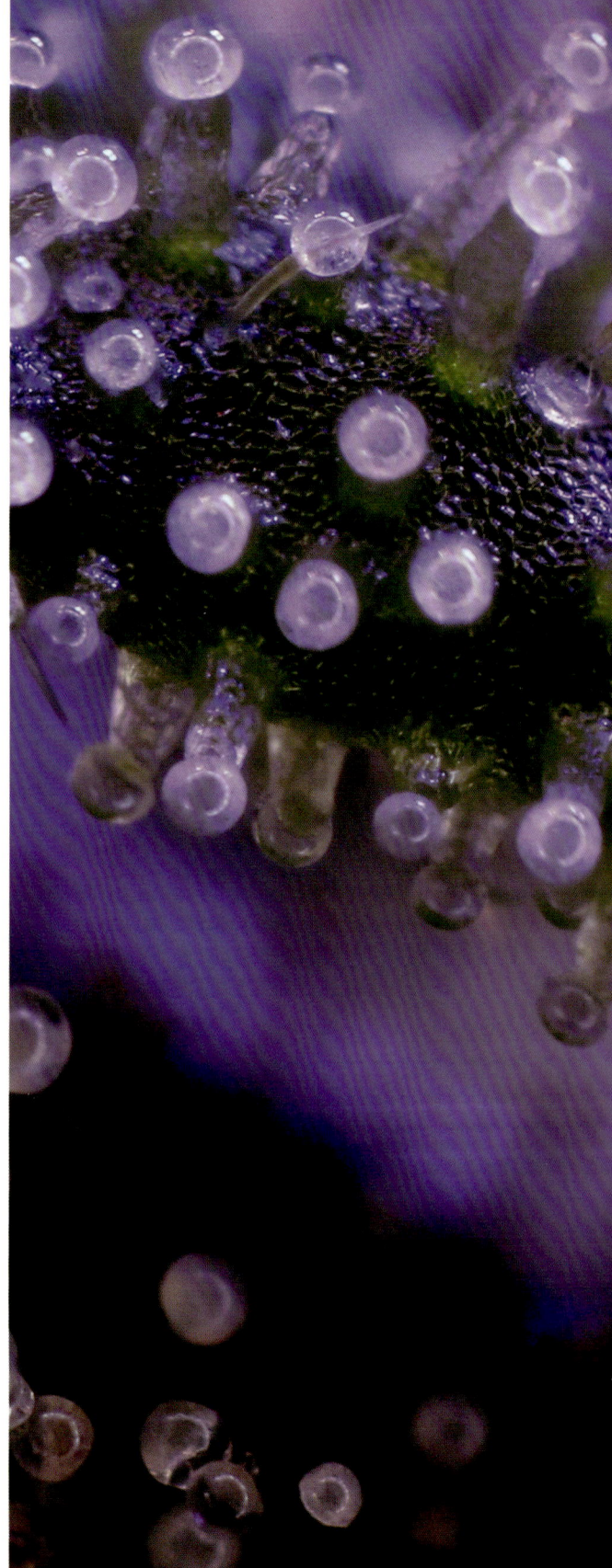

SHARE THIS KNOWLEDGE

There is nuance involved in how someone will react to a specific consumption method or why they may gravitate toward one over another including: genetics, accessibility, past trauma, metabolism, duration of experience, and so much more. As medical patients and as cannabis consumers, I encourage you to share the insights that you have personally learned from this medicine or even from this book, with your community and pass on the knowledge.

Knowledge comes from not only sharing your personal experience but also taking the time to listen and learn from someone sharing their experiences. This medicine has not always been safe to openly talk about, and many people may not trust others enough to share their cannabis use, including with their physicians, friends and family. **If someone trusts you with their story and their medicine, take it seriously and help them feel validated for their experience.**

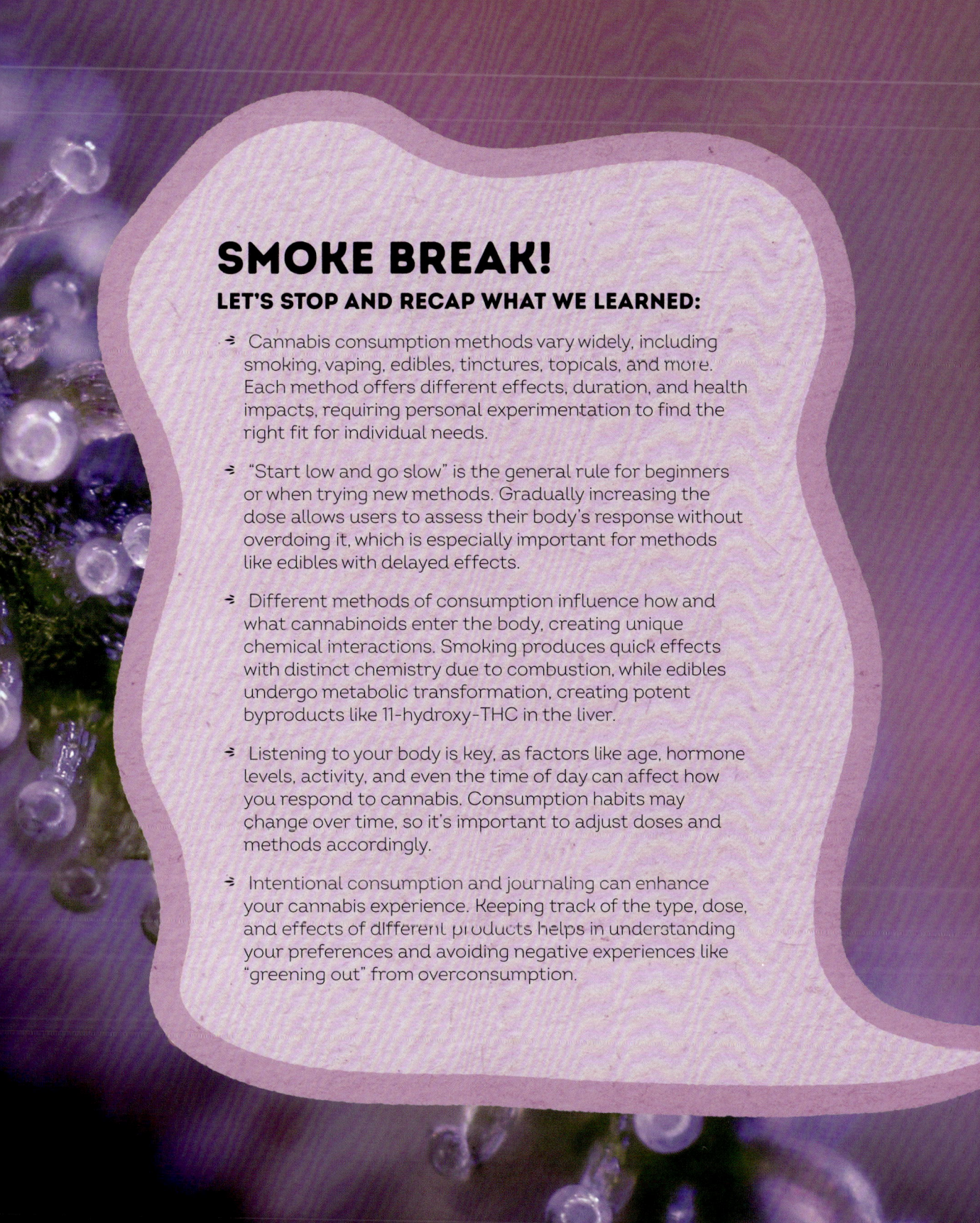

SMOKE BREAK!

LET'S STOP AND RECAP WHAT WE LEARNED:

⇉ Cannabis consumption methods vary widely, including smoking, vaping, edibles, tinctures, topicals, and more. Each method offers different effects, duration, and health impacts, requiring personal experimentation to find the right fit for individual needs.

⇉ "Start low and go slow" is the general rule for beginners or when trying new methods. Gradually increasing the dose allows users to assess their body's response without overdoing it, which is especially important for methods like edibles with delayed effects.

⇉ Different methods of consumption influence how and what cannabinoids enter the body, creating unique chemical interactions. Smoking produces quick effects with distinct chemistry due to combustion, while edibles undergo metabolic transformation, creating potent byproducts like 11-hydroxy-THC in the liver.

⇉ Listening to your body is key, as factors like age, hormone levels, activity, and even the time of day can affect how you respond to cannabis. Consumption habits may change over time, so it's important to adjust doses and methods accordingly.

⇉ Intentional consumption and journaling can enhance your cannabis experience. Keeping track of the type, dose, and effects of different products helps in understanding your preferences and avoiding negative experiences like "greening out" from overconsumption.

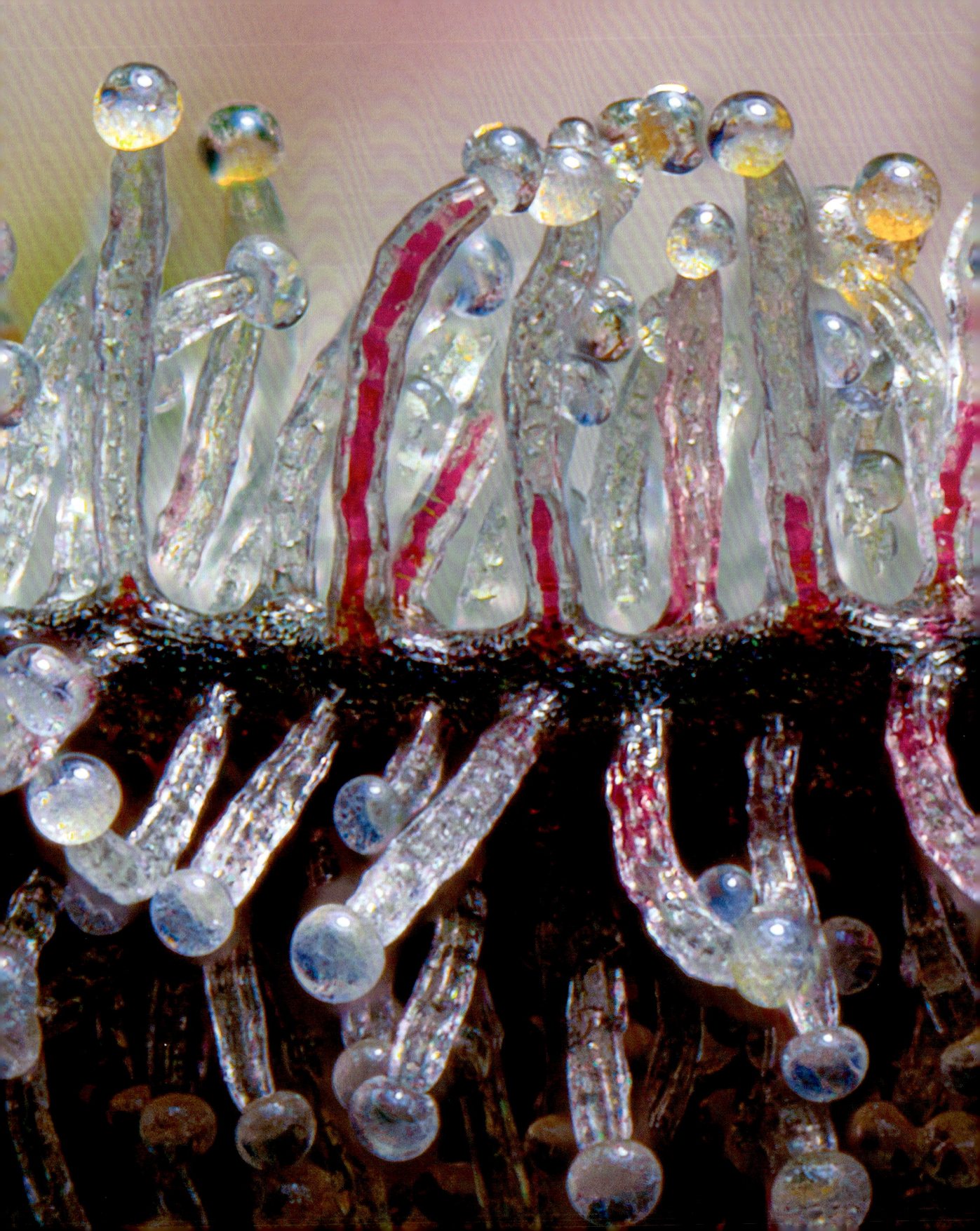

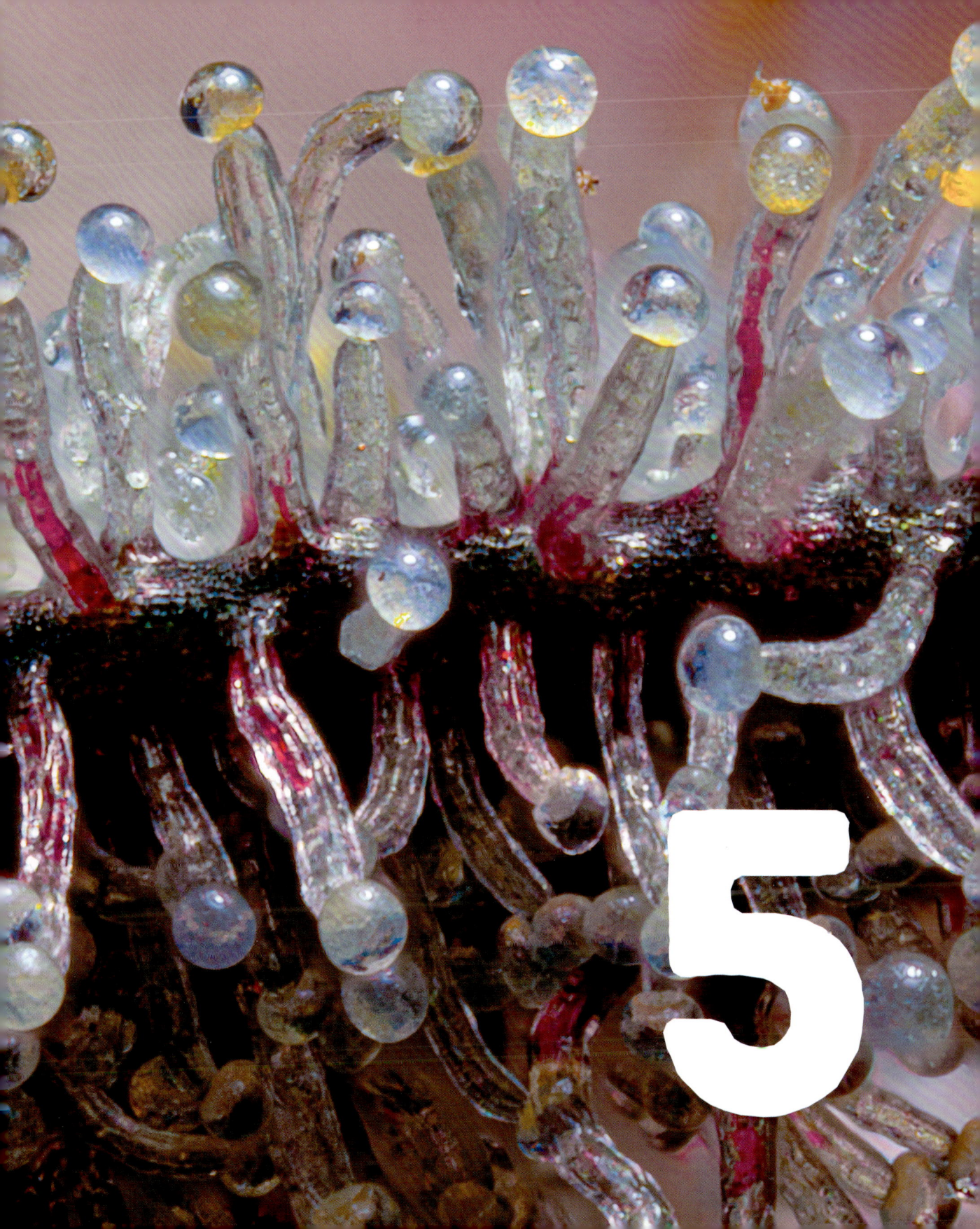

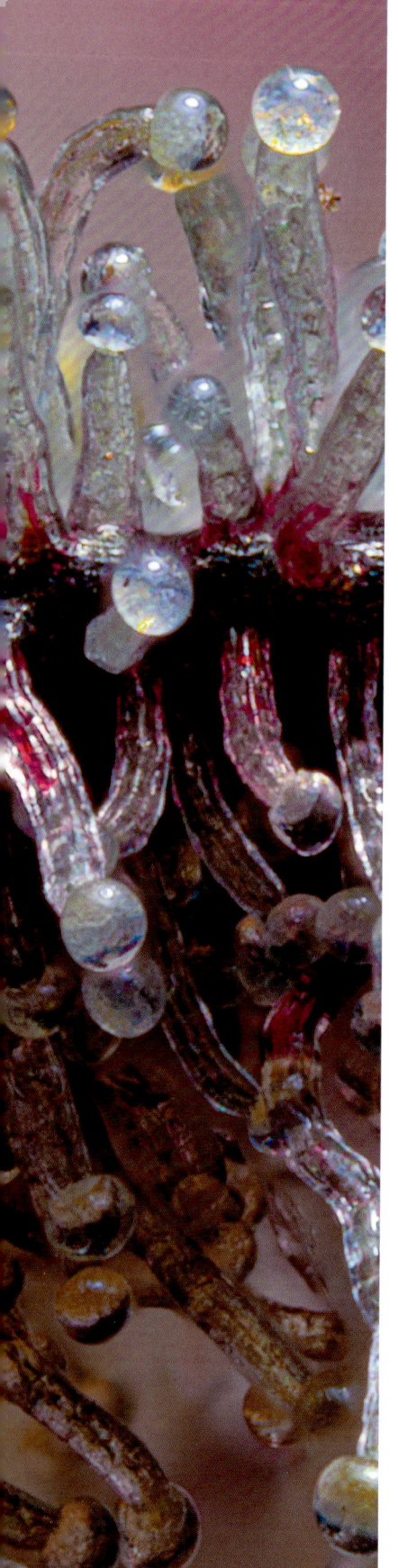

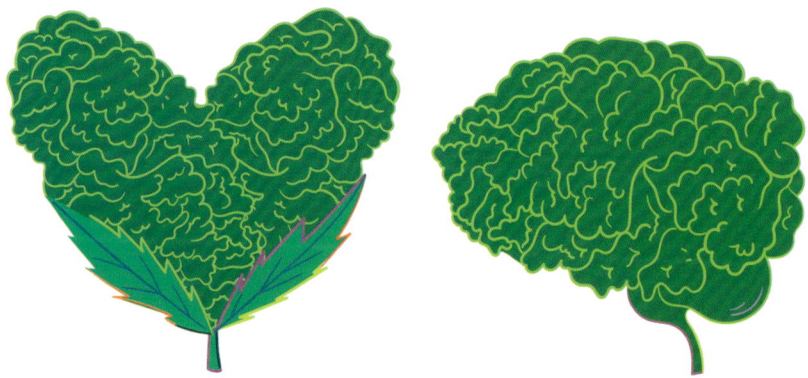

SAFETY, ADVERSE EFFECTS, AND OTHER CONSIDERATIONS

You can't die from smoking too much weed or ingesting too much THC. Cannabis alone can't kill you due to the low levels of cannabinoid receptors in the parts of the brain that control our essential functions like breathing and our heart beating. So, even if we do overwhelm our brains with too much weed, it won't kill us... it just makes us very uncomfortable for a few hours.

However, this doesn't mean cannabis is completely safe for everyone. Cannabis has such a wide range of medicinal benefits because it is a **powerful medicinal plant with many bioactive compounds**. All medicines have a therapeutic window, and if we exceed the limits of that window, we will suffer adverse effects. The window may be narrower for some and wider for others, but too much of anything is bad for you, including cannabis. You can drink too much water, you can take too much acetaminophen, and you can ingest too much THC.

While there is currently no documented evidence of a death caused by cannabis use alone, some acute or short-term complications, as well as some chronic issues, are linked to cannabis usage. These include panic attacks, severe anxiety, temporary psychosis, paranoia, convulsions, and hyperemesis.

It is estimated that someone would have to consume between 10,000 and 15,000 one-gram joints in a 15-minute period to potentially overdose from cannabis, which is likely physically impossible... but please don't try. Practice balance, be an educated consumer and know what dose you are taking, try to use cannabis with purpose or intention, keep an eye on your friends and family, and keep your weed away from children.

THC FORMULATIONS

SYNTHESIZATION

As a natural product chemist, I believe that using cannabis flower, whole plant extract products, or pressed oils (flower, rosin, hash rosin, hash, live resin, FECO) are safer options for your brain health compared to refined and isolated products like THC distillates.

Western medicine aims to separate the medicinal compounds from the parent plant to study, synthesize, derivatize, and patent. As the singular compounds are removed and isolated from the plant, we now have the ability to make potent products with 80, 90, 95, or even 99% THC. Although this can be valuable as a medicine for some—like patients with chronic pain—it no longer contains the **natural ratio** of compounds produced by the plant and is no longer the plant we've been using for millennia. Cannabis has more than 400 unique bioactive compounds and each strain has different amounts present in different ratios.

When the plant is synthesizing medicinal compounds, it doesn't just produce a ridiculous amount of THC and CBD: instead, it produces a whole arsenal of very similar but diverse molecules that are different enough to act on a variety of receptors in the body. The plant's natural ability to produce **molecules of redundancy** allows it to be more resilient and adaptive to environmental changes. When we take in whole plant medicine, it offers a more resilience and balance to our body as well.

The beauty of using a natural medicine like cannabis is that it contains unique synergies not found in refined pharmaceutical products; it is complex and still very much a mystery as far as the full potential of this plant.

Is weed the same as it was in the '70s?

If you grew up smoking weed in the '60s or '70s, you may have been used to smoking a whole joint and still feeling relatively normal. Weed had around 3% THC at that time. In 2017 that number grew to an average of 17-28% THC, a number that continues to rise as cannabis genetics get more sophisticated and breeding continues to push cultivars to produce mass amounts of THC and less of the other therapeutic compounds.

This push to offer products with high THC comes from the simple equation of supply and demand. Consumers think they're getting a better bang for their buck if they get higher THC products for less money. **Yet in reality, the highest THC products often have the least flavor, don't offer a positive spiritual experience, and honestly don't even get you that high.**

NUGS OF KNOWLEDGE

Balanced strains (1:1, CBD: THC) are difficult to find on the legal market. If you're looking for the same feeling you got from smoking weed 40 years ago, I encourage you to explore quality smokeable hemp and either mix it in with your THC flower (in any ratio you want) or try it alone. THCV- or CBG-dominant flower can be used will provide a more balanced effect and reduce the paranoia and anxiety of high-THC cannabis.

In plants, energy is the currency of life. Every molecule, every leaf, every cell is a calculation of energy. Energy is the currency of nature, and the cannabis plant has a finite amount to push towards production of therapeutic compounds; it does have to do other plant things, after all. So, if the plant is putting the majority of its energy towards producing THCA, which will become THC, it will have less energy to put towards producing the other molecules, leaving you with a less medicinally complex product.

Quality cannabis is so much more than just THC content, and oftentimes the lower the THC, the more energy the plant has to put toward other compounds, like other cannabinoids and terpenes. A greater diversity of medicinal compounds in the plant will result in a more robust and valuable product for the consumer.

There is unfortunately also incentive to excessively dry cannabis to the point where it can easily crumble. THC levels are reported by weight, so if you have a heavier flower with more water present, it will weigh more and will have a lower THC percentage than a brittle, dry bud, which by weight would contain more THC. This is another reason why you cannot rely on THC percentages alone when looking for quality flower. The strain or cultivar is just as important as who grew that plant and how it was dried and cured.

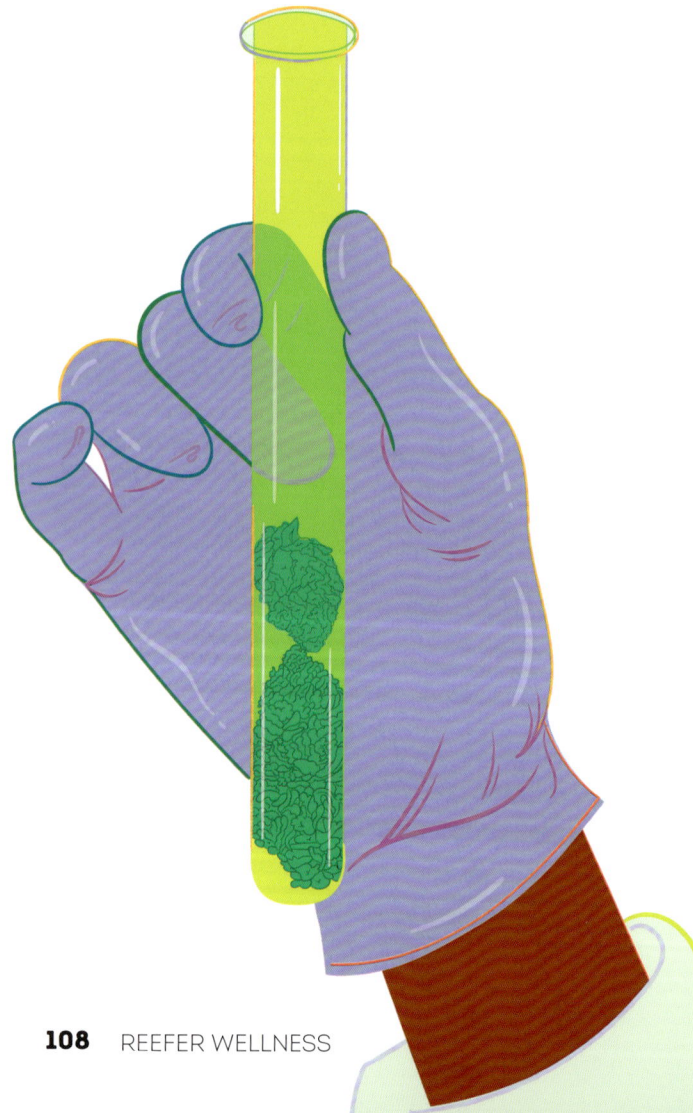

LAB TESTING OF CANNABIS PRODUCTS

Cannabis is a heavily regulated industry, and many, including myself, believe these regulations are overly strict in many cases. Much of this stems from lingering fears as we move toward a broader legal market, compounded by the fact that cannabis is often consumed for medicinal purposes—particularly through inhalation. The cannabis you purchase at a dispensary is more regulated than the groceries you purchase at a grocery store for things like bacteria, fungi, heavy metals, pesticides, and active compounds. This makes sense, as we aren't smoking our groceries. When we eat, our body has natural ways of detoxifying compounds in the liver, but we are more vulnerable when inhaling them.

One major advantage to purchasing cannabis products via legal dispensaries is that products are typically required to be tested in a laboratory before they reach your hands.

The regulations on exactly WHAT is being tested for in each product differs between product types, regions, and countries. However, in general, products are tested for active compounds (cannabinoid and terpene content), microbials (bacteria or fungi that can cause harm), water activity, heavy metals, pesticides, residual solvent (when applicable), and potential toxins.

ACTIVE COMPOUNDS

Potency testing is required by a third-party laboratory—this means that the same company that is growing the plants and making the products can't also be the one who is testing the product for potency. Despite the requirement for third-party testing, there are still many instances of artificial inflation of THC numbers[1]. As consumers erroneously associate higher THC amounts with better quality, there is incentive to inflate the numbers to get a higher price. Regardless, many testing labs report accurate numbers consistently and abide by the scientific rigor necessary for accurate data and dosing.

MICROBIALS

When we grow plants outdoors, there is a large amount of variability, like weather conditions, moisture, insects, sunlight, etc. Outdoor cannabis enthusiasts love the variability because the harsh and often unpredictable outdoor conditions force the plant to create a wider diversity of compounds—arguably increasing medicinal value[2]. However, the outdoors is highly abundant in all forms of life, including microorganisms like bacteria and fungi. Although many of these organisms are beneficial to the plant, some pathogens can be harmful to human health. These pathogenic microbes can exist in highly controlled and regulated indoor cannabis growing environments as well, and oftentimes originate from workers in cannabis facilities.

Not all microbes are bad. In fact, most are beneficial and some even necessary to our overall resistance—and same for the plant. Just like how humans benefit from having specific types of bacteria in our gut or fungi on our skin, cannabis is a living plant, and we can't expect it to be microbe-free.

In many cases, even if we were to smoke flower that contained pathogenic microbes, or ones that are bad for us, it would not cause serious harm. Typically, to cause serious damage, there would need to be high levels of the contaminant, or the person taking the product would be immunocompromised. However, it is important to test for pathogenic microbes regardless because they can cause diseases in humans. Limiting the risk associated with microbial contamination is essential for ensuring that the medicine we are putting in our bodies isn't doing more harm than good and that workers in cannabis facilities are safe.

Common pathogens that are routinely tested for are various species of *Aspergillus, E. coli,* and *Salmonella.* Some states require testing labs to report the total amount of microbes in a sample; other states are looking for specific pathogens and have limits for what is allowed. The limits for detection, and which species are tested for, are extremely variable from region to region. For instance, in some U.S. states, the product would fail immediately if there were ANY detection of certain species. But other states have specific thresholds for large groups of bacteria or yeasts/molds.

Whether we are growing cannabis at home or a multi-million-dollar grow facility, the most important way to limit microbial contamination is to control the amount of water in the bud or the final product. This is because every organism has a certain amount of water that it needs to survive, and if we can keep those water levels below the needed threshold for

these main pathogens of concern, there is a much lower likelihood of growth and contamination.

MOISTURE CONTENT

Moisture content is a more general term for the amount of water in a sample. This value is less accurate than others because it is measuring the amount of stuff that evaporates off the plant, which often includes volatile compounds in the plant other than water, like terpenes.

WATER ACTIVITY

Water activity is the measurement of free water molecules that are not bound up in the plant and are available for something like a microbe to use to survive—it is not measuring the total amount of water in the sample, just the water that is available for microbes. This measurement is the most accurate for determining the shelf stability of a cannabis product and the likelihood of microbial growth.

HEAVY METALS

Heavy metals are naturally and synthetically found all around us. Natural sources of heavy metals are found in places like sedimentary rock, volcano eruptions, and natural soil formations. Humans have also contributed to[3] the levels of heavy metals in the environment via mining, agriculture, and other sources. We require some level of heavy metals in our diet, as do plants, but this can quickly get toxic when we are exposed to high levels.

Cannabis is a plant that **bioaccumulates** heavy metals, meaning if the soil or water contains heavy metals, it will readily slurp them up and integrate them into the plant tissues. This is a great feature for cleaning up soils that may be contaminated, but also a potentially dangerous one if people are consuming the end product. If you are growing cannabis at home, you can get your soil, water, or final flower tested for heavy metals to make sure you are not exposing yourself to harmful levels after your harvest.

The way we package and store cannabis can also cause heavy metals to leach into the final product. One study from 2021[4] found that the metals chromium, copper, nickel, lead, manganese, and tin from the heating coil of vape cartridges make their way into the vape oil and can actually be vaporized and inhaled. This is particularly of concern with vape cartridges that have been sitting on dispensary shelves for long periods of time or stored in places like hot cars. So, if you're going to vape cannabis cartridges, make sure to purchase ones that were made recently from a trusted company, store them in a cool place out of sunlight, and try to use them within a reasonable amount of time. Don't hit an old vape cart that's been sitting in your car for eight months. It is not the same vape cart that it used to be—have a small funeral and let it go.

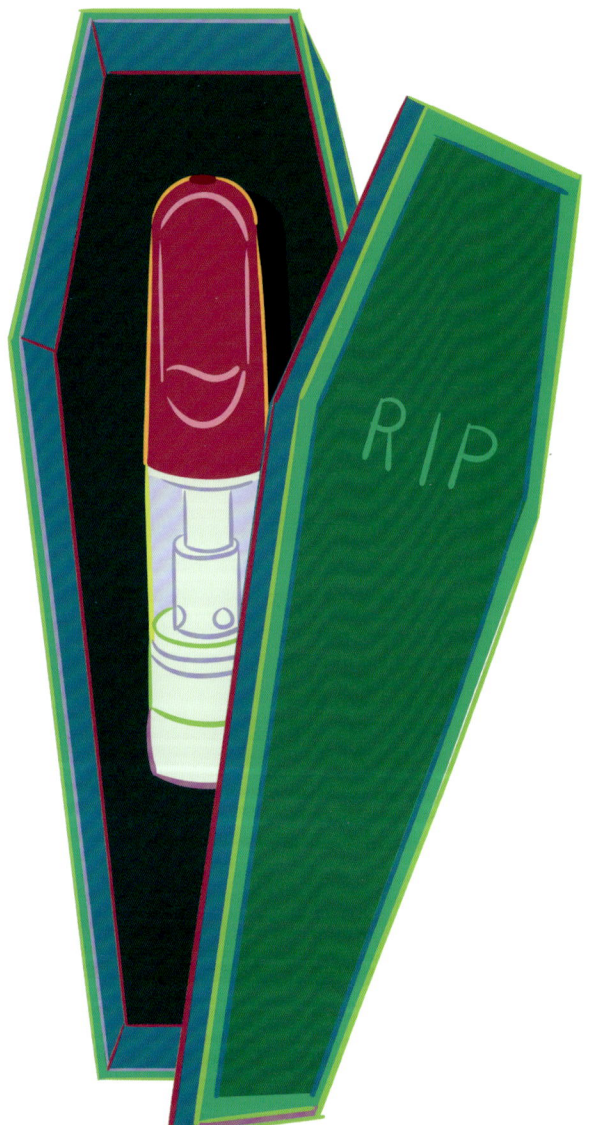

PESTICIDES

Cannabis is an agricultural crop that is susceptible to a variety of insects, mites, fungi, and bacteria that may impact its growth. Because these pests can cause serious harm to cannabis grows, many cultivators have resorted to using pesticides. There are around 200 different types of pesticides that are allowed to be used in cannabis cultivation, and again this will vary depending on what region you're growing in and what the local regulations are—and of course, if the grower is following the regulations or not.

Between 60-70% of pesticides that are sprayed on cannabis plants can transfer to the human body during inhalation[5]. This is even more concerning when we think of concentrated cannabis products, because the pesticides, heavy metals, or other contaminants are also getting concentrated during the process. Exposure to high levels of pesticides can have significant risks to humans including liver damage, cancer, and muscle damage. Repeated exposure over time OR exposure to a medically compromised patient including those with liver disease can cause significant harm. Luckily pesticide screening is typically part of the lab testing procedures, and many growers don't use them anyway and prefer organic cultivation practices.

RESIDUAL SOLVENTS

Some products at dispensaries require chemical solvents to extract the medicinal cannabinoids and terpenes from the plant. Solvents are not bad and are absolutely necessary in extracting most medicinal plants, but it is important that the solvents don't make their way into the final product because excess levels can have negative health effects. Even if products are made in a solvent-free way, residual solvents can still make their way into a final product from cleaning products or other mechanisms, but this is rare. Additionally, some of the smelly compounds in cannabis have a chemical-like flavor and may lead you to believe there are chemicals present when it is only the natural smell.

Similar to microbials, when testing for residual solvents there is typically a threshold or limit to the amount of solvent allowed, which is determined by evaluating the safety of each compound. Some common solvents used and tested for are ethanol, isopropanol, propane, and hexane. If you want to avoid solvents all together, consider solventless concentrates like rosin or using flower.

SYNTHETIC CANNABINOIDS

The cannabis plant produces more than 400 cannabinoid compounds. However, **there is still a market for synthetically derived cannabinoids due to limited access to cannabis from the U.S. government, and other governing bodies worldwide.**

Because of the specific language used in the writing of the 2018 Farm Bill—which is the bill that made CBD products legal nationwide and readily accessible from online retail stores—many states are selling "hemp-derived" cannabinoids like Delta-8 THC, Delta-10 THC, hemp-derived Delta-9 THC, HHC, THCP, and so on. Although some of these compounds CAN BE naturally occurring in the plant, they exist naturally in very small amounts. So, to get around this issue, companies take pure CBD—which is very cheap and readily available—and subject it to a variety of laboratory procedures including strong acids and bases to convert the CBD into new molecules, many of which can get you high.

There is nothing inherently wrong with the "hemp-derived cannabinoid market." In fact, many of these synthetically produced compounds have medicinal value and could be used as a medicine. However, due to the unregulated nature of these synthetic cannabinoids, there is little to no regulation as far as the purity of these products, testing standards, sourcing, etc. One 2021 study looked at ten supposedly pure "Delta-8-THC" products available on the market. The authors found almost 20% contaminants in some samples, and no sample that they evaluated was "pure" as advertised.

Synthetically-derived THC products are not required to indicate that they were made synthetically in the laboratory. Many of these product packages and advertising rely on uneducated consumers thinking that they have plant-derived THC in them.

What is most frustrating about the synthetic cannabinoid market is that it wouldn't exist if we had access to quality, legal cannabis. People would much rather use the natural product, which has been shown to be safe and efficacious for millennia. But in areas that still don't have a regulated legal market, synthetically-derived compounds are the only legal access to this type of medicine. **Our government has effectively made a safe, natural product illegal while making potentially unsafe, synthetic products legal.**

OVERUSE OF CANNABIS PRODUCTS

You can overuse and abuse anything—this includes water, coffee, blueberries, chocolate, cocaine, sex, and cannabis. In fact, it's almost human nature to explore the limits of use and abuse. Although cannabis was first thought to be completely "non-addictive," research over the past few decades has concluded that people can become dependent on cannabis—and I've seen it many times. However, it is not necessarily a bad thing to be dependent on something, as we see with many regularly used pharmaceuticals like Adderall for ADHD or Lexapro for anxiety that patients depend on daily for decades. Dependency is only an issue if the medicine is inhibiting your life either medically, financially, socially, emotionally, or spiritually.

The financial burden of cannabis is different from other substances because, although it is a medicine and is now (as of 2024) federally recognized as having medicinal potential, it still needs to be paid for by the patient instead of health insurance. Many states with legal cannabis markets still do not permit patients to grow their own cannabis; therefore, **the cost burden of this medicine is placed on the vulnerable population of patients.**

The main pathway involved in drugs of abuse such as cocaine, amphetamines, opiates, and alcohol are the mesolimbic dopamine (DA) system. This is known as the reward system in the brain, and the reason why other things like social media are also highly addicting alongside drugs. Although cannabinoids like THC don't directly act on the DA system like other drugs, cannabinoids do activate this system in indirect ways. The main function of the ECS is to control the release of neurotransmitters like dopamine, GABA, and glutamate—inhibiting the release of GABA in the brain results in secondhand action activation on the dopamine system.

Overall, the data we have on humans shows very weak evidence that dopamine is involved in cannabis addiction in humans[6], but what we do know from all human and animal studies is that cannabis is FAR less addictive and harmful than other commonly used substances like cocaine, heroin, tobacco, and alcohol.

Cannabis is not harmless, and sustained cannabis use can easily turn into a social or emotional crutch that prevents the personal healing and growth process for some or can be used as a form of **escapism** to avoid important life issues. Escapism is not a sustainable approach to using any drug; it may provide solace and escape in the short term, but if your use of cannabis (or any other substance) is inhibiting your everyday life and relationships, it's time to rethink the products you use, the consumption methods, and evaluate what other coping skills can be used.

Because cannabis has operated in the shadows of society for so long and been so highly stigmatized, **regulating the amount we use is on us as the consumer,** at least for now, and therefore requires a higher level of education and self-discipline than some other common medicines. If you are choosing cannabis over spending time with friends and family, if cannabis use is negatively impacting your mental health, or if your cannabis use is taking the place of personal growth, it may be time to rethink your relationship with the plant. This is why intention and community are reiterated so often in this book; developing a healthy relationship with cannabis can be practiced every single time you consume and should not be taken passively.

What happens when you stop smoking?

If you are a frequent cannabis consumer and suddenly stop, you will experience some withdrawal symptoms. This is not surprising, as your body has gotten used to the presence of a bioactive substance and now it is suddenly gone. Withdrawal symptoms can be especially bad when cannabis is used to initiate certain activities like eating or sleeping. For instance, if you always wait until right before bed to consume cannabis and use it as a way to initiate sleep, you have trained yourself to wait for the signal (cannabis consumption) to tell your body to sleep, and when you suddenly remove it, your body is going to need some time to adjust and acclimate. Try replacing the smoking before bed with drinking tea or reading a book to train your body with a new form of initiation to sleep.

The most common symptoms people experience after abstaining or stopping cannabis use are irritability, anxiety, muscle pain, chills, nightmares, insomnia, headaches, and decreased appetite. The symptoms are the worst two to six days after stopping and will typically resolve within two weeks[7].

Cannabis acts through the ECS, which is involved in controlling almost every physiological response, but especially those concerning mood, appetite, and sleep—these are the facets of our lives that will likely be impacted the most when cannabis use stops.

MANAGEMENT TOOLS

If you're taking a break from cannabis, rather than abruptly stopping, consider taking a week or two and every day using less and less cannabis. Taking a slower and more gentle approach allows your body time to respond to the lower levels of THC and helps your body prepare for change through a slow introduction, rather than an abrupt switch.

While your body is transitioning to a new state without any supplement of THC, you can help your body adjust by supplementing with naturally occurring cannabinoids in your body. Although these compounds are always being produced because they are necessary for almost every function in the body, there are ways to increase them with notable effects on the mind and body. **Exercise is one of the best ways to increase levels of naturally-occurring endocannabinoids.**

The "high" feeling that you get when you have a good pump of exercise is due to your body releasing endocannabinoids. This feeling was originally thought to be from your body releasing naturally occurring opioids (endorphins), but more recent research unveiled the real source to be the endocannabinoid system. Beyond vigorous exercise, meditation and yoga are other ways to encourage your body to release naturally occurring equivalents of THC to reduce the withdrawal symptoms.

LISTENING TO YOUR BODY

Aging... is your body telling you that you don't need THC anymore?

One trend that I've noticed in the cannabis community is that as people age, they often start to gravitate away from high-THC products and toward more CBD-dominant products. Often, this aversion to cannabis is sparked by bouts of anxiety after smoking or consuming cannabis around the age of 35. The same amount of cannabis that someone used to smoke in their twenties now gives them debilitating anxiety. When people come to me with these issues, they often say, "I don't know what's wrong with me"—and the answer is often nothing!

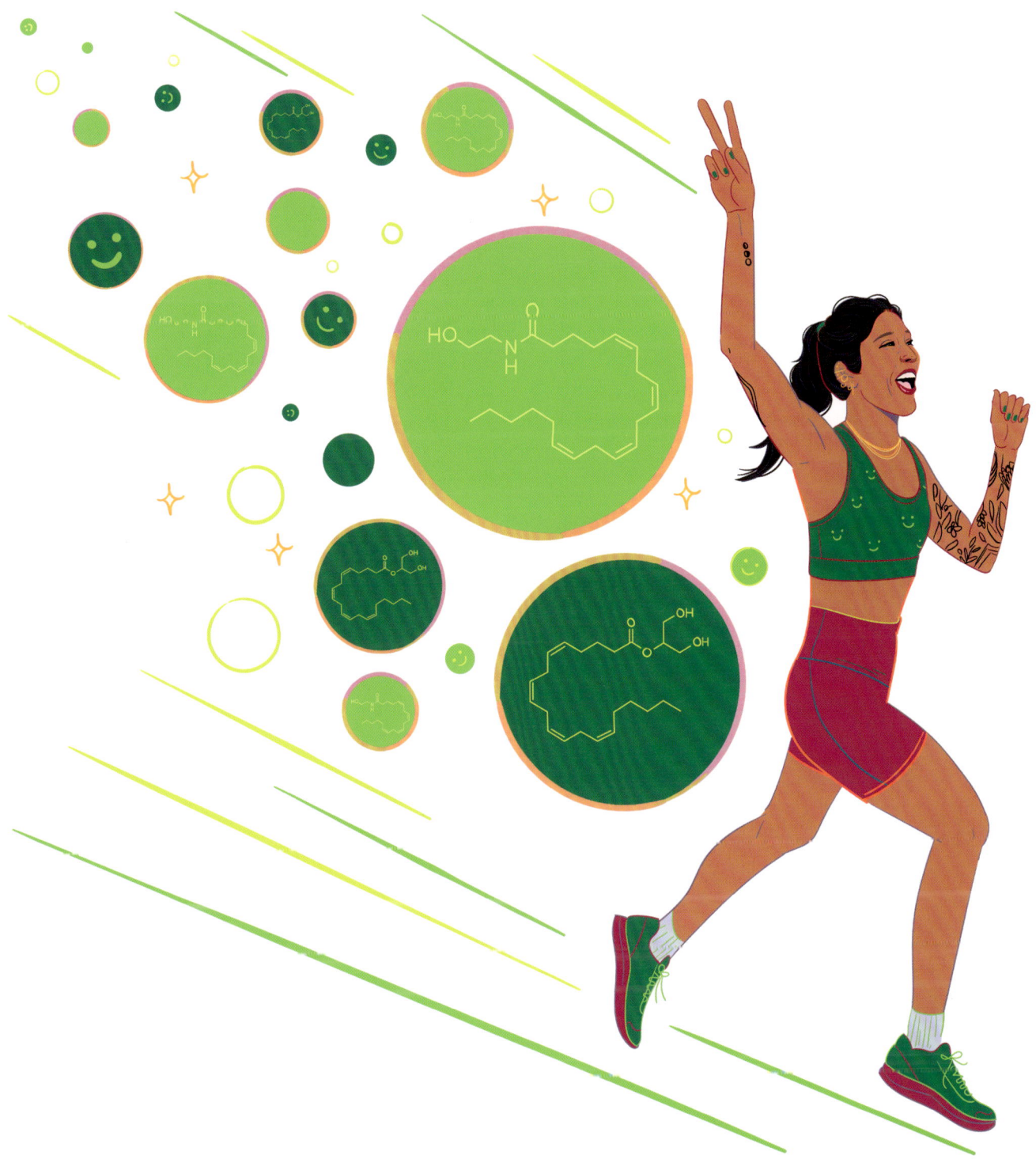

As we age and our hormones change, our entire body is changing. If cannabis is giving you anxiety, maybe your body no longer needs the medicine or no longer needs the products or doses that you are providing it. Some people decide to completely stop using cannabis and others start using far less THC and switching to CBD-dominant products.

Additionally, as we age, our bodies often need more anti-inflammatory medicines, especially on the joints and back. Cannabis can be a great preventative medicine in many different forms. Topical products can be applied to localized areas to help with pain, and smoking or vaping CBD flower (hemp) has many anti-inflammatory therapeutic benefits—providing a much more mellow experience and avoiding the anxious response.

Part of responsible cannabis use, and aging, is learning to listen to your body and not forcing it to live in the past. Change your use habits as you age and listen to what your body has to say.

What happens if I take too much THC?

If you overdo it on THC, you will not die, but it's not going to be a fun time either. A common slang term for using too much cannabis is **greening out**—a play on the term blacking out used to describe heavy alcohol consumption. There are no studies I can cite on greening out, but from personal experience and community stories, I know too well what it is like.

I once accidentally overconsumed THC when making infused butter. I had made the infused butter and had a good guess of how much THC it contained based on the flower that I used, but when I went to taste it, I tried it with some really delicious perogies. In fact, the perogies were so delicious that I ate about six more than I was originally planning on eating, and cooked and dipped them all in cannabutter. Thirty minutes later I was in outer space. I started to feel sick almost immediately. The room started spinning and I ended up throwing up from the experience. I had to sit on the couch with a cool, wet rag on my head and a weighted blanket. I was still a bit high and extremely groggy when I woke up the following day. This definitely was not a positive experience and has completely changed how I go about making products at home—and solidified that edibles were not my preferred method of consumption in general.

CANNABINOID HYPEREMESIS SYNDROME

Cannabinoid hyperemesis syndrome (CHS) is an adverse effect from cannabis consumption that affects a small portion of cannabis consumers and was first reported in 2004. CHS is characterized by cyclic episodes of nausea and vomiting after chronic, and often high, doses of cannabis. CHS is extremely painful and often debilitating as patients are vomiting dozens of times per day.

Many people with CHS who don't know about the condition end up using MORE cannabis once they develop symptoms because cannabis is one of the best antiemetic drugs to exist, meaning it can stop you from feeling sick and vomiting. However, in the case of CHS, cannabis will only make the nausea and vomiting worse.

CHS has three stages:

1. Prodrome: This phase can last for months before any chronic vomiting starts. This phase is often characterized by increased anxiety, morning nausea, increased thirst, sweating, and flushing of the face and body. If you are experiencing these symptoms and think it may be CHS, stop using cannabis products immediately.

2. Hyperemetic: As the name suggests, this phase is characterized by excessive vomiting that does not typically resolve with antiemetic drugs, severe abdominal pain, nausea, and vomiting.

3. Recovery: This starts as the symptoms lessen and the body starts to heal from the excessive stress and vomiting.

Although we still are unsure exactly what causes CHS, we have evidence that there is likely a genetic component to the condition, meaning not everyone is equally susceptible to developing CHS[8]. Additionally, there seems to be a link between the use of high-THC concentrates and the development of CHS—but the cannabis community has hypothesized everything from pesticide use to irradiation of cannabis products being the source of illness.

There are some cases when people either take too many edibles, take a MASSIVE rip off their bong, or just use too much cannabis and end up vomiting. This is not CHS. CHS is a debilitating condition where patients are experiencing cyclical vomiting up to fifty times per day. When patients go to the emergency room, CHS is often misdiagnosed with other conditions like CVS (cyclical vomiting syndrome) or another GI disorder.

Some of the telltale signs that you have CHS are: (i) you are a heavy cannabis consumer, AND (ii) ONLY hot showers and/or capsaicin cream alleviate stomach pain. These methods are effective because both hot peppers and high temperatures activate the **TRPV1** receptor—which is thought to be involved in the pathology of CHS.

Although CHS is getting more common, it is still relatively uncommon among the millions of cannabis consumers and should not be a reason to limit the accessibility or doses of cannabis products. However, cannabis consumers and medical professionals should be educated on this condition for early diagnosis and harm reduction to the patient.

COMMON ADVERSE EFFECTS
DRUG-DRUG INTERACTIONS

There are both physical and mental complications that can occur with cannabis use, and many of these complications are a product of sensitive populations using the wrong dose or product type.

It is important to remember that cannabis is much safer and more efficacious than many medicines that we use in our everyday lives—including acetaminophen, which very likely would not pass FDA guidelines if presented today because of liver toxicity.

Cannabis contains hundreds of powerful compounds that have a multitude of medical benefits. This plant is extremely safe for how bioactive it is, but anything with this level of medicinal benefit can also have adverse effects. Although the majority of adverse effects are attributed to THC, it is important for consumers of CBD, especially at high doses, to be aware of drug-drug interactions which can occur with both THC- and CBD-dominant products.

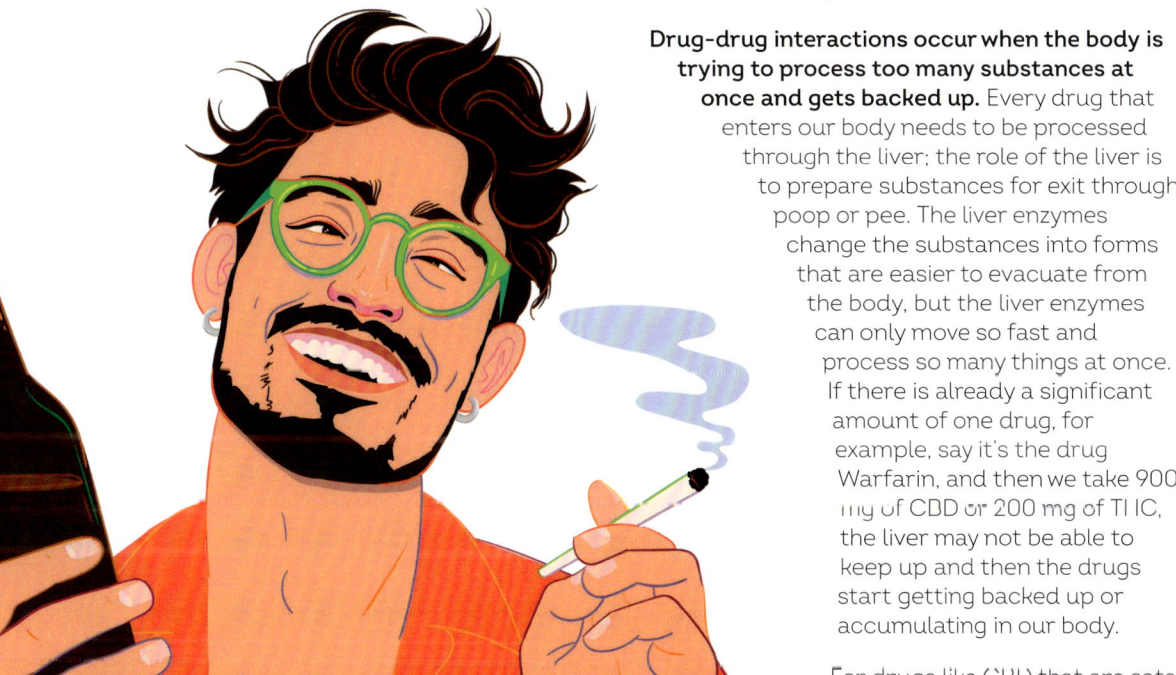

Drug-drug interactions occur when the body is trying to process too many substances at once and gets backed up. Every drug that enters our body needs to be processed through the liver; the role of the liver is to prepare substances for exit through poop or pee. The liver enzymes change the substances into forms that are easier to evacuate from the body, but the liver enzymes can only move so fast and process so many things at once. If there is already a significant amount of one drug, for example, say it's the drug Warfarin, and then we take 900 mg of CBD or 200 mg of THC, the liver may not be able to keep up and then the drugs start getting backed up or accumulating in our body.

For drugs like CBD that are safe at relatively high doses this isn't much of an issue, but if the other drugs like Warfarin or acetamenophin (that have a much narrower therapeutic window) aren't getting processed quickly, it is possible to have a dangerous level accumulate in the body. This is why it is important to check with your doctor before trying anything new, or at the very least, research the drugs you're taking on a website like drugs.com and see if there are interactions with other drugs, or research whether the same liver enzyme processes the drugs, you're on and THC/CBD. The specific types of liver enzymes that process cannabinoids are CYP2C9, CYP2C19, CYP3A4, UGT1A9, and UGT2B7[9].

INTERACTIONS WITH ALCOHOL

Another common adverse effect to THC is feeling dizzy or lightheaded. This happens because THC is a vasodilator, meaning consuming THC makes your blood vessels wider, which can drop the blood pressure in the body[10]. However, the cardiovascular effects of THC are complex. While it can cause vasodilation and lower blood pressure, it may also lead to increased heart rate and, in some cases, elevated blood pressure. These varying effects depend on factors such as dosage, individual physiology, and method of consumption. Think how much more difficult it is to sip a drink out of a thick straw versus a thin straw—your body is working with a thicker straw when your blood vessels widen. The risk of passing out or feeling dizzy is significantly exacerbated when combined with alcohol because alcohol is a blood thinner and makes it even more difficult to move blood around.

Additionally, although you may be comfortable with feeling drunk and comfortable with feeling high, it does not mean you will be comfortable with feeling both at the same time. Being drunk and high at the same time is called being **cross-faded, and can result in feeling the spins. The spins feel like your entire room is spinning around you and very often leads to a vomiting episode.**

CANNABIS AND NEUROCOGNITION

ACUTE PSYCHOSIS

Cannabis can cause acute symptoms of psychosis. This often presents in features like paranoia, hallucinations, depersonalization, and confusion[11], and typically occurs when people take abnormally high levels of THC and do not dose or titrate properly. It can be very scary for the person experiencing the symptoms and for friends or family who may be involved as well. This situation is particularly concerning when someone has taken a high dose of edibles or tincture, as those result in a long-lasting journey in the body.

Some evidence suggests that chewing on peppercorns can help balance out the effects of too much THC by providing the body with additional terpenes that can balance out the effects, or that taking CBD can help balance the brain as well. These practices may work for some people, but staying calm, comfortable, and hydrated will likely be the best way to get through this episode.

GENETICS AND SCHIZOPHRENIA

There have been a variety of studies that have tried to link specific genes with an increased likelihood of developing schizophrenia or increased likelihood of being someone who uses a lot of cannabis (a stoner gene of sorts). Some of these genes include the COMT gene, which codes for an enzyme involved in dopamine metabolism, the AKT1 gene, which codes for an enzyme activated by the cannabinoid receptors; and the genes for BDNF[12] or brain derived neurotrophic factor, which is involved in dopamine transportation. These data are not conclusive but are promising for the future; if we are able to develop genetic screening to help identify people who may be at higher risk for developing mental health conditions related to cannabis consumption, that should be a priority in cannabis medicine. However, we are not there yet.

Interestingly, there is evidence that the endocannabinoids that our body makes are also linked to symptoms of schizophrenia. The levels of anandamide (AEA) are higher in schizophrenic people. Because the increase in AEA is seen in the very early stages of schizophrenia and noting that patients with the lowest AEA in the body have the worst symptoms, it is hypothesized that AEA acts as a protective molecule in the brain against the symptoms of schizophrenia. This also builds on the theory why some people with schizophrenia find such value in using cannabis to help with minor symptoms, as THC acts similarly to AEA in the brain[13]. Obviously take this research with a grain of salt because this situation can be different for different people and change with severity of symptoms.

So, is there risk?

There have been multiple studies that have tried to link cannabis as a causative for mental health conditions like schizophrenia, but in all cases, there were too many confounding factors to say that cannabis use alone was the main factor for psychosis. Multiple studies have presented evidence that cannabis use at a young age can result in episodes of psychosis occurring earlier than they would without cannabis use. For example, if you are genetically susceptible to schizophrenia, and the average age of onset is 20, you may experience symptoms at 17 rather than 20 (average of 2.7 years earlier).

Because schizophrenia and many other mental health conditions are genetic, it is important to remember that the risk for developing schizophrenia is greater when there are already genetic ties—meaning someone else in your family also has this condition. **It is not like the common cold; cannabis use alone will never be sufficient to "cause" schizophrenia, but it can be a risk factor for some vulnerable populations.** If you have a genetic predisposition to serious mental health conditions, understand the risks of using any psychoactive substances and talk to your mental health professionals. In general, if you aren't already using cannabis and you are schizophrenic I would advise staying away from any mind-altering substance.

Is it safe for teenagers to use cannabis?

Using cannabis before the brain has a chance to fully develop and before a child's social and emotional skills are developed can be harmful to a child's mental health. This is the same for every drug. But being a teenager is difficult emotionally and physically, and many young teens look to substances to numb the pain, look cool, or simply explore the limitations of our brains. Cannabis works in the body to bring balance or homeostasis—during puberty the body goes through some pretty incredible changes. This leads to spikes in hormones and mood; I don't find it surprising at all that many teens find value in cannabis for bringing regulation to their bodies.

One survey I took on social media with over 14,000 respondents revealed the average age of first cannabis use to be about fourteen-and-a-half years old. At that age, when many teens are starting high school, education about cannabis and other drugs is critical. Programs like D.A.R.E. or sex education often try to preach abstinence as the only option, when in reality any form of abstinence can be difficult to impose. I believe in teaching harm reduction and trying to educate kids on the dangers of drugs and any safety precautions to be aware of with different substances. After all, the decision of teens using cannabis is often not cannabis or sobriety—it's cannabis or a much more dangerous drug.

For cannabis, I believe the best harm reduction method is combining CBD with THC and staying away from concentrated products at a young age. To start, combining CBD with THC reduces the amount of THC administered per use. CBD also has documented antipsychotic effects and has shown to be more efficacious and safer than other antipsychotic drugs[14]. Although I do think that cannabis concentrates have a place for many medical patients, I do not believe they are healthy for a developing brain and should be avoided until older.

I first started using cannabis in high school, as most people do. I wouldn't say that my parents encouraged the use of cannabis, but it was clear that my parents viewed cannabis as a method of harm reduction. Rather than going to random pit parties in rural Maine or driving around with drunk friends, we chilled at home, played Guitar Hero, and ate cookies. Aside from keeping us out of far more trouble, cannabis also helped me, my brothers, and my parents get along. Prior to cannabis use, we would fight over the smallest things or nothing at all. With three teenagers in the house and raging hormones there was no winning. From high school to this day, cannabis is an integral component of peace in our house.

Although this isn't researched with peer review, one of the major advantages to cannabis is that it makes many people nicer and easier to be around–an effect that can transform relationships.

REPRODUCTIVE HEALTH

Is cannabis safe to use while trying to conceive, while pregnant, or while breastfeeding?

When you start trying for a family, you want to make sure all parties involved are as healthy as possible. Most of the data that we have on this topic concerns sperm health and sperm movement–not the female egg–and is most relevant to men who may already have underlying fertility issues. For men who are heavy cannabis users, there is a concern of having a lower sperm count, changes in the shape of the sperm, reduced movement of the sperm, and decreased fertilizing capacity of the sperm.

With anything in life, it is a balancing act of pros and cons. If you are trying to conceive and cannabis is the only thing that sparks your libido and gets you in the mood, then the pros may outweigh the potential cons for conception.

Cannabis has been used for a variety of women's health conditions for centuries. This includes relieving pain during childbirth and menstruation, treating uterine hemorrhage, and increasing labor contractions[15].

In general, one role of our ECS is to help us endure[16], balance, forget, and carry on. Cannabinoid receptors are found throughout the uterus, and it is thought that AEA may dull the pain of childbirth and help women forget it later.

A study on maternal health of more than 7,000 women in Canada showed that 3.1% of respondents reported using cannabis during pregnancy and 2.6% while breastfeeding[17]. I know personally from the hundreds of messages I've received that women are regularly using cannabis while trying to conceive, during pregnancy, and while breastfeeding. However, they almost never share their experiences with friends, family, or physicians because of the fear of their baby being taken away, losing access to their medicine, or being publicly reprimanded for their decisions. This is part of the reason why we have very little data on the safety of cannabis during pregnancy, because (i) it is obviously unethical to test drugs including cannabis on pregnant women, and (ii) most women aren't honest in surveys due to fear and mistrust in the system.

Several longitudinal studies (following mothers and children over time) have found negative implications in children's neurodevelopment, behavior, and mental health[18] when the mothers used cannabis during pregnancy. However, the largest study[19] (12,424 pregnancies) did not find any significant association between cannabis and low birth weight, shortened gestational period, or other deficits after controlling for other confounding variables–like the use of other substances while pregnant, socioeconomic class, access to medicine, etc. Other limitations of these studies are the missing data on cannabis type, dose, method of consumption, and more.

CANNABIS AND PREGNANCY

Most mothers do not want to consume while they are pregnant, but the nausea and other mental and physical changes their bodies are going through are extremely difficult to endure. It is often not a matter of whether to use a drug of any sort or not, but rather which is safest for mom and baby. For medical patients, it's important to remember that you are still a medical patient when you are pregnant and will likely continue to need the medicine through your pregnancy journey. Almost all physicians are going to tell you to not use cannabis while pregnant, and if you can abstain that is the best option. However, for those who can't, there are ways to reduce harm if you are consuming while pregnant.

Women experience varying levels of sickness during pregnancy. Some women have moderate morning sickness, and some women suffer from a condition called **hyperemesis gravidarum**–which is a very serious condition consisting of intractable vomiting leading to weight loss and often resulting in hospitalization. Chronic vomiting is not only concerning for the mother and baby because she is unable to hold nutrients down, but it is also incredibly stressful on the body. Maternal stress has been linked to many adverse outcomes like preterm birth, issues with neurocognition, behavioral disorders, issues with the endocrine system, and motor development issues for the child.

There are multiple pharmaceutical drugs that are deemed safe enough to use for chronic vomiting during pregnancy including a combination of pyridoxine-doxylamine, dopamine receptor agonists like promethazine, and if needed, serotonin agonists like Zofran. All drug use during pregnancy has risks associated with it, including pharmaceutical use in which all these drugs have limited studies on safety. But in general, the use of these medications, and in my opinion cannabis as well, is a safer option compared to chronic uncontrolled vomiting.

Almost all data on cannabis and pregnancy and breastfeeding is in regard to THC exposure—almost no data has been collected on CBD exposure to a developing fetus. Research shows that THC can readily cross the placenta and be exposed to the fetus's developing brain, although at levels significantly lower than the mother's exposure. The National Academy of Science Engineering and Medicine performed a review on data collected on cannabis and pregnancy and made the following conclusions[20]:

1. There's limited evidence of any statistical association between material cannabis smoking and pregnancy complications to the mother.

2. There is substantial evidence between maternal cannabis **smoking** and lower birth weight of the child.

3. There is insufficient evidence for the association between maternal cannabis smoking and later outcomes in offspring like sudden infant death syndrome, cognition issues, academic achievements, and later substance use/abuse disorders.

Smoking anything—whether it be cannabis, tobacco, or other products—is linked to a statistically lower birth weight in the newborn. It may not be the molecules present in the plant or substance that are impacting birth weight, but the actual smoke itself. For this reason, it is highly recommended that if you choose to consume cannabis while pregnant, do not smoke the herb. A secondary option could be a one-hitter dry herb vape that allows immediate relief while still avoiding the compounds produced via smoking. Additionally, using **the therapeutic minimum dose** of cannabis while pregnant should be the goal with consumption. This means taking in the minimum amount necessary to relieve the symptoms and concerns and not overconsuming. It is irresponsible to use cannabis in a recreational or fun manner while pregnant, and this is not how most women choose to utilize cannabis during pregnancy.

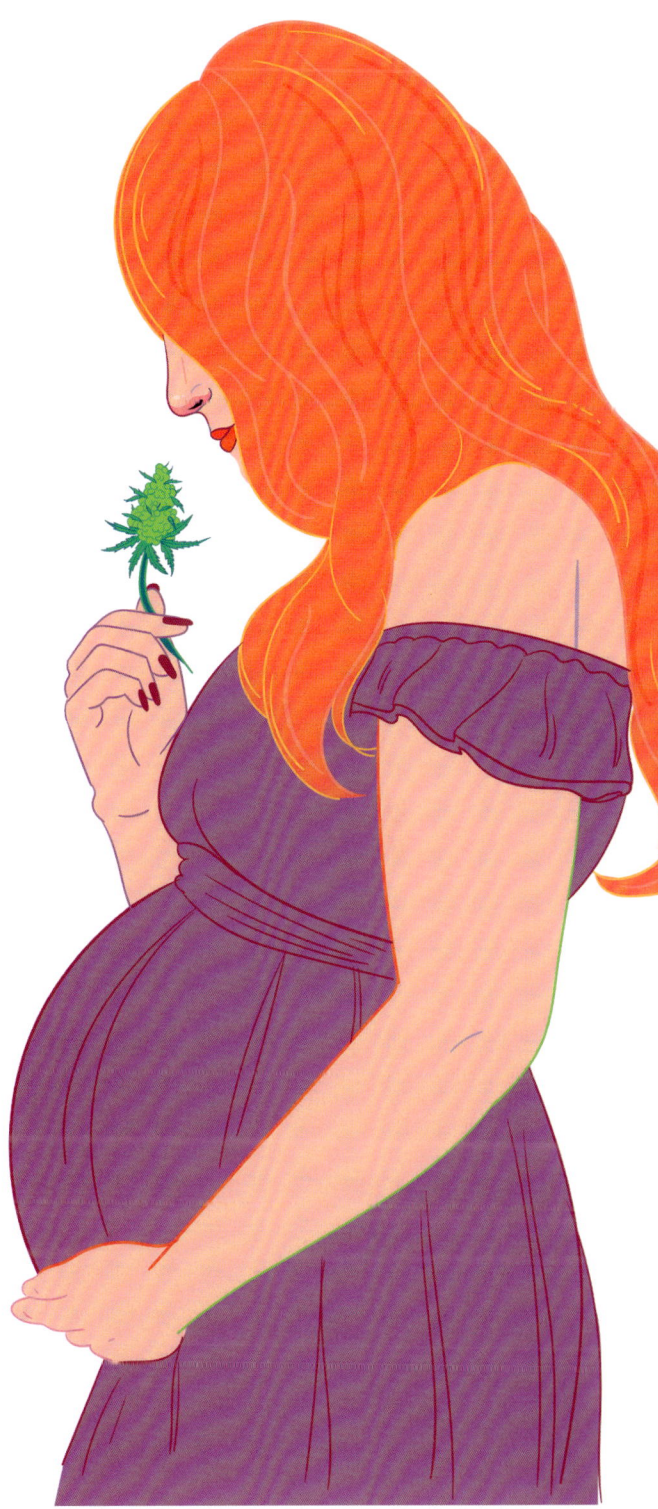

CANNABIS AND BREASTFEEDING

Cannabis is the most commonly used recreational drug among breastfeeding women[21] in the U.S. Phytocannabinoids, when consumed by the mother, can be exposed to the baby through breast milk. Multiple studies have investigated the amount of THC exposed to the baby versus the mother's dose and the numbers range from 0.08% to 2.5% of maternal dose per kg of bodyweight. So yes, the baby is exposed to levels of THC from the weed mom is using, but in pretty small amounts. The concentration of THC in breast milk peaks after one hour, and due to their fatty nature, cannabinoids are detectable in the breast milk for up to six days after use.

There are some hypotheses that moderate cannabis consumption during lactation could potentially increase the mother's milk supply or help with babies who are unable to develop the latch response. However, these theories are based around the fact that THC acts similar to our bodies' endocannabinoids—as **the endocannabinoid 2-AG helps newborns establish their first suckling response by activating the system needed to get milk pumping via the CB1 receptor**[22]. As Dr. Dustin Sulac writes in *Handbook of Cannabis for Clinicians*, "Appropriate maternal consumption directed at correcting a physiological disturbance in the mother could theoretically convey more ideal cannabinoid activity to breastmilk."

Using cannabis should not stop you from breastfeeding and most physicians don't recommend "pumping and dumping" unless you are consuming LARGE amounts of cannabis. Similar to the conversation around cannabis use while pregnant, if you have to use cannabis while breastfeeding, use the minimum therapeutic dose, try to avoid smoking, try to use cannabis as far away from breastfeeding sessions as possible, and avoid high doses of THC.

Lastly, never smoke or vape next to a newborn, child, or anyone who doesn't want to be near it. There are still some adverse effects from secondhand cannabis smoke that little lungs should not be subjected to.

CANNABIS AND DRIVING

Cannabis has been shown to impair motor skills for short periods of time. Cannabis use leads to impairments in eye movement, tracking, reaction time, increased weaving, larger spacing between vehicles, and decreased speed[23]. In general, the impairments seen from cannabis consumption while driving compared to alcohol while driving are much less pronounced, but combined they are very dangerous. Interestingly, studies have found that cannabis consumers are more aware of their intoxication while medicated and express a general unwillingness to drive while under the influence compared to alcohol consumers who tend to feel unstoppable and act in riskier ways while driving[24]. We'd rather look out the window and enjoy the scenery than partake in a *Fast and Furious* journey down the highway.

EVALUATING INTOXICATION

There is currently a massive amount of grant funding available for any researcher that can figure out how to test that someone is "too high to drive." This seems like an easy task, as we've done it before with other commonly used drugs like alcohol, benzodiazepines, and opiates. However, there are distinct differences with cannabis that make it a much more challenging task.

Cannabis stays in your system far longer than most other drugs; therefore, it is difficult to test "acute intoxication" or real-time intoxication. Cannabinoids like THC are lipophilic (fat-loving molecules), so they stick to fat and slowly release over time. THC can be detected in blood several hours after consumption for occasional users and days after the last use in chronic consumers[25] even though they no longer feel the "high" effects. This is in contrast to other drugs like cocaine that are used and flushed from our bodies within a few days of use. Because cannabis lingers in the body for so long, we don't have accurate data on how many motor vehicle accidents involve cannabis intoxication, and we will continue to lack this data until we have the ability to test for acute intoxication. However, U.S. states that have experienced a significant increase in legal cannabis

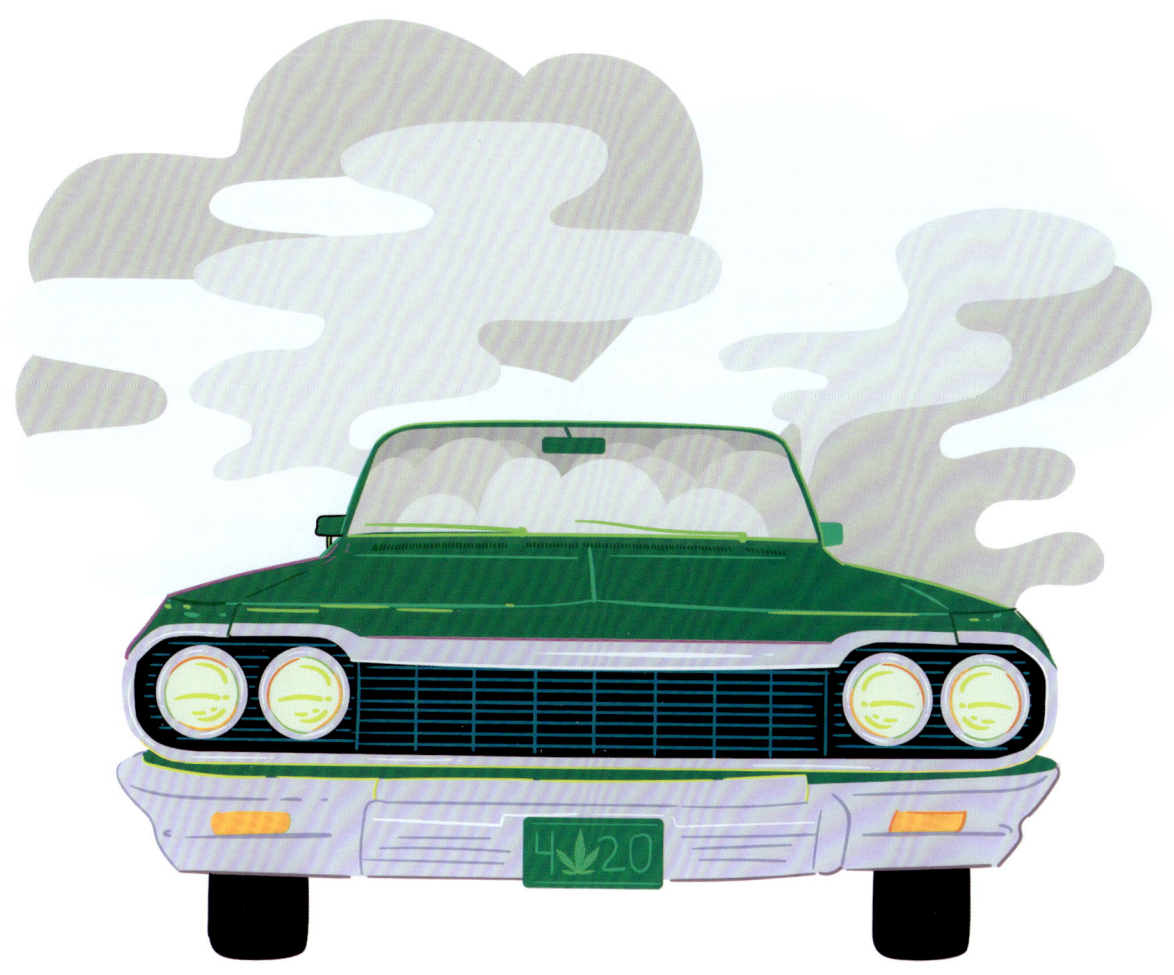

sales and medical card patients have not seen a proportional rise in traffic fatalities. Better still, most states have experienced a decline in fatal accidents[26] post legalization.

Another challenge is that different forms of cannabis are processed in the body at different rates. To accurately grasp levels of intoxication, we would need studies on smoking, vaping, edibles, suppositories, etc. and driving. A recent study tested participants' ability to operate a simulated vehicle after taking their normal dose of a THC edible. The study found people still felt the effects six hours after dosing (which is much longer than smoking or vaping). Participants drove slightly slower while high,

but there were no changes in other metrics used to measure good driving. Additionally, there was a lower amount of blood THC than predicted, revealing it would be challenging to use THC in the blood as an accurate predictor of intoxication[27].

CANNABIS TOLERANCE

When we think about drinking alcohol and testing for it in our body, it is a relatively linear relationship. The more drinks you have, the more messed up you feel, the higher your blood-alcohol levels, and therefore the more dangerous it is to drive. Cannabis has some similarities, but cannabis users can build tolerance to the substance. Our bodies get acclimated to more and more THC by lessening the number of cannabinoid receptors in our brains so there aren't as many targets for the THC to bind to.

Alcohol also works on receptors... kind of. Alcohol has activity on GABA-A receptors in the brain and prevents some neurons from signaling, but beyond that, it indiscriminately acts as a poison. Alcohol easily passes through almost all our organs and is metabolized into reactive chemicals that damage cells, limit energy in the body, deprive tissues of oxygen, cause inflammation and, especially at high doses, dilute blood and impair motor function.

The effects of cannabis are targeted at the ECS. When a chronic cannabis user builds up a tolerance to THC in their body, they are also developing a tolerance to the neurocognitive-impairing effects on task performance[28] like driving.

Not all cannabis consumers are safe to drive—in fact, most are likely not. New cannabis consumers who have not built up a tolerance and are unfamiliar with the effects from cannabis should never drive while medicated. Studies have evaluated cannabis consumers who have a tolerance to THC and those who are naive to the substance while driving. Not surprisingly, consumption from the naive cannabis consumers had a significant impact on their motor function. However, seasoned cannabis consumers who had developed a tolerance to THC did not.

I have also collected data through my cannabis research nonprofit, the Network of Applied Pharmacognosy. In a pool of approximately 4,750 participants, we found that 91% of participants were daily consumers and 64% of participants drove while high. Medical patients consume cannabis multiple times a day and often have a significant tolerance to THC. Their lives are already affected with their chronic medical conditions that often present physical and mental obstacles. To say that these patients can never drive a vehicle because they have THC in their system is egregious and unjust, and the science doesn't support that they are dangerous to society.

Remember, everyone has a different response to THC. Some people can take 100 mg of THC in edible form and feel nothing. Some people can smoke full joints and feel functional and normal, while others are knocked out from one puff of a joint or 2 mg of an edible. All our bodies are different, have lived through different experiences, have different metabolisms, different levels of liver enzymes, and different tolerances to THC.

Ultimately, cannabis use while driving is especially dangerous when other substances like alcohol are present, because the effects are often exacerbated and unpredictable[29]. It is especially unsafe if you are not accustomed to something like an edible because you may slowly start to feel the effects during your drive. You need to be an educated consumer and understand your body and your tolerance. Having another person as a designated driver is always the safer option. But I strongly believe those who consume cannabis multiple times a day and understand their dosing and their bodies are not a danger on the roads. They may even be better drivers without the chronic pain, anxiety, and rage overtaking them on the road.

PETS AND CANNABIS PRODUCTS

All animals have endocannabinoid systems. There are obvious differences between our pets and us that we do not see with the naked eye. Our pet's nervous systems are different from how our nervous systems are designed and distributed within the body. **It is not safe to assume that a dose of THC that is therapeutic for your problems can translate to your pets' experience.** Even if you correct for weight, the distribution of receptors in your pet's brain, is different, so they will feel different effects.

Although not all animals have been studied to understand the exact distribution of CB1 receptors in the brain, dogs' cannabinoid receptors have been studied by the U.S. government and other research institutions in great detail. The research found that dogs have a higher abundance of cannabinoid receptors in the hindbrain, cerebellum, brainstem, and medulla oblongata compared to human counterparts[30].

Between these research studies and the unfortunate regular occurrence of dogs accidentally being dosed with THC products, it has been shown that there is a unique neurological reaction that occurs when dogs take in large amounts of THC called "static ataxia," which is essentially temporary paralysis. This condition is thought to be due to the high concentration of cannabinoid receptors in a dog's cerebellum—the portion of the brain that controls functions like balance, posture, motor control, and bladder control. If your dog does end up accidentally getting into your cannabis products, it can often become very disoriented, lose bladder control, and be temporarily paralyzed (worst case scenario). Most veterinarians will recommend getting comfortable and waiting it out. Give your dog some water, a nice bed to sleep on, monitor their reactions, and wait it out. Don't hotbox your vehicle with your dogs in it, blow smoke in your cat's face, or give your dog THC oil to relax.

Not all cannabis is bad for animals, however. You will often see bacon-flavored CBD oils, CBD-infused dog treats, salmon CBD tinctures, and a multitude of other creations meant for your pets. CBD has been scientifically shown to be well-tolerated in dogs at doses of 4 to 20mg/kg of body weight per day for 6 to 12 weeks. Cannabis flower also won't make your animal sick. The bud needs to be heated up or smoked to get the psychoactive effects. If your animal eats a nug of weed, it won't harm them; and they probably won't want to eat it anyway (although you never know). Conversely, products like edibles are the most dangerous for your animal, especially if it is something like a chocolate or brownie—because chocolate is harmful to dogs as well as THC.

We are greatly lacking scientific data on other relevant animals, like horses, cats, and rabbits. In general, it is always recommended to discuss changes in your pet's diet and supplements with your veterinarian. However, if your animal has joint inflammation or pain, they may respond well to CBD.

If you are introducing CBD for the first time, introduce the product slowly and note how your pet responds. If they need a higher dose, try more the next day. Many CBD products have up to the legal limit of 0.3% THC present. This microdose will likely be fine for your animal, but it is not recommended to increase the dose of THC more without further consultation.

CONCLUSION

Cannabis is not a simple medicine—weed is not just weed. There are almost infinite combinations of active molecules, ratios, consumption methods, doses, and genetics that personalize our experience.

Before you puff on something or ingest an edible, make sure you know what you're taking. If your friends brought the weed, ask them what strain it is and if they know how strong it is. These questions will allow you to become a more educated consumer, start to learn what products work for you. and can help you gauge your dose before you consume.

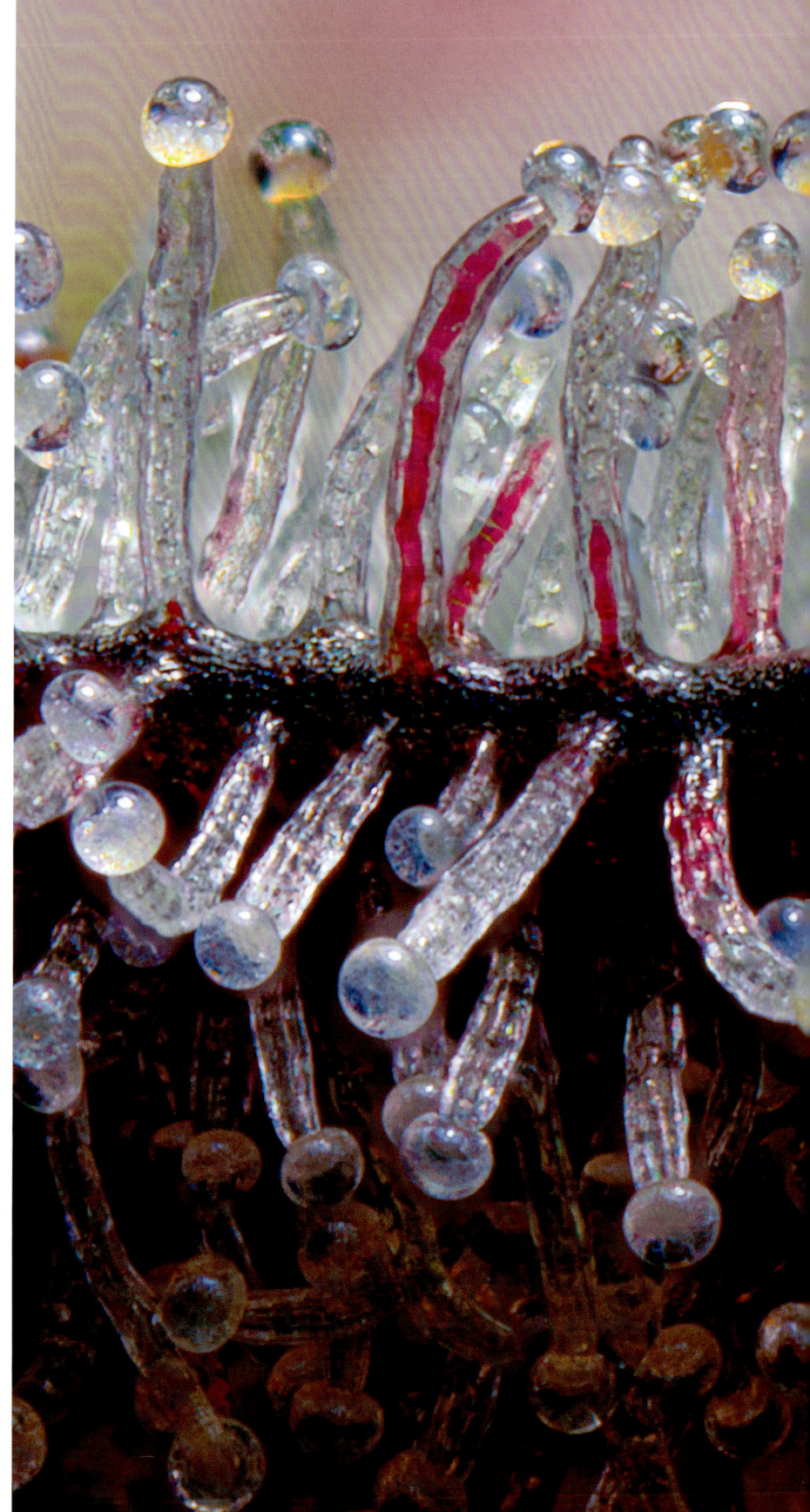

SMOKE BREAK

LET'S RECAP WHAT WE LEARNED:

➤ Cannabis can't cause a fatal overdose, but overconsumption can lead to temporary discomfort such as anxiety, panic attacks, paranoia, or hyperemesis. Practicing balance and understanding individual limits is key to avoiding negative experiences.

➤ The rise of high-THC products has shifted cannabis potency compared to the past, often sacrificing the natural balance of cannabinoids and terpenes. Whole-plant extracts or balanced products (with CBD) are recommended for safer and more balanced effects.

➤ Lab testing for contaminants (e.g., microbials, heavy metals, pesticides) in legal cannabis markets ensures higher safety standards for consumers, though issues such as the artificial inflation of THC percentages and long-term product degradation can still occur.

➤ Potential drug interactions with cannabis should be considered, especially with substances processed by the same liver enzymes. Combining cannabis with alcohol can lead to increased dizziness, slowed reaction times, and a higher risk of negative effects.

➤ Cannabis use during pregnancy, breastfeeding, and with pets remains a debated topic. While limited data exists, it is recommended to use the lowest effective dose, avoid smoking, and consult with healthcare professionals before making decisions. Pets can tolerate CBD but should avoid THC.

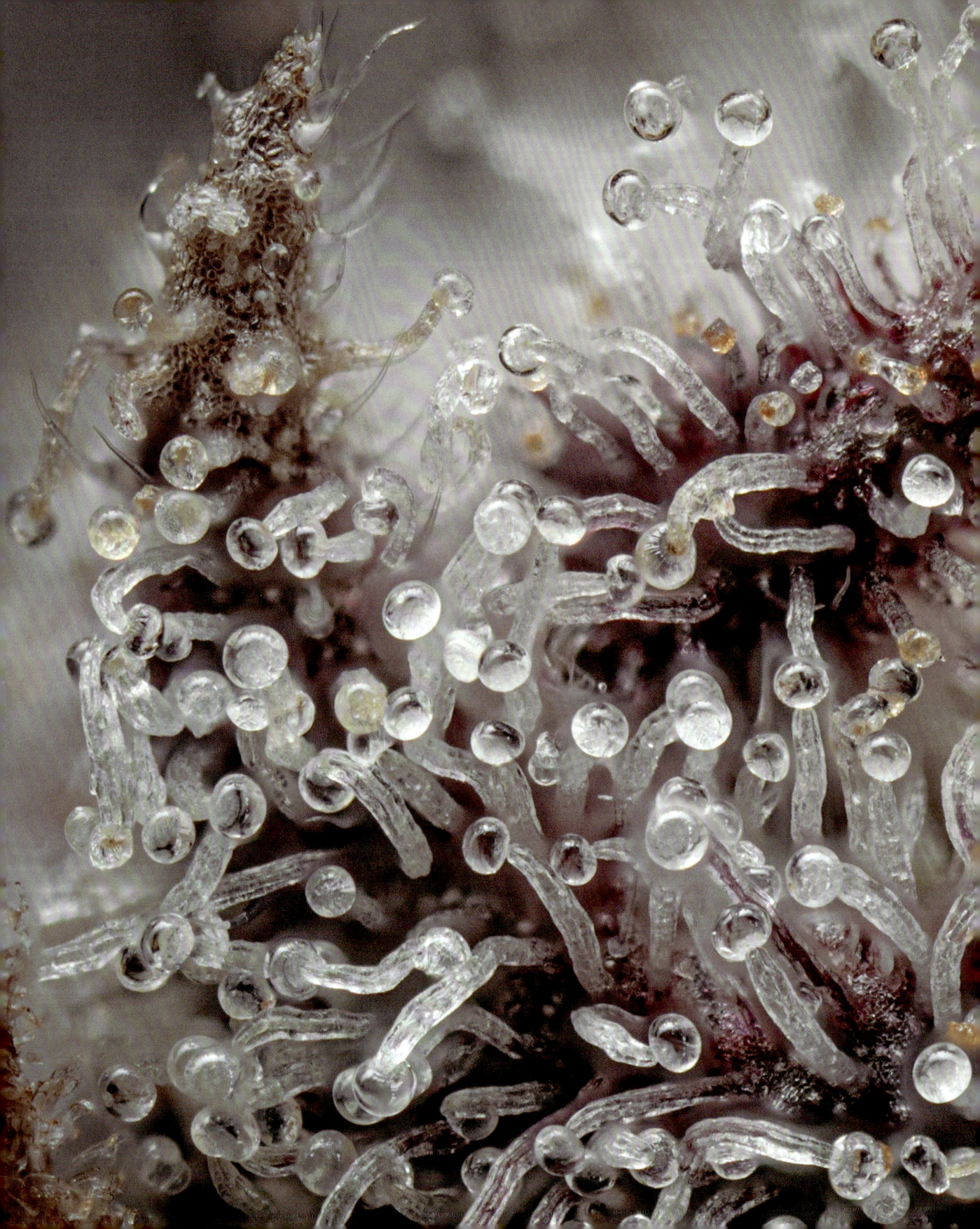

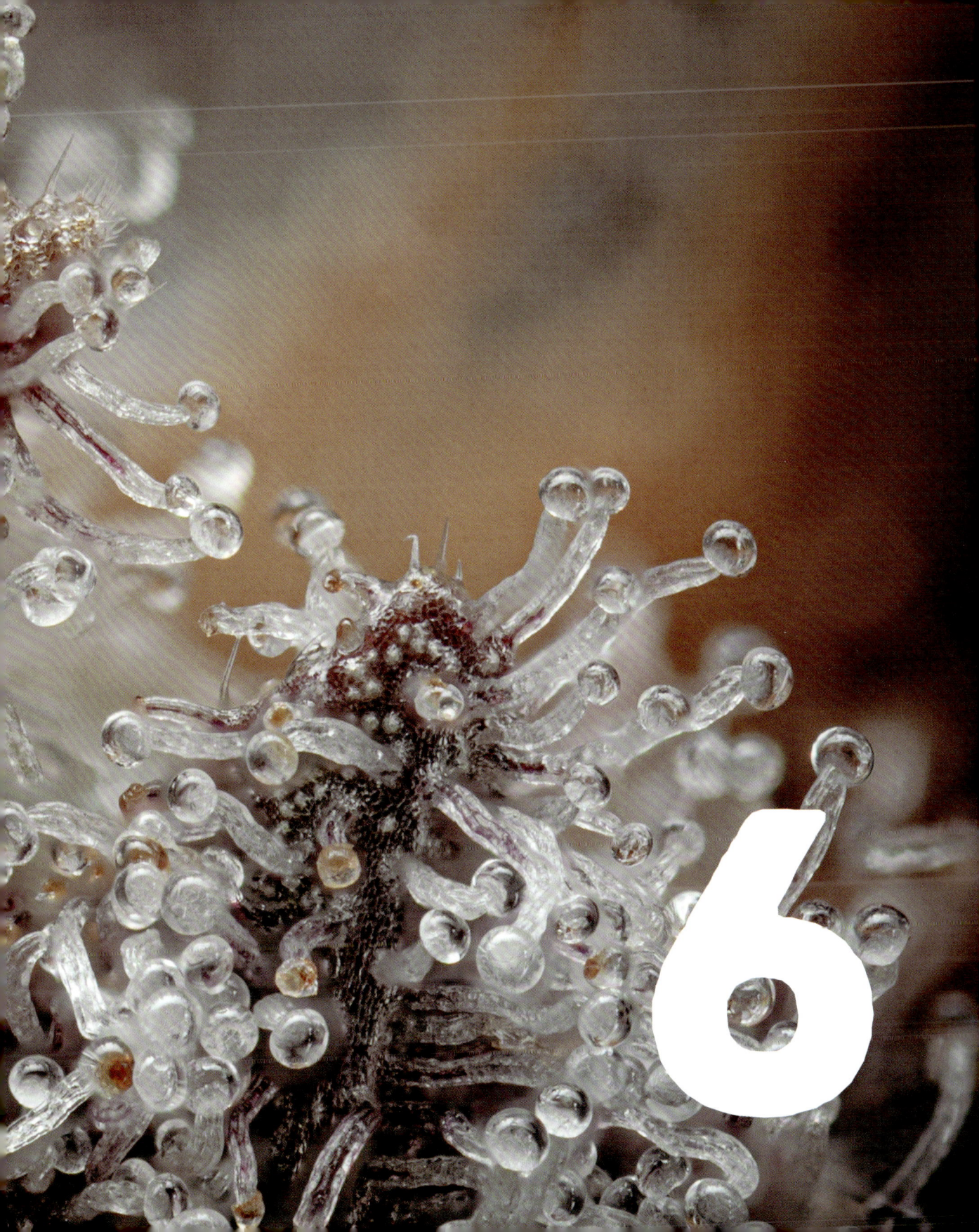

6

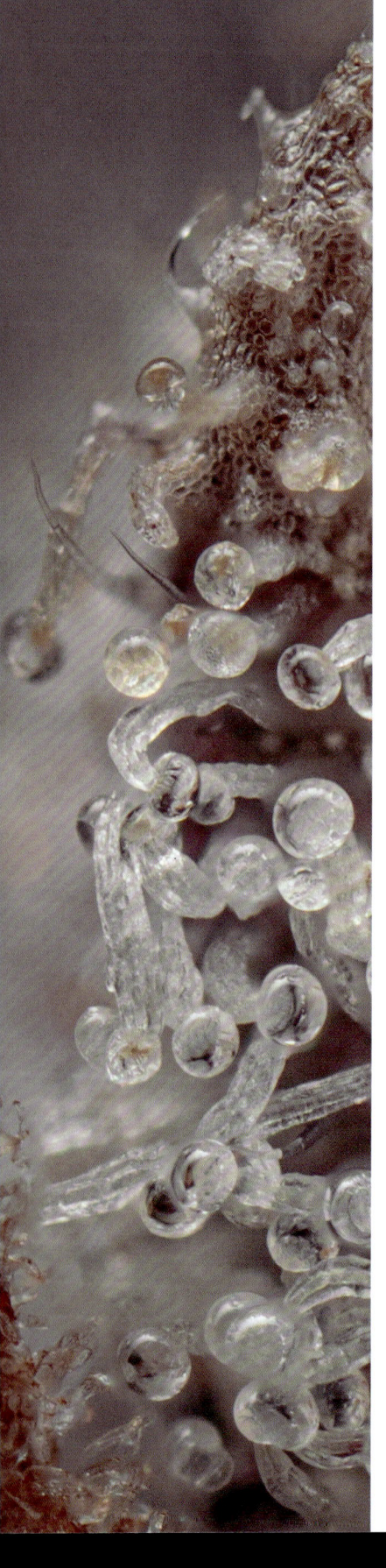

THE MANY MEDICINAL USES OF CANNABIS

Throughout this book I've emphasized that cannabis is a personalized medicine. Whether through controlling the dose, determining what consumption method to use, or choosing active compounds, we can cater cannabis and cannabinoids to our individual needs.

The wide range of therapeutic benefits from cannabis come from the unique way in which cannabis interacts with the master regulatory system in the body, called the Endocannabinoid System (ECS). The role of the ECS is to maintain balance or homeostasis in the body. If the body becomes dysregulated in some way, whether that it's sending too many neurotransmitters or inflammatory signals, activation of the ECS can halt the signals and bring them back to baseline. The unique interaction of cannabinoids on the endocannabinoid system provides almost limitless potential as a therapeutic target.

In this chapter we are going to discuss a variety of medical conditions for which cannabis can provide beneficial relief. These are validated by research and lived experience within the cannabis community. Although the mechanism is similar in all cases, with cannabinoids acting via activation of the ECS, it can be helpful for medical patients and providers to understand some underlying mechanisms to help determine the best method of consumption, dosing, and other important factors.

In some specific cases like for fibromyalgia, migraines, and inflammatory bowel syndromes, it has been hypothesized by Dr. Ethan Russo that these conditions (and likely many more) are a product of people not producing enough endocannabinoids. The theory is called **Clinical Endocannabinoid Deficiency, or CED,** and was first introduced into the literature in 2001. If someone was not producing enough endocannabinoids, it could lead to a variety of treatment resistant inflammatory conditions that often overlap with chronic pain. Evidence for migraine, fibromyalgia, and irritable bowel syndrome (IBS) are presented in a 2017 publication, and likely many others will be added to the list in the coming decades.

The location of the cannabinoid receptors in the body is important for pairing therapeutic options with medical conditions. Although the endocannabinoid system exists throughout the entire body, the cannabinoid 1 receptor (CB1) receptor is more abundant in the central nervous system, which is the brain and spinal cord, and the cannabinoid 2 receptor (CB2) is more present on the immune cells and peripheral sites throughout the body.

CANNABIS AND ANESTHESIA

If you're undergoing surgery and you're a cannabis user, you must be honest with your medical professionals or you may not be given enough anesthesia. Although this can be uncomfortable, for safety reasons it is necessary information.

Propofol is a common general anesthetic drug that works directly via the GABAA receptor and indirectly through the cannabinoid 1 receptor. Propofol administration increases the levels of the endocannabinoid anandamide and can prevent the enzyme that degrades this endocannabinoid in the body (FAAH), keeping it around longer. The increase in anandamide levels causes activation of the CB1 receptor, which is part of the way that this drug works as an anesthetic.

Chronic cannabis users with a tolerance to THC will have lower levels of CB1 receptors and therefore may require higher doses of Propofol to get the anesthetic effects. Most surgeries will suggest a minimum of 72 hours of abstinence from cannabis prior to surgery, although many suggest a full week of abstinence to reset the tolerance of the CB1 receptors prior to surgery. Medical professionals may choose a different dose or a different type of anesthetic that doesn't interact with the ECS if you are a cannabis consumer.

CANNABIS AS A PREVENTATIVE MEDICINE AND WELLNESS TOOL

INFLAMMATION

Inflammation is a necessary process in the body—the body's natural inflammatory response can be activated by infections, toxins, allergic response, and trauma. This inflammation should be short lived, but as we age and as inflammation becomes more chronic, it can eventually play a role in the development of cardiovascular disease, autoimmune conditions, neurological conditions, and cancer[1].

All components of the ECS (endocannabinoids, enzymes, and receptors) are expressed on most immune cells[2], but immune cells express CB2 receptors up to 100 times more than CB1 receptors[3]. Cannabis contains several compounds that activate the CB2 receptor including the cannabinoids cannabichromene (CBC), delta 9 tetrahydrocannabivarin (THCV), as well as the terpene beta-caryophyllene (BCP), and THC. Activation of CB2 receptors can prevent the release of compounds that cause inflammation and can

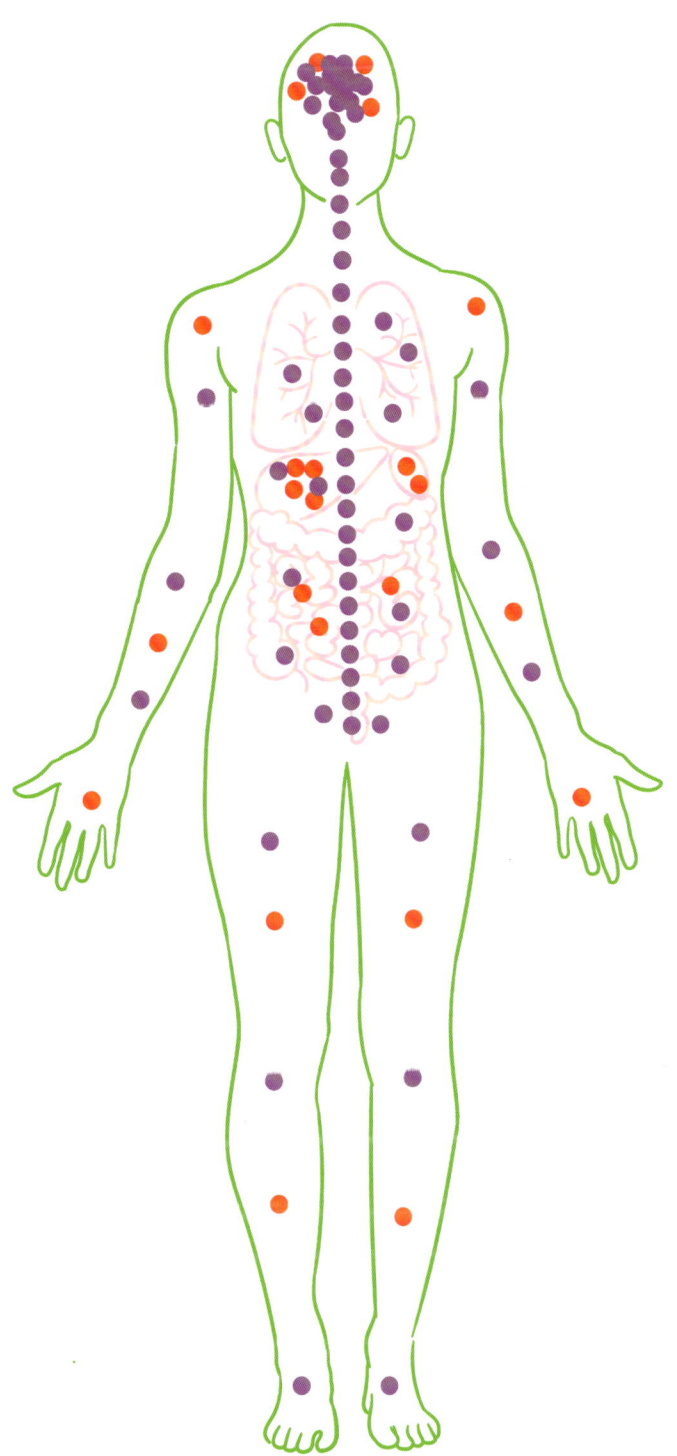

initiate the release of molecules that reduce inflammation[4, 5].

Cannabis contains many compounds capable of reducing inflammation, many of which act through different pathways. CBD extracts reduce skin, gut and brain inflammation[6]. Similarly, THC reduces inflammatory markers in HIV patients and reduces skin[7], gut, and brain inflammation.

STRESS

Cannabis's ability to mitigate stress is one reason why many chronic users of cannabis continue to medicate[8] daily. Most studies on cannabis and stress focus on short-term or acute effects and have noted that THC lowers the response of the amygdala—the part of the brain that responds to stressful stimuli. This effect is dose dependent, with low doses relieving stress and higher doses causing a stressful response[9].

However, this data pertains to acute or short-term stress relief. Chronic or long-term cannabis use is associated with changes in cortisol levels as well as the adrenocorticotropic hormone—another hormone that regulates cortisol production—and reduced emotional reactions to unpleasant images[10].

Although cannabis can be effective as a tool in stress management, remember that cannabis is not a cure-all—there are other components of preventative medicine like exercise, a healthy diet, hydration, creative outlets, and good company that also contribute to overall health. Although cannabis doesn't directly improve all of these, many people use cannabis as a general wellness tool to help morph into the right headspace.

PLAY

Play is technically defined as doing something that is not "serious" or "work". It may seem like a trivial thing that we do as children, but play is a vital component of neurodevelopment for humans and other animals. Not only is play critical for children but it is also a major component of well-being for adults. Play doesn't need to be playing kickball with your friends, but it can be. It can also be as simple as doing a puzzle, writing poems, painting, golfing, or whatever you enjoy that is not work or taken too seriously.

I'm not aware of specific studies proving that cannabis enhances play, but I'm 100% certain it does. From my own experience, my friends and I—well into our 30s—will light up a joint and play four square for hours, throw absurdly themed parties, or go on fun dates at pick-and-paint pottery shops. Countless people, especially parents, have told me that cannabis helps them relax, have fun, and truly enjoy spending time with their kids in the moment.

Parents who use cannabis are still good parents, and in many cases, cannabis makes them better parents. Allowing them to have tea parties, dress up, play Rapunzel, race trucks, sing songs, or simply take the time to enjoy their kids' company without feeling annoyed or irritated. Whether you're coming home after 10 hours of answering emails from Stephanie in sales all day or staying at home to take care of the kids while your partner is at work, childcare is objectively exhausting. Many parents use cannabis to engage and have fun with their children and play.

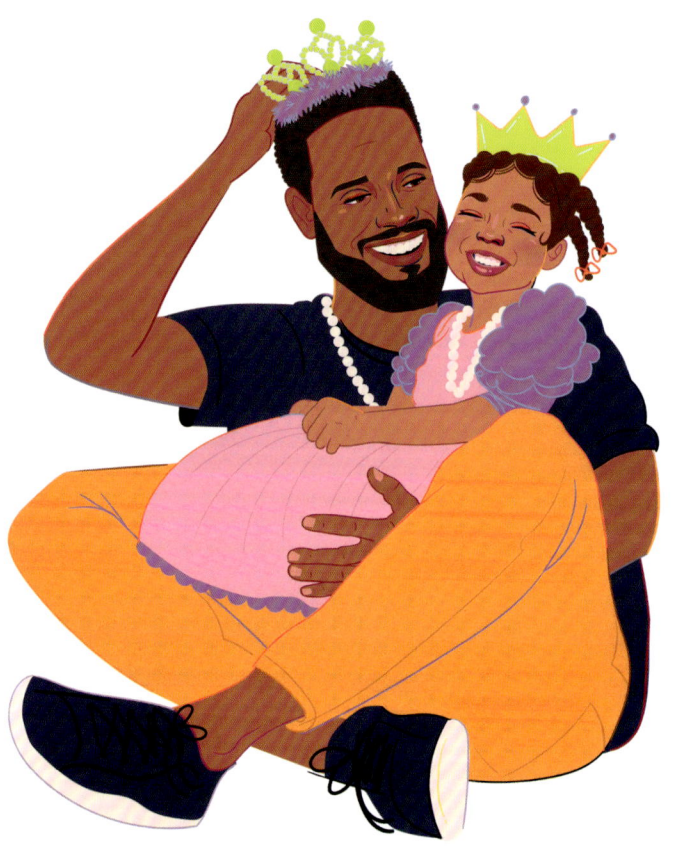

REPLACING WITH HERB

OPIOIDS

Cannabis is not a perfect drug—there are side effects—but cannabis is orders of magnitude safer than any opiate. Opioids are molecules often prescribed for pain which have immense therapeutic value in clinical settings. Opioids like morphine and codeine were first isolated from the poppy plant (*Papaver somniferum*) and were later altered chemically to work faster and stronger in the body, leading to the birth of heroin and other opioid derivatives. Opioids are used clinically as pain relieving drugs, and many people who become addicted to opioids are first introduced to these drugs in clinical settings through a prescription. These drugs can be especially addictive because they are meant to take away pain and work rapidly. This often leads to seeking more pain-killing compounds after the initial prescription expires from the pharmacy, ultimately leading to illicit sources of oxycontin, oxycodone, heroin, or fentanyl.

There is limited systemic support to wean off opiates or alternative effective pain treatments. The current "gold standard" treatment for opioid dependence—controlled-release opioids in a regulated manner—is clearly not effective, as the rates of opioid use and dependence remain relatively unchanged[11].

CANNABIS AS AN ALTERNATIVE

People in chronic pain need some sort of treatment, but if they have previously struggled with opioid addiction or don't want to risk it, these medications are not an option. Cannabis has been linked to reductions in use of alcohol and prescription[12] drugs, largely because it has fewer adverse effects, works better at relieving pain symptoms, and is less addicting/causes less withdrawal[13]. Cannabis has been studied for acute and chronic pain as well as supplemental treatment with other opiates, reducing the amount of drug needed for the pain-relieving effect. In the U.S., states with legal accessible cannabis report considerably fewer opioid-related deaths[14] compared to states still in active prohibition.

When THC is co-administered with morphine, one quarter of the dose of morphine is required to reach a significant reduction in pain[15]. THC has also been shown to displace or essentially knock off opiates from the opioid receptor (mu opioid receptor) as well as affect the ways the receptors signal in other ways[16], which could add to the harm reduction effects of cannabis for opiate use disorder.

Furthermore, CBD-forward products can help with the anxiety, jitters, and inflammation that may be contributing to pain. CBD is well tolerated in high doses up to 800 mg per day, but likely requires far less than 800 mg when paired with small doses (0.3%) of THC, like those found in full spectrum hemp products.

> ### PRO TIP
> If you are struggling with alcohol use and are exploring cannabis as an alternative, look into infused drinks. They often come with 2.5 mg, 5 mg, or 10 mg of active cannabinoids like THC, CBD, or both. These are a great option if you are in a social situation where everyone is drinking, and you want something to sip on to relax but don't want alcohol.

CANNABIS AND CANCER

CAN CANNABIS USE CAUSE CANCER?

There is often the question as to if smoking cannabis causes lung cancer, and multiple large, controlled studies have investigated this topic and have found **no statistically significant increase in lung cancer with cannabis smokers[17], unlike the harrowing statistics with nicotine products**. There have been several theories on why this isn't the case, including increased activity about the immune system in lung cells when exposed to cannabinoids, or the anti-proliferative (growth) effects cannabinoids have on some cell types.

Other studies found that some cannabinoids can also prevent the growth of cancer cells or act as a preventative medicine. Regardless, smoking in general is associated with decreased lung health and can cause chronic inflammation and free radical damage. If you have a preexisting condition or start to experience any issues with chronic phlegm, itchy throat, or discomfort, it is advised to stop inhalation methods.

ANTICANCER POTENTIAL

The ECS is involved in the process of regulating cell growth and division within the body. As cancer is, in simple terms, dysregulated cell growth, it is no wonder that activating the ECS with cannabis may help for some types of cancer[18].

Endocannabinoids have been implicated as a preventative mechanism for the growth of some cancer cells like breast and prostate cancers[19]. Additionally, dysregulation of the ECS receptors and endocannabinoids has been observed in various cancer cells[20]. Terpenes found in cannabis have also shown anticancer activity. Interestingly, one famous anticancer natural product is also of terpene origin—taxol or paclitaxel from the Pacific yew tree. In cannabis, limonene demonstrated anticancer effects for pancreas, stomach, colon, skin, and liver cancers[21]. Pinene has demonstrated the ability to prevent cancer cell growth in skin cancer melanoma cells[22] and prevent some of the pro-inflammatory compounds[23] from recruiting. The terpene beta caryophyllene can sensitize melanoma cells to other anticancer agents like doxorubicin by preventing drug resistance[24].

Cannabinoids like THC have shown to have anticancer effects, and cannabis users in general have been linked to having an increase or decrease in some instances of specific cancers. In the case of bladder cancer, cannabis use was associated with a 45% decrease in bladder cancer[25] rates. Beyond cannabinoids, flavonoids, such as cannflavin A[26], were also shown to inhibit bladder cancer growth. Interestingly, cannabis consumers may be at higher risk for some cancers like testicular cancer, in which cannabis can be an indicator of increased risk[27].

Additionally, cannabinoids have been used during chemotherapy treatment to help with adverse effects such as pain, nausea, weight loss, constipation, anxiety, trouble sleeping, and vomiting.

CANNABINOIDS AND PALLIATIVE CARE

For end-of-life care, cannabis is used not only to improve appetite, and decrease nausea and pain, but to do so in a way that allows the person to live their last days as true to themselves as possible. Many end-of-life medications turn people into a shell of what they used to be mentally and physically. For the sake of both the family and the person transitioning, the last memories with a loved one should involve being as pain-free, happy, and relaxed as possible. Many patients on palliative care will utilize multiple mechanisms of cannabis consumption including vaping for instant relief and edibles, drinks, patches, and suppositories. Even if someone has been notoriously anti-cannabis for their entire life, it is still worth offering the medicine for one last opportunity, as oftentimes people's mental state changes as they near the end of life

CANNABIS AS PAIN RELIEF

HOW DOES CANNABIS HELP WITH PAIN?

Pain relief is one of the top reasons why people consume cannabis. Pain is a product of our brain cells or neurons being stimulated to send chemical messengers that tell the brain there is something painful happening—**drugs for pain including opioids and cannabis work by reducing the pain signaling to the brain.**

In the body, our ECS is activated when something painful starts happening. This causes the synthesis of the endocannabinoids 2-AG and anandamide—there is also an upregulation of cannabinoid receptors in the dorsal horn, which is the pain center of the body. When the body needs to press the breaks on pain signaling, the endocannabinoids bind to the CB1 receptor on the neuron; Binding to the CB1 receptor halts the production of some of the pain signals and reduces your pain. As this mechanism of pain relief is centered around CB1 activation, **THC and CBN are the best cannabinoids for chronic pain**. However, CBC, or cannabichromene is another promising cannabinoid that helps reduce pain either synergistically with THC or through alternative mechanisms like reducing inflammation, increasing levels of endocannabinoids, and binding to other pain-related receptors like the TRPV1 receptor[28].

Activation of CB2 receptors by other CB2 agonists like tetrahydrocannabivarin (THCV), or beta-caryophyllene (BCP) can also help with reducing pain likely through **reducing pro-inflammatory compounds**[29] **and increasing anti-inflammatory compounds**. Beyond the cannabinoid receptors, CBD offers additional pain-reducing benefits through activation of the TRPV1 channels[30] and reduces pain-related anxiety via serotonin 5HT1A receptor activation.

Terpenes that should be targeted for analgesic effects are linalool, myrcene, and beta-caryophyllene, which have shown to produce pain-relief on their[31] **own**[32] **or in combination with cannabinoids like THC, CBD, CBC, and CBN.**

CHRONIC PAIN

It is estimated that 20% of the world's population suffers from chronic pain[33]. There are various types of pain that can happen in the body, and some people suffer from multiple types of pain. Acute pain is temporary, but chronic pain is pain that lasts more than three months.

Chronic pain is usually persistent because the body continues to send flushes of pain signals to the brain. Those signals can arise from past injury or trauma in a specific area of the body–this type of chronic pain is called **nociceptive pain**. Pain signals can also arise from within the nervous system itself, from damage to the nervous system–this is called **neuropathic pain**.

Cannabis can help alleviate symptoms of chronic pain; however, cannabis can sometimes make acute pain worse by making the body hyper-aware of accelerated blood flow to painful areas. Many chronic pain patients use a multitude of

consumption methods to help manage their pain, although smoking is still the preferred method among most. Activation of the ECS through cannabis use not only reduces pain signaling but also alters the perception of pain and dulls the emotional reaction to pain[34].

Pain patients often find products with CBD and THC the most beneficial for symptom management[35]. If the pain is localized to a specific area, topicals are a great option to locally relieve pain and inflammation in a sore area like the knee, hip, elbow, or foot. Oftentimes, chronic pain patients require higher doses of THC compared to non-pain sufferers. Dabs are a great way to get higher levels of THC in the body with instantaneous relief and fewer carcinogens compared to smoking the equivalent level of active compounds. Edibles provide long-lasting relief for events or sleep, and suppositories are a great tool for below-the-waist pain like endometriosis or IBS.

NUGS OF KNOWLEDGE

Don't limit yourself to one consumption method. Knowing the average duration and effects allows you to combine different product types and doses. Stacking consumption methods or dose layering products and delivery methods could look like taking a dab while you wait for your edible to kick in after rubbing a salve on your arm.

EFFECT / TIME

● edibles
● inhalation

CANNABIS AND ENDOMETRIOSIS

ENDOMETRIOSIS

Endometriosis is a condition where tissue similar to the uterus lining grows outside the uterus, and it is estimated that about 10% of women have endometriosis. Endometriosis is very painful, especially around the time of menstruation. The pain associated with endometriosis is called endometriosis-related chronic pelvic pain (CPP), and the term encompasses period pain, pain during sex, general tiredness, pain on bowel movements, and pain during urination. There is a high overlap between endometriosis and irritable bowel syndrome (IBS), rheumatoid arthritis, chronic fatigue syndrome, psoriasis, anxiety, and depression.

Part of the pathology of endometriosis is changes in the efficiency of estrogen and progesterone, which ultimately leads to progesterone resistance, excess estrogen levels[36], and an inflammatory response. The current treatments for endometriosis are surgeries, pain management medications (opioid and non), hormonal treatment, and medications that reduce nerve activity[37]. The treatments are not effective in a large portion of women, and there are substantial side effects associated with each option.

How can cannabis help with endometriosis?

The ECS is deeply integrated within the reproductive system, of women and men. Cannabinoid receptors have been found throughout all female reproductive tissue, and medical cannabis has been shown to alleviate some of the pain associated with endometriosis through activation of CB1 receptors. Beyond pain, the ECS also controls other mechanisms involved in endometriosis like inflammation, building new blood vessels, cell death and growth, and wound healing[38].

One study found that levels of the endocannabinoid AEA, 2-AG, and OEA are increased in women with endometriosis, specifically in the S phase of the menstrual cycle, which is progesterone dependent, compared to women with no evidence of endometriosis[39]. Additionally, there was a correlation between increased endocannabinoids and decreased cannabinoid receptors in people with endometriosis. It is thought that these three endocannabinoids may be involved in activation or desensitization of the TRPV1 receptor in some endometrial cells and could be related to hypersensitivity to chronic inflammatory pain[40]. These data suggest that CBD may be a good candidate to desensitize CB2 receptors paired with THC to help with pain via activation of the CB1 receptors[41]. Other CB2 agonists are beta-caryophyllene, cannabichromene (CBC), THC, and delta 9 tetrahydrocannabivarin (THCV) which could all be of benefit in various forms of consumption.

Although we have some data on cannabis and endometriosis, I wanted to include a segment from an author, educator, and endometriosis warrior, Lara Parker. Lara wrote the book, *Vagina Problems: Endometriosis, Painful Sex, and Other Taboo Topics*. Here she gives some practical advice on consumption methods, strains, and dosing for other women to use:

"On bad days when I need quick relief from all-over pain or a barbed wire around my abdomen feeling, nothing works as well for me as smoking cannabis does. Depending on the severity of my pain, it can impact the way I choose to consume. For example, when I am in a particularly painful flare, it can be quite difficult to grind cannabis, pack it into a bowl or bong, and then light it. For this reason, I almost always have pre-rolls or pre-ground flower on hand. Not only does smoking provide the quickest relief for me (next to dabbing), but it's the most flavorful option for me and for some reason I have always been the type of consumer who loves to taste/smell the plant. It's why I prefer smoking cannabis to almost all other forms of consumption.

Depending on the type of symptom I am hoping to address, I will reach for a few different types of cannabis. For deep pain: I love heavier body high strains such as Papaya, Gorilla Glue, Banana OG. For nausea or help eating (one of my most common symptoms is lack of appetite/ nausea/ pain and bloating with eating): I love GSC (Girl Scout Cookies), Ice Cream Cake, Gelato, GMO Cookies. I LOVE Cookies strains for this in particular.

For the type of pain I describe as 'rock in your shoe' pain (you can function, but it really starts to drive you crazy after a bit) I love: Sour Diesel, Blue Dream, Chemdawg, Bubba Kush.

I reach for edibles for more overall preventative pain management and not immediate relief. I enjoy 'micro-dosing' edibles meaning I'll take 2.5 to 5 mg doses at a time 3 to 4 times a day and this keeps me going with some pain relief, appetite help, mood help, but without the full on 'Wow, I am stoned' feeling. My favorite edibles of all time are the Wonderbrett Solventless Rosin fruit chews. I've never had such a consistently great all-around high with other edibles. I also find that they are easier for traveling when I can't easily smoke.

In addition to smoking cannabis during a hefty pain flare, I also reach for salves and topicals often. I love a cannabis balm (I usually go for CBD/CBG since I already consumed THC) and apply it directly to my abdomen and lower back. From there, I will apply heat. It's so soothing.

One of the most effective forms of cannabis usage for specifically pelvic pain—related to period cramps, orgasm pain, or the like—are CBD or THC suppositories. Like with salves, I usually reach for CBD-only suppositories since I almost always have THC already in my system. Foria is my preferred brand, but I also recommend Hello Again."

Some other notes from Lara:
"When I first began consuming, I relied heavily on budtender recommendations because I had no idea what I was doing, I had never smoked at all prior to 2014. From there, I began keeping track of strains and how I felt on them with various symptoms. I began to explore different ways of utilizing the plant. I feel like I have a solid grasp on what works well for my body and mind at this point, but it requires patience, money, and access to this plant. I have always said that I don't believe cannabis is the answer for everyone with pelvic pain, but it's been life-changing for me to have access to this medicine, and I believe in access above anything else. It may not be a perfect solution, but it's a possible avenue that everyone should have the option to explore.

While things have been very difficult for me over the years, it would have been much harder without the assistance of cannabis, a plant that somehow allowed me to feel at home in my body after so long."

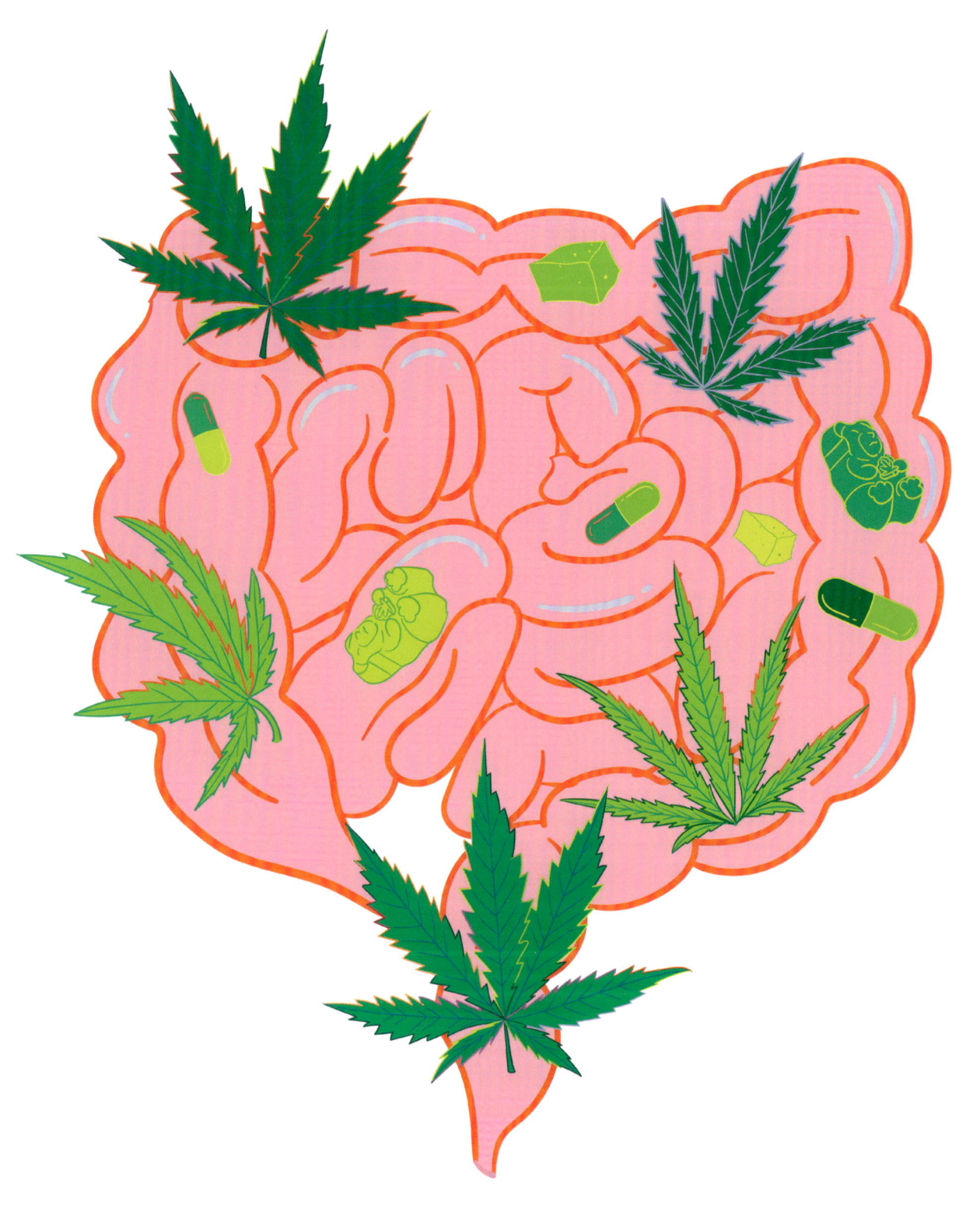

CANNABIS AND INFLAMMATORY GUT CONDITIONS

Cannabinoids have shown promise for a variety of inflammatory gut conditions like inflammatory bowel disease (IBD) and irritable bowel syndrome (IBS). IBD is an autoimmune disorder which causes chronic inflammation of the intestinal tract and includes ulcerative colitis and Crohn's disease, while IBS is characterized by abdominal pain, constipation, and diarrhea.

THE ECS' ROLE IN THE GUT

Gastrointestinal (GI) movement, secretion, and inflammation are all altered and controlled by the endocannabinoid system, providing rationale for cannabinoid as therapies for inflammatory gut conditions[42].

CB1 receptors are localized in the colon smooth muscle tissue and colon epithelium tissue, and CB2 receptors can be found in the immune regulating cells of the intestinal mucosa and submucosa, as well as the plasma cells[43] in colon tissue and in the epithelium of colonic tissue. **Both receptors are targets for inflammatory gut conditions, as these conditions often require pain management via activation of the CB1 receptor and a reduction in inflammation from activation of the CB2 receptor**[44].

Cannabinoids have shown to help with the pain, inflammation, and permeability in the gut that can lead to decreased symptoms in these gut conditions. Endocannabinoids levels fluctuate based on the current metabolic and inflammatory status and endocannabinoids and phytocannabinoids have an opposite effect in gut permeability. The endocannabinoids AEA and 2-AG seem to increase gut permeability, while THC and CBD reduce gut permeability[45], which indicates phytocannabinoids may be useful in "leaky gut" conditions[46].

Models of colitis research have found that levels of the endocannabinoid anandamide but not 2-AG were significantly increased[47]. Anandamide is also increased in colon biopsies from patients with ulcerative colitis. In mouse models, CB1 expression is upregulated and blockage of CB1 receptors worsens the condition. CB1 activation has also been shown to slow gut motility[48], prevent ulcer formation, and reduce inflammatory cytokines[49].

CB2 receptor expression is also increased in the intestinal tissue of patients with IBD[50], and especially during inflammatory[51] flares[52]. Interestingly, CB2 antagonists, or compounds that turn off the receptor, have decreased some inflammatory markers[53] and CB2 receptor agonists have shown to decrease inflammation caused by other sources[54].

Apart from the cannabinoid receptors, there was more than a three-fold increase in TRPV1-immunoreactive nerve fibers in IBS sufferers' biopsies compared to controls, which may contribute to the visceral pain sensitivity, another target for cannabinoid therapies[55].

CBD USAGE

There is evidence that CBD may be effective at managing symptoms of inflammatory gut conditions. Similar to the relationship with endometriosis and TRPV1 receptors, it is hypothesized that CBD's activity on TRPV1 receptors may help desensitize the receptor and help reduce GI inflammatory and pain symptoms. One study found that CBD use alone was not effective for Crohn's disease; the same group found that type 1 THC-dominant cannabis, however, provided clinical benefits[56]. Capsules with balanced ratios of THC/CBD have also shown to be effective.

CANNABIS AND FIBROMYALGIA

Fibromyalgia is poorly understood but is typically characterized by musculoskeletal pain, tiredness, and tenderness. It is thought to occur from **abnormal pain processing in the brain** and has high overlap with other CED conditions like migraines[57] and IBS[58]. Additionally, like most chronic pain conditions, there is also a relationship with depression and anxiety, and is more common in women than men.

Hyperalgesia, or the increased sensitivity to pain, is linked to dysfunction of the ECS, as the ECS plays a central role in pain processing in the brain[59]. Nabilone, a pharmaceutical equivalent of THC, showed significant improvements in fibromyalgia pain and sleep at as little as 1 mg dosed for four weeks[60]. In additional studies with inhaled and ingested cannabis products, patients with fibromyalgia showed improvements in mental health, pain, and quality of life[61].

One study that examined the types of cannabis that work for fibromyalgia evaluated type 1 cannabis (THC-dominant), type 2 (balanced THC:CBD), and type 3 (CBD-dominant) flower and placebo. The data suggested that CBD combined with THC may prevent some of the pain-relieving effects, and that inhaling CBD with THC increased the THC concentrations in the participant's body but reduced the pain-relieving effects of THC[62]. Commercially available supplements for the endocannabinoid Palmitoylethanolamide (PEA) have also been shown to reduce symptoms of fibromyalgia[63].

CANNABIS AND MIGRAINES

MIGRAINES

Migraines are characterized as complex conditions with genetic influences that come about as periods of severe head pain, often accompanied by nausea, light sensitivity, and sound sensitivity. They can last hours to days and are a serious neurovascular event[64].

Migraines are more common in women than men. There are many different types of migraines, some with aura (sensory signs that a migraine is approaching), without aura, abdominal migraine, ocular migraine, and others[65].

Triptans, anti-inflammatory drugs, opioids, antiemetics, and others have been used to treat migraines, as well as antidepressants, anticonvulsants, and beta-blockers used to try to prevent migraines. Triptans are drugs that act on the serotonin receptors and are the first-line treatment for migraines—they work by constricting blood vessels to relieve pain by reducing blood flow and pain markers. However, the effects of drugs on the vascular component of migraines can't be the only endpoint considered because the different phases of migraines can cause both vasoconstriction and vasodilation. For many patients, migraines are still treatment-resistant either because of the inability of the drugs to help with symptoms or because of the negative side effects from the drugs.

Migraines are linked to clinical endocannabinoid deficiency, or CED—an umbrella term for conditions that are thought to be caused by people having lower levels of endocannabinoids or low endocannabinoid tone. Cannabis and migraine drugs both act to lower plasma glutamate levels[66], and some endocannabinoids and phytocannabinoids have shown activity on various serotonin receptor subtypes.

DOSING FOR MIGRAINES

Surveys with medical cannabis patients found that most people prefer inhalable methods for migraine relief, which makes sense as rapid relief is required. Smoking was the primary method followed by vaping then dabs[67]. CB2 agonists like the terpene beta-caryophyllene are likely beneficial at reducing the inflammation associated with migraines and could help alleviate pain in that way[68]. One study found that low doses of cannabis helped alleviate migraines while higher doses could trigger them.

I have suffered from migraines for about 5 years and have found some migraines can be helped with cannabis and others can be worsened with cannabis. Effects may depend on the migraine type or other variables, like the cannabis product or the dose of the cannabis product.

Where cannabis helps the most (for me) is in reducing nausea associated with migraines, helping me feel less pain, and ensuring I am more easily distracted from the pain. In other cases when I've tried to use cannabis to help, it has gone from a bad migraine to a terrible migraine where I was more aware of the pain and felt as if my heartbeat was going to explode from my temple.

I have noticed to avoid strains with very uplifting effects and astringent smells and to **gravitate towards the rich, savory varieties.** My favorite is GMO, and now I make sure to grow GMO every year because it is my go-to for migraine relief. Smoking is the only method that I have found that works for my migraines, even dry herb vaping GMO does not do the trick.

While tension headaches, which form more of a band of pain around the head, are not the same as migraines–they are still applicable in this section.

CANNABIS AND SLEEP

INSOMNIA

About 30% of the population struggles with insomnia, which can lead to a variety of conditions such as diabetes, weight gain, high cortisol[69] levels, high blood pressure, heart disease, stroke, arthritis, and mental health issues[70]. Current treatments for insomnia include benzodiazepines, antidepressants, and antipsychotics, all of which have pretty intense and sometimes dangerous adverse effects like dizziness, brain fog, weight gain, and the potential for addiction[71].

The ECS plays a vital role in regulating the circadian rhythm, control of sleep[72], and memory consolidation[73] during sleep.

THC, CBN, AND SLEEP

It is important to find the right cannabis product because some cannabis products can be stimulating and will keep you up in bed thinking about what color to paint your cabinets and others will knock you out in minutes. Various clinical studies suggest that THC and CBN are the best compounds to help get to sleep and stay asleep.

THC and CBN act in similar ways as partial agonists on the CB1 receptor, meaning they can partially turn on the receptor. CBN is kind of like diet THC; it is about ¼ as strong on the CB1 receptor, so its effects are much weaker. Activation of the CB1 receptor is how our body initiates its sleep cycle–our body naturally produces endocannabinoids as this signal, and consumption of phytocannabinoids from the plant can also help send this sleep signal.

I've heard it said a few times that "THC helps you get to sleep and CBN helps you stay asleep," and the research does support both claims. THC reduces the time it takes to fall asleep, increases the total sleep time, and decreases the amount of time a person spends awake after initially falling asleep[74]. CBN is missing a significant amount of published data on sleep, but one study found that 20 mg of CBN was effective at reducing the number of times someone wakes during the night.

THC affects your short-term memory, likely because of the effects that THC has on REM (Rapid Eye Movement) sleep. During REM we process our memories from the day as well as consolidate memories[75]. Multiple studies have shown that THC decreases REM sleep, and it appears that THC may affect REM most for short-term cannabis users. In fact, some evidence suggests REM may even increase as someone develops a tolerance to THC[76].

Because sleep is thought to be partially facilitated through the CB1 receptor, CBD is not a promising candidate for a sleep medicine. In fact, for many CBD has shown to be stimulating, especially in high doses and in combination with THC and may even cancel out some of the sleep promoting effects of THC[77] and CBN. Other older studies have found that CBD may have a biphasic effect on sleep, causing stimulating effects at low doses and sedating effects at higher doses[78] (160 mg).

DOSING FOR SLEEP

CBN is not naturally being produced in the plant at high levels–it is mainly produced either in a lab or from THC naturally breaking down into CBN. If products are formulated as gummies, tinctures, or capsules, the CBN used to create them was likely synthesized in a lab. There are many labs that produce high quality CBN isolate that is great for manufacturing at scale or at home for personal needs. If you're purchasing a CBN product, make sure to check the COA for purity before consuming, or purchase from your local dispensary.

Naturally, people who smoke or vape at high temperatures are producing and inhaling CBN because it is being converted from THC during the heating process. This is why I recommend using high-temperature vaping for a nighttime routine. With smoking or high temperature vaping, not only are you getting more CBN produced as temperature increases, but you are also able to more readily evaporate the heavy terpenes, called the sesquiterpenes, which in general have more sedating effects, like beta-caryophyllene, humulene, nerolidol and bisabolol. Whereas the lighter monoterpenes are often known for their more uplifting effects and are less drowned out at lower vape temperatures. Other terpenes to look for in flower are the monoterpenes myrcene and linalool. Linalool is the terpene responsible for the sedating[79] and calming effects of lavender and has been shown to potentially counteract some of the memory impairing effects of THC[80].

For people who struggle with both getting to sleep and staying asleep, I usually recommend combining consumption methods for overlapping and diverse effects. Starting with a sedating type of flower, look for varieties with mainly THC and little to no CBD, and terpene profiles with myrcene, linalool, beta-caryophyllene, humulene, or bisabolol. These are going to be your Indicas, or sedating varieties.

When you smell the flower, you want it to hit the back of your nose–avoid weed that smells like it would be good at cleaning something. Try varieties that lean towards earthy, rich, spicy, clove, floral, autumn, rich scents. I have found that the purps (purple weed) or the darker cannabis in general are typically more sedating.

MANAGING THE HIGH

With inhaled cannabis the effects tend to be almost instantaneous, and will peak after about 10 minutes[81]. The effects are felt rapidly but also go away pretty quickly. This is why I recommend not only inhaling something THC-dominant before bed but also taking an edible or tincture to help you stay asleep with the long-lasting effects. The effects of edibles can last between 4 and 12 hours[82]–if you are a slow metabolizer this is something to consider because many people feel groggy or like they have a "weed hangover" if they consume cannabis too close to bed or at too high a dose. Smoking or vaping is not necessary; using a specially formulated product like a fast-acting sleep gummy may help in getting around the inhalation step for initiating sleep and may be able to get you to sleep and stay asleep.

If you're new to cannabis, start with as little as 2 mg of THC and each night increase by 1 to 2 mg until you find a good dose. If you struggle with waking up in the middle of the night, don't be afraid to combine

consumption methods for longer relief, like smoking right before bed, then taking an edible which will kick in right when the smoking effects wear off.

I know many patients who struggle with insomnia keep a vape on their bed stand and they keep it locked and loaded with flower or concentrate, depending on preference. This way, if they wake up during the night, they can hit the vape and try to get back to sleep as fast as possible.

Also note, if you are already on sleep medications like benzodiazepines, using cannabis can increase the sedative effects and increase the risk of a fall or other complications. It is best to talk to your physician before starting cannabis to ensure it is safe to taper off the other medications.

DREAMING AND NIGHTMARES

Cannabis is commonly used to treat symptoms of post-traumatic stress disorder (PTSD). PTSD is a condition that emerges for some people after exposure to trauma and results in intrusive symptoms of trauma re-experiencing like flashback and nightmares, numbing, avoidance, hyperarousal, and negative moods.

Both human and animal studies have confirmed the role of the endocannabinoid system in PTSD, with CB1 being a pivotal component of unlearning negative memories[83]. Additionally, brain imaging studies have found more CB1 receptors and fewer endocannabinoids in patients with chronic PTSD, providing evidence that the ECS is involved in the symptoms and pathology of PTSD[84].

People with a traumatic background don't necessarily dream of monkeys and unicorns when they fall asleep–it can be intense, scary, and debilitating to have to relive experiences through dreams. Because activation of the CB1 receptor can affect REM sleep cycles, cannabis consumers who consume before bed **typically don't experience dreams because of this disruption of REM sleep.** For people who suffer from PTSD, the lack of dreaming is one of the main medicinal benefits[85]. One study with Nabilone, which is synthetic THC, found that 34/47 patients with PTSD who took Nabilone before bed experienced total cessation or significant reduction of nightmares[86].

Cannabinoids can also play a critical role in balancing the stress-induced emotions common in people who experience PTSD[87].

TOLERANCE BREAKS AND SLEEP

If you are a heavy user of cannabis and decide to take a short break, called a tolerance break, to reset your body, there is a high likelihood that you will experience issues with your sleep—especially if you typically use cannabis before bed. One study reported that 76% of people who abruptly stopped using cannabis reported strange dreams, insomnia, and/or poor sleep quality[88].

When I took a tolerance break, the insomnia I experienced for the first few days was insane. I simply would not get tired. I was reading books, working, and watching TV literally all night long. Since then, I've learned a few tricks to help reduce the sleep issues. Tolerance breaks do not need to be abrupt—if you are a heavy cannabis user, you should use similar precautions to people weaning off other drugs like antidepressants or stimulants. If your body is used to smoking before bed, without smoking, your body won't have a signal to know when to initiate sleep. Replacing the signal with something else like a cup of tea, meditation, reading a book, playing a game, etc., can help. As your body readjusts, the worst period for sleep disturbance will be the first 3 nights, but effects can last up to 6 to 7 weeks[89].

MENOPAUSE AND SLEEP

Sleep issues are very common in women experiencing menopause, with over half of women surveyed around the world experiencing sleep disorders from night sweats to insomnia[90]. Women who use cannabis for menopause symptoms also report using it for a variety of other symptoms beyond sleep, like joint and muscle pain, anxiety, depression, irritability, and hot flashes[91].

Menopause symptoms are caused by fluctuations in estrogen and progesterone. Evidence suggests that estrogen levels may be affected by the ECS and vice versa, and that cannabinoids can help relax the blood vessels which can help alleviate hot flashes and night sweats[92].

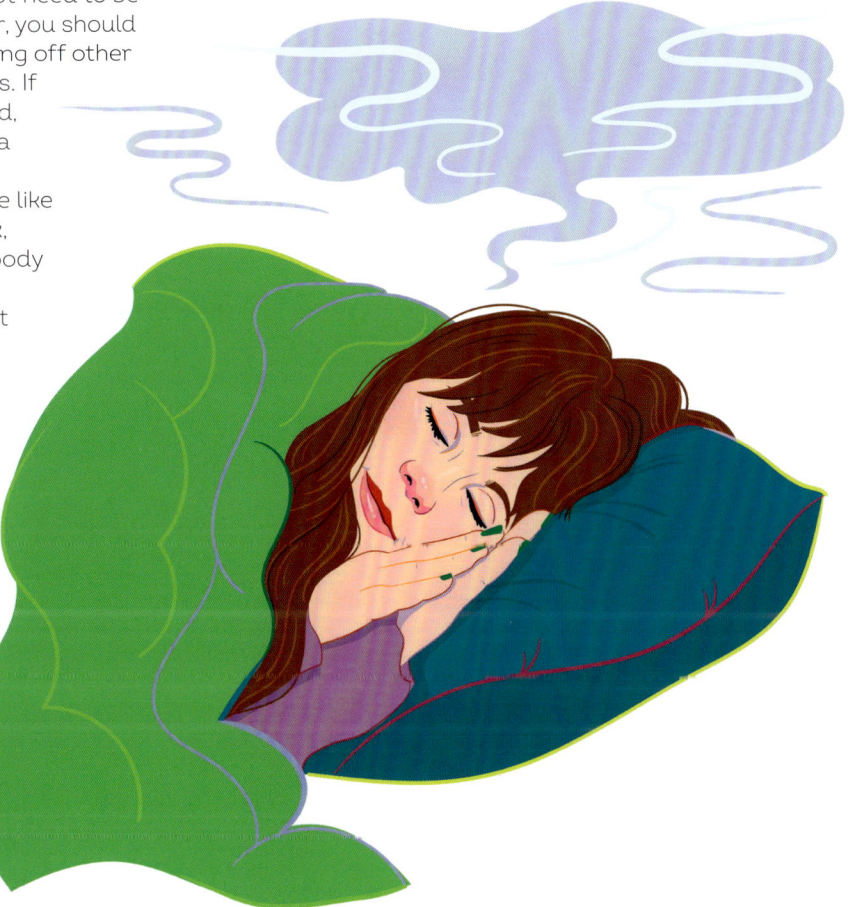

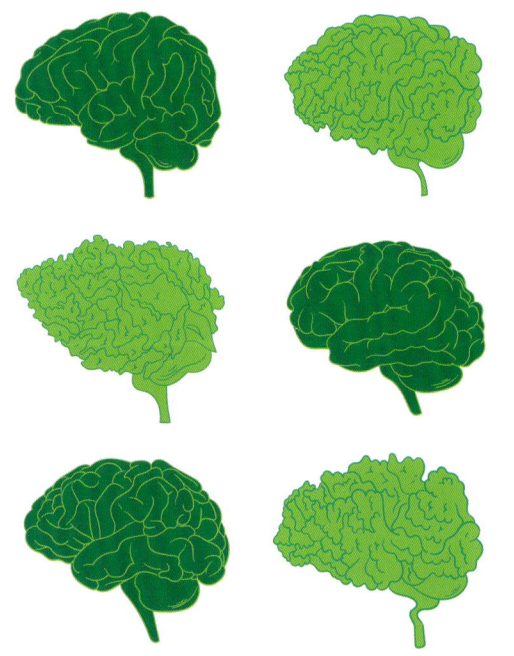

as 1 to 2 mg may be a good place to start. For high responders, even the microdose of THC present in hemp products, which legally needs to be below 0.3%, may be sufficient. Studies have shown that doses below what make you high are still effective at reducing anxiety[93].

Studies with pure CBD on anxiety show that doses of 200 mg were effective at reducing acute anxiety, but higher doses of 600 mg and lower doses of 150 mg were not effective[94]. These doses would likely be lowered when using full-spectrum-type CBD products that contain microdoses of THC and other active cannabinoids rather than extreme levels of pure compound.

Cannabis and depression is complex and multifaceted. While some people experience heightened mood and euphoric feelings regularly from cannabis, others have experienced worsening symptoms with chronic THC use and felt as if they were falling deeper down a depression hole[95]. I have seen cannabis as a helpful tool in helping people with the expression of emotions with friends or counselors; I hope in future years to see cannabis as an accommodation in some therapy settings.

Do not ignore the impact of set and setting while consuming cannabis. Your physical location, what's around you, the lighting in the room, the noise level, and who you're with all play a role in how you react to a substance. If you are an anxious person, take the time to cultivate your space so it reduces anxiety. Whether that is cleaning up dirty dishes or turning off the big light and putting on a lava lamp, make it comfortable.

If you're a flower lover, the terpenes to gravitate towards for reduced anxiety are linalool and bisabolol. Smelling lavender through linalool has shown to restore the expression of more than 500 stress-induced genes[96] which are involved in neurotransmitter transmission, brain peptides, and other hormones. Bisabolol acts on the GABAA receptor—likely at the same receptor subtype that mediates the effects of benzodiazepine drugs.

You can add dried lavender, which contains linalool, or chamomile, which contains bisabolol, directly in with your flower while dry herb vaping to increase these levels of terpenes—just make sure it's organic

NEURODIVERSITY

Neurodiversity is an umbrella term to describe a diversity of types of brains that diverge from societal standards. This encompasses an extremely large variety of brains including ADHD, autism, PTSD, dyslexia, synesthesia, schizophrenia, OCD, epilepsy, Alzheimer's, bipolar disorder, seizures, anxiety, eating disorders, and more.

Because many divergent brains are the result of different levels of neurotransmitters, trauma experiences, or genetic variabilities there is biochemical and societal evidence that cannabis is a powerful therapeutic for helping people regulate their brains. My favorite way to describe cannabis for neurodivergent people is as a "weighted blanket for the brain".

ANXIETY AND DEPRESSION
THC and CBD

THC has a well-known dose-dependent effect on anxiety. This biphasic response results in anxiety being relieved with THC at low doses, but high doses of THC can cause anxiety and/or make it worse. "Low doses" or "high doses" may be different for different people. If you are susceptible to anxiety, doses as low or grown yourself so there are no extra chemicals present and it's safe for consumption.

Other terpenes like α-phellandrene and pinene have also shown antidepressant activity[97]. Terpenes to potentially avoid if you suffer from anxiety are pinene and terpinolene, which are known to be uplifting and produce the most sativa-like effects.

AUTISM

Autism is usually characterized by hypersensitivity to a variety of stimuli, language and social barriers, and sometimes presents in other ways like aggression, anxiety, sleep disorders, and GI issues[98]. Many of these key indicators of autism are related to the functions of the endocannabinoid system in regulating emotional response, behavioral reactions, sleep cycles, seizures, and social interactions[99].

Clinical evidence suggests that the endocannabinoid system may be altered in autistic people—autistic children have lower levels of the circulating endocannabinoids anandamide (AEA), oleoylethanolamine (OEA), and palmitoylethanolmaine (PEA[100]). Interestingly, THC works like AEA in the body and, while OEA and PEA do not act on cannabinoid receptors, they may have similar activity in the body to CBD—suggesting that both CBD and THC may have therapeutic benefits for autistic people.

How can those with autism benefit from cannabis?

The goal with cannabis use isn't to "treat" autism; it is to make some of the environmental and mental stressors more manageable for autistic people. Miyabe Shields, my close friend and co-founder of our research nonprofit, is autistic and greatly benefits from cannabis. Miyabe says, "I didn't try CBD until I was 26 years old, even though by then I had been self-medicating with high-THC cannabis for mental health, chronic pain, and GI issues for over a decade. I didn't try CBG until I was 31. By experimenting with my own ratios (my go-to blend is 40/40/20 CBG/CBD/THC flower) and being more conscious about my dosage and dose schedule needs, I gained a more reproducible and intimate relationship with cannabis as my medicine. Understanding different ratios and different ways to use cannabis—like edibles versus inhaling flower or concentrates—enables cannabis to be personalized

to meet your individual needs which can be different day to day or even throughout a single day.

But by far the biggest shift in my perspective came from finding community. While research often focuses on children and pathologizes autism and other forms of neurodivergence, there is a significant population of neurodivergent adults who benefit from medical cannabis for **anxiety, sensory overstimulation, mood regulation, and memory processing and integration that is not well-represented in scientific and medical studies.** We often have complex and overlapping issues that challenge our ability to live a high quality of life, like migraines, PTSD, and irritable bowel syndrome, and cannabis is unique in its ability to help address so many different pieces of this quality-of-life puzzle. For this community, cannabis is truly a gift and is an alternative option where the existing medical system is limited and often falls short. While there will always be risks to everything in life, making informed and conscious decisions about medical cannabis has improved its therapeutic uses for me and has had a clear net benefit on my quality of life."

Dosing Considerations

A CBD product is usually recommended for a first time use for autistic children or adults, especially CBD products that contain small amounts of THC. The dose of CBD or ratio of THC:CBD can gradually be increased until a preferred effect and balance are met. If you can afford it, working with a cannabis nurse, pharmacist, physician, or naturopath for your child's medical needs is always recommended.

ADHD

Attention deficit hyperactivity disorder (ADHD) is a neurotype that is characterized by difficulty paying attention to certain tasks, impulsivity, and general hyperactivity. It is more common in children than adults and often has overlap with sleep issues and alterations in mood/anxiety[101]. The first-line therapy for ADHD is stimulant medications, but they can have adverse side effects like heart palpitations and addiction, especially with chronic use.

Many internet forums have noted cannabis relief for symptoms of ADHD, even working better than some medications. One clinical trial noted that a THC:CBD oral spray had no statistical benefit for ADHD[102]. From community stories and personal experience, I believe the story is much deeper than CBD or THC. For instance, CBG, which is the only known cannabinoid that activates the a2-adrenoceptor, may be another good option for people with ADHD as it acts similarly to other ADHD drugs in a stimulating way without the intoxicating feeling of THC-dominant products. Different types of cannabis produce different chemical profiles. Some are uplifting and others are sedating. Although the amount of THC can be relatively consistent from indica to sativa, the terpene profiles are vastly different. ADHD brains react very well to stimulants and compounds with uplifting effects. I and most other people I know with hyperactive brains prefer the uplifting, stimulating varieties much more than the sedating varieties.

My recommendation for someone with ADHD is to look for upper-type cannabis with terpene profiles that smell bright, citrusy, or astingent, with notes of Pinesol or other chemically/gassy notes. I gravitate toward varieties that tickle the front of my nose. This is going to correlate with terpenes like terpinolene, limonene, and pinene that will give the most uplifting effects. While it may not affect someone with ADHD in a stimulant way, it will still help their brain calm down and focus. However, if you're joining a sesh of someone with stimulating cannabis and you don't have an ADHD brain, you may experience anxiety or paranoia from the same strain that calms a hyperactive brain. Additionally, these "upper" varieties can often be consumed by people with ADHD brains right before bed with no stimulant effects but would keep another brain up for hours. My absolute favorite strain for cleaning the house, writing this book, or completing any other big task is Jack Herer–it keeps me locked in and focused and feels similar to Adderall on my brain.

PTSD AND TRAUMA

The ECS is altered when someone experiences trauma, and different alterations in the ECS are observed depending on whether someone experiences trauma as a child vs. as an adult. Childhood trauma results in decreased levels of endocannabinoids and cannabinoid receptors; whereas adult trauma results in decreased levels of endocannabinoids but increased cannabinoid receptors[103]. Disturbances in neuronal, hormonal, and inflammatory systems have been identified in PTSD and shown to be modified with administration of cannabis products.

Many patients report finding relief with medical cannabis for PTSD, not only for dream/nightmare suppression, but also for general relaxation, anxiety, and hyperarousal. Medical cannabis patients are reported to experience as much as a 75% decrease in symptoms of PTSD[104].

If you are using cannabis for PTSD, it is highly recommended to use balanced products with both THC and CBD. THC is great for avoiding nightmares and aiding with sleep, but at high doses can cause anxiety, which can result in an unfavorable headspace. Additionally, a 2013 study found that CBD helps with the extinction of fear memories, similar to THC, noting the impacts of these findings for people with PTSD and anxiety[105].

EPILEPSY

Medical cannabis gained attention for anti-seizure properties in 2013 when a story came out about a CBD-dominant variety of cannabis that helped a four-year-old girl stop her treatment-resistant seizures–her name was Charlotte and the strain was named **"Charlotte's Web"** after her.

Beyond this variety of hemp, CBD is used in clinical settings for rare and severe seizure disorders as the pharmaceutical drug Epidiolex, which is pure CBD. A main goal with anti-seizure medications is to control abnormal signaling or electrical activity in the brain. The things that are causing the electrical activity are typically excitatory neurotransmitters like glutamate. CBD is a great anticonvulsant drug because it acts as an antagonist on the GPR55 receptor which is located on these excitatory neurons that are hyperactive during seizures[106].

Additionally, CBD acts as a negative allosteric modulator on the CB1 receptor, which is the receptor that THC binds to. While small amounts of THC have shown to help with convulsions and prevent seizures, high levels are pro-convulsant and should be avoided[107]. Combining CBD with THC is highly recommended to protect the brain from overstimulation and seizure genesis. Lastly, the terpene beta-caryophyllene has displayed anticonvulsant activity in seizure models and may be a beneficial terpene to consider in inhalable formulations[108].

APPETITE

THE MUNCHIES

Pharmaceutical THC was originally approved to treat the weight loss associated with AIDS, also known as AIDS wasting syndrome. Many cannabis consumers know the appetite-stimulating effects of THC from personal experience, which we typically call the munchies. **The munchies** are caused by cannabis's influence on the hunger hormones in the body. For example, ghrelin is a hunger hormone that is produced in the gut. When the stomach is empty, ghrelin signals to the brain that you should go find food. THC triggers the release of ghrelin and causes more to be released, making you want to eat more.

Cannabis also affects a group of neurons in the brain called the POMC neurons, which help control hunger and appetite, by causing them to start producing endorphins that increase appetite further. Lastly, both when you eat sugary, fatty, delicious food and through secondhand mechanisms when you use THC products, there is increased dopamine released in the brain, making things taste extra good when you're high.

Despite the often-increased appetite with cannabis, from a population perspective chronic cannabis

users typically have a lower body mass index (BMI) compared to the general population.

The use of cannabis for anorexia or other eating disorders is very complex because food is very addicting. On one hand, one of THC's documented benefits is helping patients with anorexia eat, but on the other hand, getting the 'munchies' from THC products can also elicit binge eating behavior that may be difficult to control, especially if you're feeling high. Food tastes extra good when you're high, and it is easy to have regret and think obsessively after the fact.

If you are trying to avoid the munchies when you consume cannabis, there are some ways to help. In no way is this meant to be a diet tip, but more of a way to help with impulses if you do struggle with the munchies or binge eating. Cannabis varieties that have the molecule tetrahydrocannabivarin or THCV have shown to reduce appetite. This is because THCV essentially binds to the CB1 receptor in the opposite way that THC does. So, rather than 'turning on' the molecular switch for hunger in the body, THCV can help turn it off.

One of the most well-known THCV rich varieties is Durban Poison, and hemp varieties are now bred to produce high amounts of THCV that can be added into "salads" while smoking or vaping. Additionally, THCV tinctures, gummies or other products can be used in combination with other products to curb appetite or alone.

EATING DISORDERS

The ECS is known to regulate energy and food intake, which we can sometimes directly feel the effects of when we get the munchies after consuming. Because of this association between the ECS and food intake, it is thought that ECS dysfunction may be involved in what causes anorexia, bulimia, and other eating disorders. One study evaluated blood ECS biomarkers in women with and without eating disorders and found that were increased levels of anandamide and leptin (fat hormone involved in energy balance) in patients with anorexia and binge-eating disorder but not in women affected by bulimia nervosa—these findings suggest that

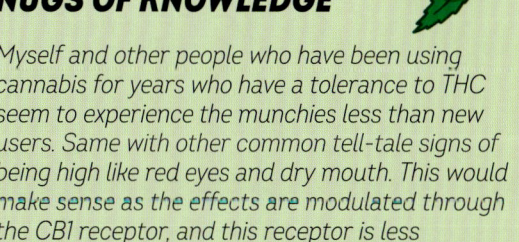

NUGS OF KNOWLEDGE

Myself and other people who have been using cannabis for years who have a tolerance to THC seem to experience the munchies less than new users. Same with other common tell-tale signs of being high like red eyes and dry mouth. This would make sense as the effects are modulated through the CB1 receptor, and this receptor is less abundant in heavier users of herb. Additionally, we have now gotten used to this state and it is essentially our new norm. I find that when I use cannabis similar to when I use psychedelics, I crave quality food like fruits and nuts and not filler foods like candy or chips.

decreased leptin could be related to increased levels of anandamide[109].

OBESITY

Obesity is also partially modulated by the endocannabinoid system, and a general positive association is seen between overproduction of endocannabinoids, or overexpression of cannabinoid receptors and obesity. The heightened levels of endocannabinoids are thought to be due to decreased activity of the FAAH enzymes responsible for metabolizing the endocannabinoids. Additionally, anandamide levels have been found to correlate with body mass index, waist circumference and fasting insulin levels[110].

The pharmaceutical industry tried to create a cannabinoid drug to treat obesity called Rimonabant under the premise that, if THC made you feel hungry, a drug that operated in the opposite manner would make you feel less hungry. The drug did work for hunger, but unfortunately was taken off the market because it also made people very suicidal. Luckily, THCV is a CB1 antagonist and does not act in the same way as Rimonabant, which is an inverse agonist rather than antagonist on this receptor.

Early evidence also showed that CBD reduced food consumption in rats, potentially due to CBD's antagonistic activity on the GPR55 receptor–which is associated with reductions in food intake and alterations in the GPR55 gene are linked to increased risk of anorexia[111].

AUTOIMMUNE DISEASES

The evidence that the ECS plays a vital role in immunomodulation by decreasing the activity of the immune system–which can be beneficial for a variety of autoimmune or chronic inflammatory conditions–is vast. Cannabinoids can decrease the production of antibodies and have a clear role in cell growth and death, as demonstrated by CBD and anandamide increasing T-cell cell death and THC and anandamide decreasing cell multiplying[112]. Other immune cells like macrophages also express cannabinoid receptors, and activation of the CB2 receptor can block the migration of immune patrol agents like monocytes[113].

Various cannabinoids and terpenes have anti-inflammatory action. Both THC and CBD prevent the release of IFN-gamma, IL-6, IL-1, and TNF-α which are pro-inflammatory compounds. Different autoimmune conditions have different pathways in the body, therefore may require different cannabinoid medicine targeted at various molecular pathways, or in some cases no cannabis at all.

Remember, before starting cannabinoid treatment for autoimmune conditions, check with your doctor because the activity of THC on the immune system as well as other CB2 agonists can decrease resistance to pathogens and infectious agents, similar to the side effects of other immunosuppressive drugs for autoimmune diseases[114].

RHEUMATOID ARTHRITIS

Rheumatoid arthritis is an autoimmune condition characterized by inflammation of the joints. The inflammatory markers best associated with rheumatoid arthritis are increases in the inflammatory cytokines TNF-α, IL-1, and IL-6, as well as increases in IL-10 which is an anti-inflammatory compound. The cannabinoids THC, CBD, and CBG all reduce levels of TNF-α and CBD reduces IL-6. The terpenes D-limonene, α-phellandrene, terpinolene, borneol and linalool have all been shown to lower the expression of these pro-inflammatory cytokines[115].

MULTIPLE SCLEROSIS

Multiple sclerosis (MS) is an autoimmune condition where the immune system attacks the myelin sheath of nerve fibers resulting in damage to the central nervous system. THC and other compounds that act on the CB2 receptor have shown promise as a therapeutic treatment. The CB1 receptors are highly involved in chemical release in the brain, and medical cannabis helps patients with MS-associated spasticity[116]. Synthetic THC has been approved to treat some symptoms of MS, such as muscle stiffness and neuropathic pain.

This allows patients the ability to regain control of hand movements and gain more autonomy over their life. Beyond regulating neurotransmitter release, the pro-inflammatory cytokine IFN-y is known to be a driver of MS, suggesting THC may have beneficial effects as an anti-inflammatory and immunomodulatory compound as well[117].

The role of the ECS in MS has been demonstrated in studies that show that clinical remission of MS is seen in mice with lower FAAH levels[118]–and mice without CB2 receptors have worse clinical scores than controls.

NEURODEGENERATIVE DISEASES

The ECS has neuroprotective properties against neurodegenerative diseases and acts to prevent the damage from acute sources of toxicity, help regulate neurotransmitter release, reduce neuroinflammation[119], regulate dysfunctioning mitochondria, reduce oxidative stress, and reduce toxic excitability and protein misfolding. CB1 agonism is associated with neuroprotective effects and cannabis can improve quality of life by targeting a variety of symptoms associated with neurodegenerative diseases—such as agitation, aggression, lack of emotion, sleep issues, and GI symptoms.

Dosing is important with sensitive populations who may already have issues with memory. Low doses of THC have been shown to be effective in reversing age-related cognitive issues[120]. This dose is easily achieved in full spectrum hemp products that contain around the legal limit of 0.3% THC but would not be present in a CBD isolate product. High doses of THC may result in additional confusion and should be avoided or worked towards slowly.

PARKINSON'S DISEASE

Parkinson's disease (PD) is a neurodegenerative disease mainly affecting mobility due to the loss of dopamine-producing neurons. The ECS has been studied as having a protective role in PD[121]. The terpene beta-caryophyllene may have neuroprotective effects—as shown in mice models of PD[122] where beta-caryophyllene was able to improve motor function, protect the dopamine producing neurons, and reduce inflammation in the brain.

If you want to read up on some research papers but don't know where to start, or you have a medical condition and want to know if there is any research on the ECS or cannabis head to the website https://pubmed.ncbi.nlm.nih.gov/. In the search bar, type in your condition AND cannabis or endocannabinoid system—for example, if I had fibromyalgia I would type "fibromyalgia AND the endocannabinoid system." Look for the top cited papers or papers that were published within the past few years. The full papers can be a bit intense, but a good place to start is the abstract and the discussion sections.

If the paper is behind a paywall and costs money to read, I would recommend contacting the email of the author who is listed LAST on the publication (the email will be provided in the paper). Let them know that you are a medical patient and would like access to the manuscript and 99/100 times, they will send you the pdf with no further questions!

CONCLUSION

This chapter outlines some of the main therapeutic uses of cannabis and cannabinoids for a variety of medical conditions. This is not a comprehensive list of conditions that have pathologies overlapping with the endocannabinoid system. After all, the endocannabinoid system is the master regulator in the body and responsible for maintaining balance or homeostasis. If portions of the ECS are disturbed, cannabis can help supplement this system and bring regulation or balance. In states like New Hampshire, patients no longer need to meet a strict list of qualifying conditions to obtain a medical cannabis card. Physicians now have the flexibility to assess patients on an individual basis, recognizing the wide range of therapeutic benefits cannabis can offer. This shift reflects the growing understanding of cannabis' broad medical potential, allowing doctors to tailor treatments based on their patients' unique needs rather than being confined by a predefined list of conditions.

Although the laboratory studies cited in this section are important in understanding the pieces of the puzzle when it comes to cannabis medicine, it is important to understand the limitations of research. Most of these studies are utilizing isolated compounds on a specific target or receptor in the body. The human picture is more complicated than a laboratory model. Not only are we often ingesting whole plant medicine, but we metabolize chemicals and turn them into new chemistry; we eat foods that are bioactive and could interfere with drugs, many of us are on pharmaceutical medicines that could interact with cannabinoid medicine; and ultimately our bodies, like nature, operate as cohesive signaling networks rather than as isolated systems. Each paper published is a snapshot of what is happening in the body, but is often manipulated by a variety of other factors. Documenting human experience paired with scientific studies can help us gather a more nuanced look into the practical uses of complex natural products.

Regardless of the condition, if you are trying a new product, strain, consumption method, etc, it is important to take it low and slow. Although the benefits of cannabis are expansive, there are absolutely some cases in which cannabis should be avoided, or cannabis could worsen the symptoms. Some examples of this are with some mental health conditions like schizophrenia, anxiety, or specific types of migraines.

Cannabis is absolutely not right for everyone. If you consume cannabis with other people, you will quickly see how diverse the reactions of different brains are to cannabis. With 6 people standing in a circle, sharing a joint, they will have 6 unique experiences. You cannot make assumptions on expected experience based on physical factors like someone's height and weight as we often do with other substances like alcohol. I'm a 5'2", 120 lb woman who can smoke more than most large men that I've met. Our reactions are based on a variety of factors including our tolerance, genetics, hydration level, and so on. If you find yourself no longer benefiting from cannabis, it may be your body's way of telling you to lay off it for a while or to change your routine.

At the end of the day there are many consumers who don't fit into any of the buckets listed above. Many people consume cannabis for general enhancement of their quality of life, using cannabis as a wellness tool to enhance their likelihood of exercising, socializing, eating healthy, going outside, and so on. Many people use cannabis to feel more like themselves or feel comfortable in their own skin, be able to express themselves sexually, or to relax after a long day. These are not topics often studied in the peer review or prioritized in modern medicine, but for many, cannabis can be the difference between just living and having a life.

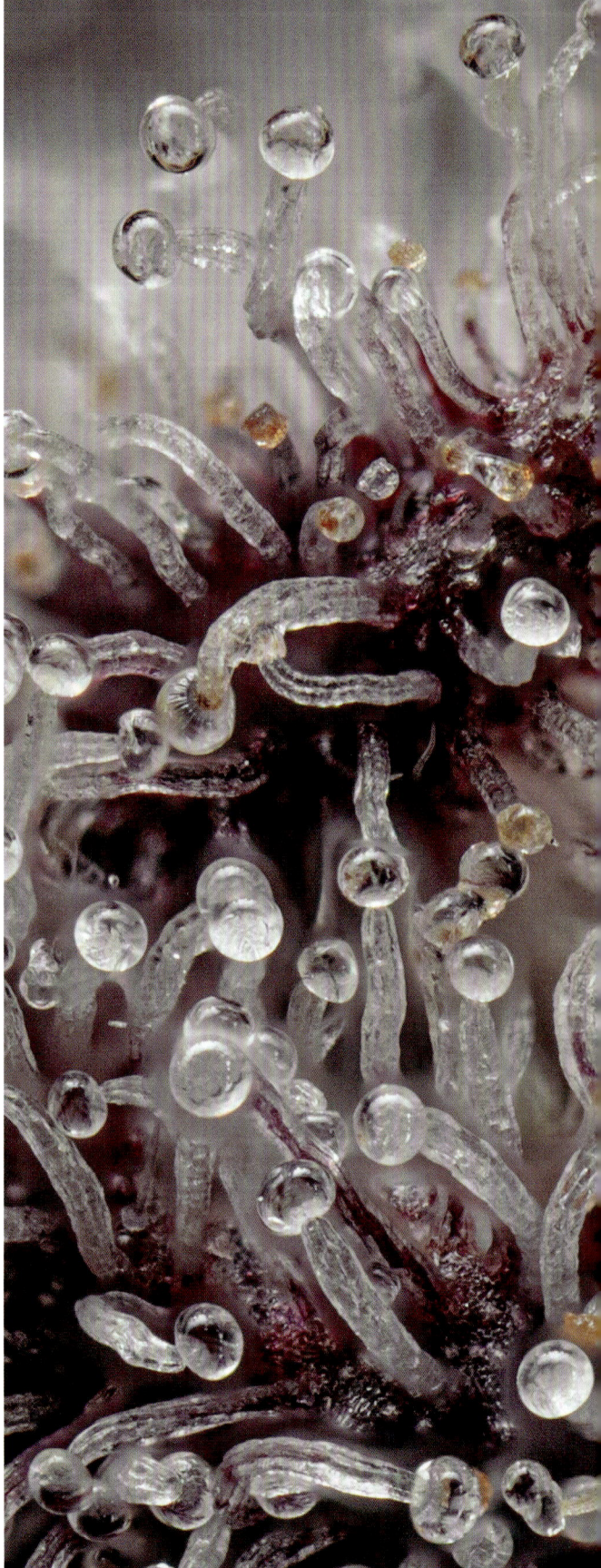

SMOKE BREAK!

LET'S RECAP WHAT WE'VE LEARNED:

⇥ Cannabis is highly personalized medicine due to its interaction with the endocannabinoid system (ECS), which helps maintain balance in the body. It offers therapeutic benefits for numerous conditions, including inflammation, stress, and chronic pain, by regulating neurotransmitters and reducing inflammatory signals.

⇥ Clinical Endocannabinoid Deficiency (CED) is a proposed theory by Dr. Ethan Russo, suggesting conditions like fibromyalgia, migraines, and IBS may arise from insufficient endocannabinoid production, leading to treatment-resistant inflammation and chronic pain.

⇥ Cannabis as an alternative to opioids has shown promise in managing chronic pain, reducing opioid dependence, and even preventing withdrawal. It has fewer side effects than opioids, and states with legal cannabis report fewer opioid-related deaths.

⇥ Cannabis and cancer care involves both prevention and symptom management, with cannabinoids showing anticancer potential. It is used to alleviate chemotherapy side effects, such as pain, nausea, and appetite loss, and studies suggest it may prevent the growth of certain cancer cells.

⇥ Cannabis for sleep and neurological conditions highlights the use of cannabinoids like THC and CBN to aid sleep, reduce nightmares, and help manage neurodivergent conditions like ADHD, autism, and PTSD. Low doses are generally more effective for promoting relaxation and reducing anxiety.

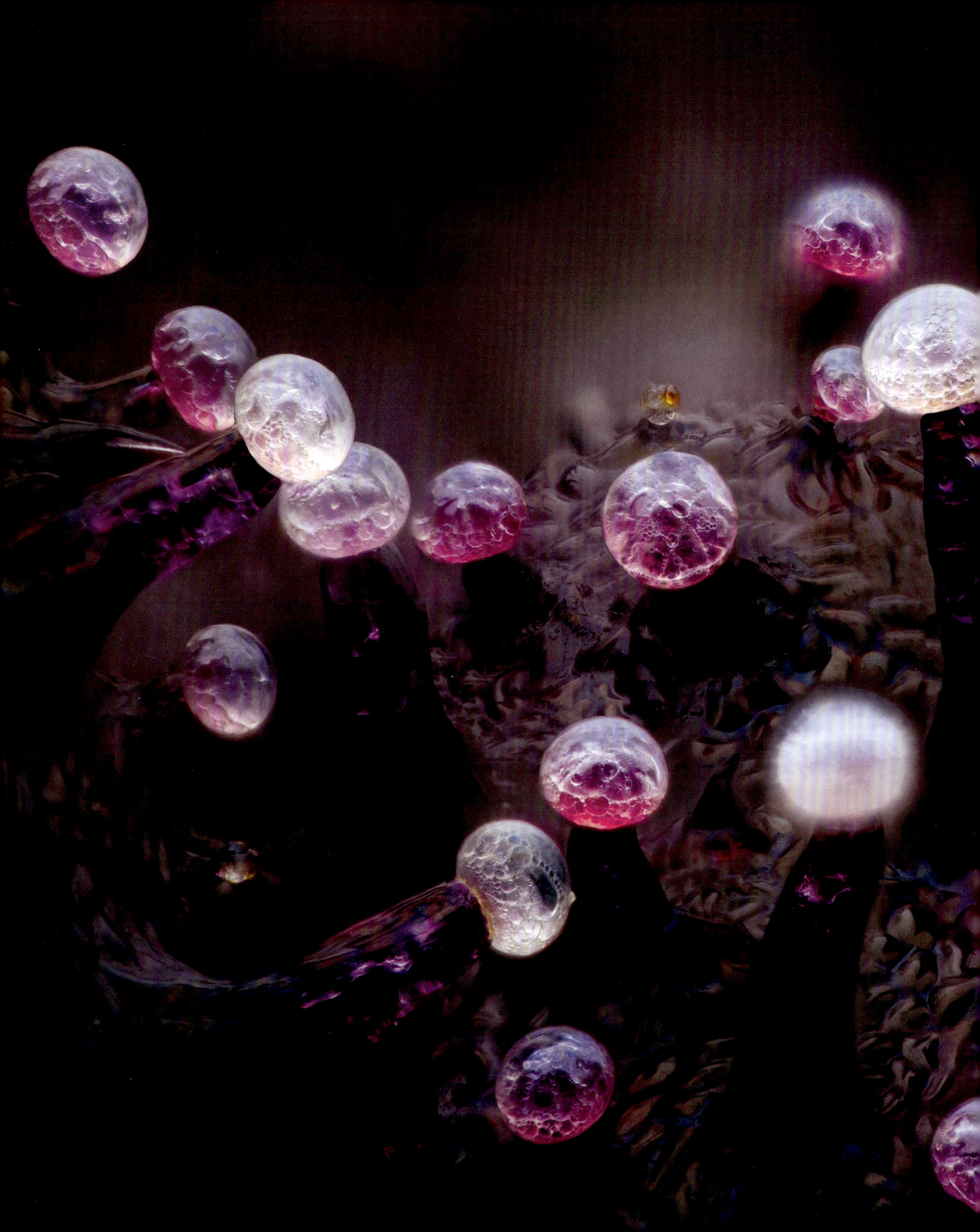

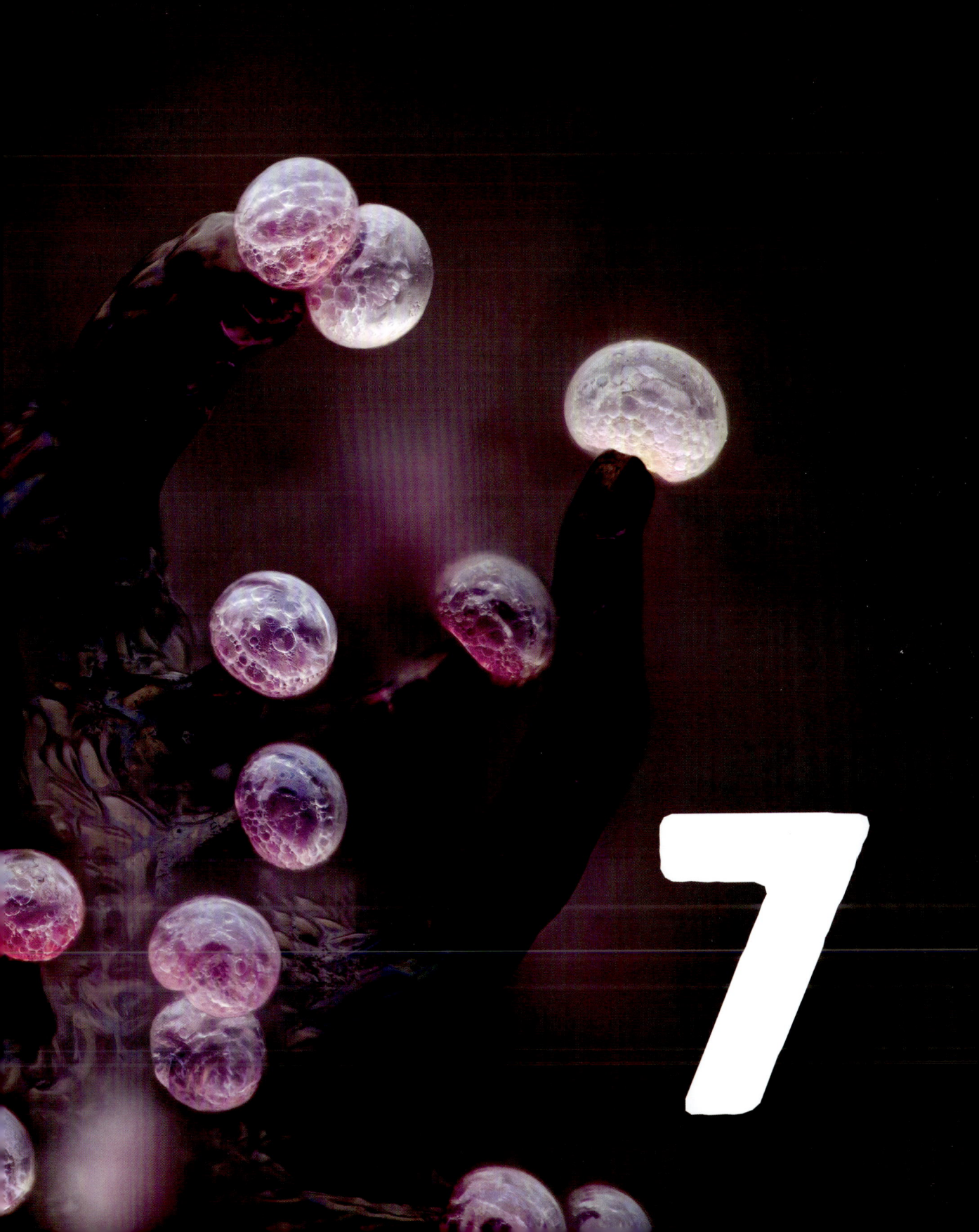

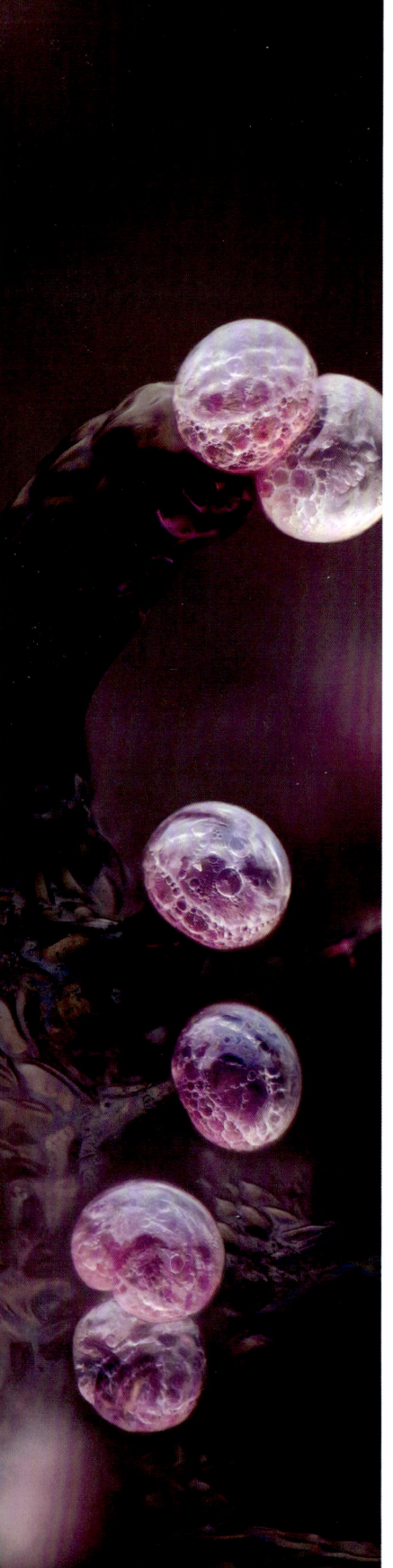

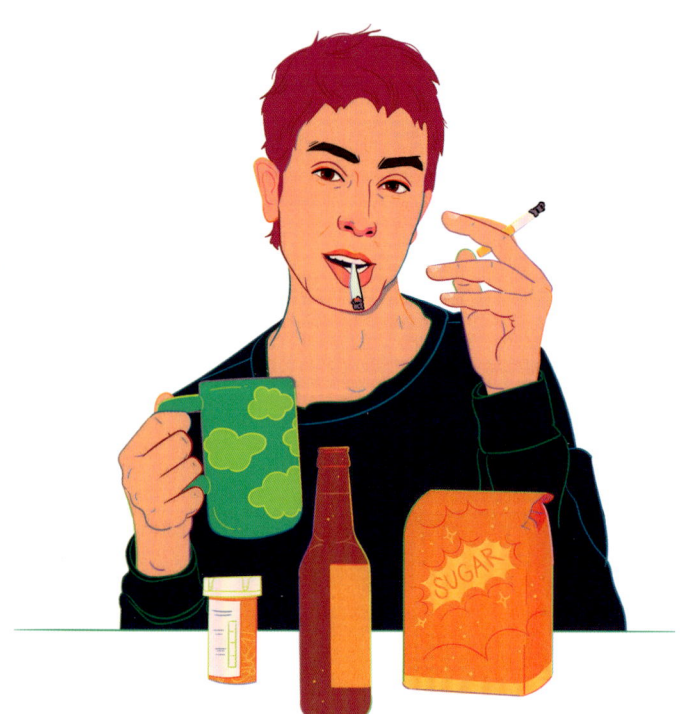

TOLERANCE

Imagine this: with every cup of coffee, cigarette, or edible you consume, your body is silently recalibrating, adjusting to the effects of caffeine, nicotine, or THC. If you consume any bioactive substance, your body will begin to build a tolerance to it. The more you indulge, the more your system becomes accustomed, reshaping itself to handle these substances with increasing efficiency—meaning as you build tolerance, it will require more and more to feel the same effects.

WHAT THC TOLERANCE LOOKS LIKE

Tolerance is happening at the receptor-level in the body. When the body is operating without any sort of drug involved, the different parts of the body are communicating by sending signaling molecules that travel and activate receptors to the brain. For instance, with cannabis the endocannabinoid system (ECS) sends signals in the form of endocannabinoids AEA or 2-AG to the cannabinoid 1 (CB1) receptor, which then control neurotransmitter release and other functions in the body. Typically, when the CB1 receptor is activated, the body sends very deliberate signals at relatively low concentrations. However, when we start using cannabis, THC and other compounds activate the CB1 receptors in a global manner across the brain in doses that are higher than what our bodies would typically be making.

The body begins to compensate for this frequent high-level activation and starts to remove some receptors—if the receptors are constantly being activated, the body doesn't need to produce or expend so much energy into a great number of receptors. The two main ways that the body compensates is through:

1. Receptor desensitization: Under receptor desensitization, your receptors are less sensitive to activation. Normally, after a compound like THC binds to a receptor, it causes a series of downstream effects. With receptor desensitization, it's more difficult to initiate the response, and it often is dose dependent.

2. Receptor downregulation: Receptor downregulation is where some receptors are internalized into the cells that are expressing them. This means the receptors are essentially gobbled up by the cell, and are therefore unavailable for activation on the outside of the cell.

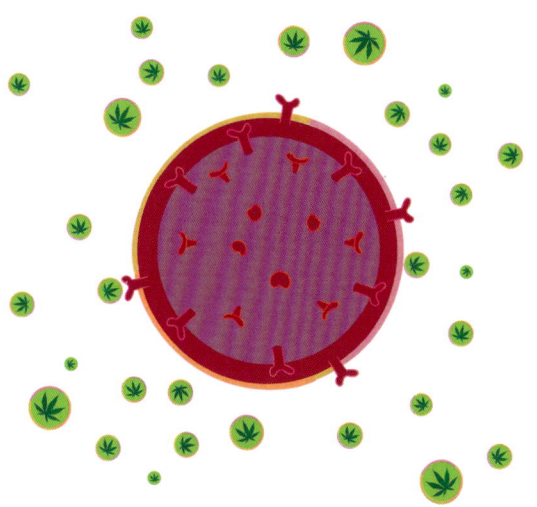

THE IMPACT OF REDUCED CB1 RECEPTORS

CB1 receptors are crucial for a wide range of bodily processes, including appetite, mood, anxiety, and pain thresholds. Developing a tolerance and reducing CB1 receptor levels can have varied effects, potentially being positive, neutral, or negative depending on the individual's **endocannabinoid tone** or the level of receptors, endocannabinoids, and enzymes.

There is evidence that many chronic conditions are related to elevated CB1 receptor levels, and **developing a tolerance may benefit some people**. For instance, PTSD: one study[1] found that people with PTSD had a higher amount of CB1 receptors in the brain in the regions associated with fear and anxiety compared to people without PTSD, and PTSD sufferers had lower levels of the endocannabinoid anandamide. These data suggest that the symptoms of PTSD may be due to an imbalance in the ECS, and providing the body with supplemental cannabinoids from the plant while also developing some tolerance to reduce levels of CB1 receptors may be part of the reason so many PTSD patients react positively to cannabis.

CB1 receptor expression levels are linked to pain reduction, especially in cases of hypersensitivity. Lower CB1 receptor levels are associated with decreased appetite and can offer benefits for autistic or neurodivergent individuals, where chronic consumption may lead to improved social interactions, reduced irritability, and enhanced sensory sensitivity.

THE CONS OF TOLERANCE

Building a tolerance to THC can negatively impact health and well-being. Beyond the financial strain of consuming large amounts of cannabis, a high tolerance can sometimes diminish the therapeutic potential of the medicine. Maintaining a lower tolerance allows the body to respond more effectively to smaller doses of active compounds like THC and CBD without altering receptor dynamics. For medical patients who rely on THC's effects through CB1 receptor activation, excessive tolerance can reduce the plant's overall efficacy.

From my personal experience as a daily consumer of cannabis, I manage my tolerance by figuring out the amount of cannabis that works best for me. For example, I will often use my dry herb vape many times throughout the day, but I'm typically only adding in 100 to 250 mg of flower, in comparison to a full joint which is about 1,000 mg (1g). This will fluctuate based on how I'm feeling and if I'm in social situations or by myself, but in general I try to either consume small amounts or mix in some CBG or CBD flower to balance out the cannabinoid profile.

With a high tolerance, it takes more and more cannabis to feel the effects, so you may have to smoke two joints, or take huge dabs to feel the same way your friend does after a couple of puffs of a joint. With a high tolerance you may also find that you're feeling more and more dependent on cannabis and feel the urge to smoke more often. This can easily lead to a negative relationship with cannabis over time.

WHEN YOU CONSUME

The majority of medical patients consume first thing in the morning, and there is a biologically validating reason for this. Endocannabinoid levels change throughout the day. Levels of anandamide are highest earlier in the day, and 2-AG peaks around midday and is lowest in the early morning and late evening. Because 2-AG is similar to THC but not very abundant in the morning, there is less competition at the receptor level when you consume cannabis in the morning and therefore the effects hit harder and are more pronounced.

Consuming first thing in the morning, aka **the wake n' bake**, can hit HARD and cause you to feel more high and more euphoric than normal. Not to mention, you have no other substances in your body at this time, and the cannabinoid receptors have not been activated for a few hours while sleeping so the receptors are primed and ready for activation.

A majority of cannabis users prefer to medicate at night, seeking relief for sleep issues, anxiety, pain, or simply to unwind after a stressful day. However, a drawback of regular cannabis use is its impact on short-term memory, which can be particularly problematic for students preparing for exams or individuals in memory-intensive jobs. THC affects REM sleep, a critical phase for memory consolidation and dreaming. Disturbances in REM sleep can alter our ability to recall memories. Fortunately, evidence suggests that as we develop tolerance to THC, its effect on memory diminishes and REM begins to return to normal.

To prevent the memory-impairing effects of cannabis, I have found it helpful to avoid consuming right before bed. This is not for everyone—as we know in cases with trauma, avoiding dreaming is the goal of medication before bed. However, for others, consuming even an hour or two before bed rather than directly before can provide your body the ability to get more REM sleep and promote memory consolidation. Additionally, cannabinoids like cannabichromene (CBC) and terpenes like pinene and linalool have been shown to counteract the

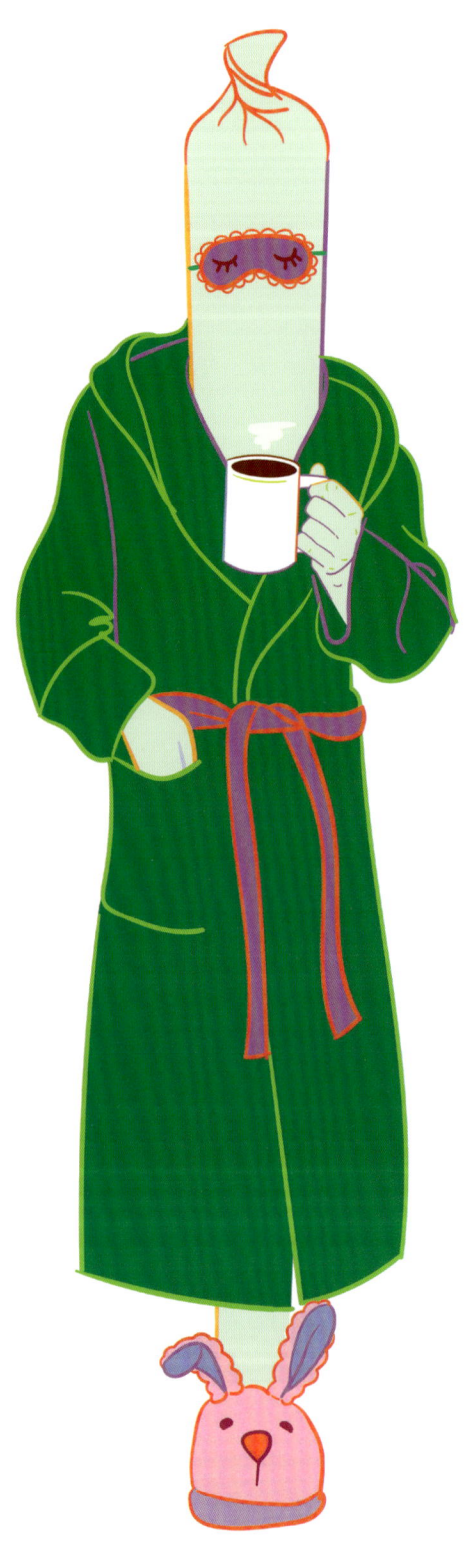

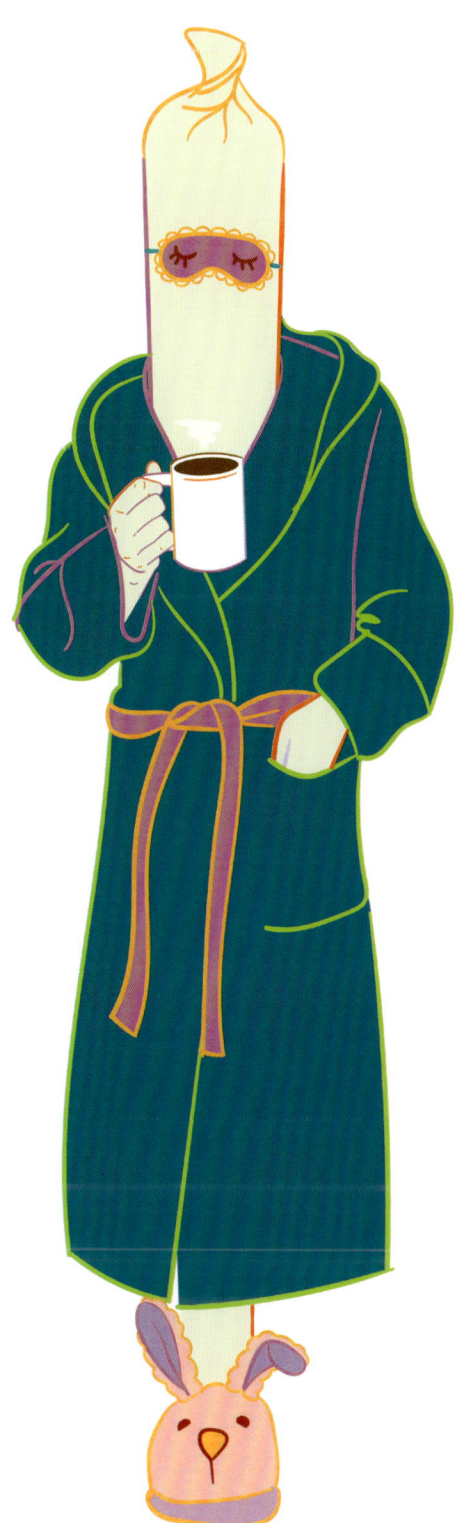

memory impairing effects of cannabis and should be considered for nighttime formulations. Think of strains like Skywalker OG and G13 for nighttime or Jack Herer and Amnesia Haze for daytime memory help.

TOLERANCE BREAKS

A tolerance break is taking a break from cannabis until you feel that your tolerance has been reset. Tolerance breaks can also help you maintain a positive relationship with the plant, lower the threshold to achieve the medicinal value of the cannabinoids, save you money, prevent dependence, and more. However, **tolerance breaks are not for everyone,** and there are ways to take tolerance breaks that don't result in a cold turkey stop for weeks at a time. For those using cannabis for therapeutic purposes, **regularly changing consumption methods or strains can help maintain a lower tolerance while still achieving effective relief.**

With any new substance, supplement, food group, or drug that is regularly used, the best way to start and stop using a substance is the tapering method. The tapering method simply involves a gentle increase or decrease in use until you reach a steady state.

Even if you're not addicted to something, your body will struggle if you suddenly remove a substance it's accustomed to. In the case of cannabis, if you are a daily consumer and consume multiple times a day, the tapering method might involve: (i) halving the amount that you consume for a few days, (ii) then only consuming twice a day, (iii) then only consuming once a day for a period, and (iv) then potentially moving towards consuming zero times a day.

Reducing tolerance is not an all-or-nothing game. If you have a very high tolerance, consuming less THC in general is going to help, but it doesn't need to be cold turkey. A tolerance break could also constitute replacing THC cannabis for CBD-dominant cannabis. This way you are still microdosing THC, getting the medicinal benefits of CBD, and supplementing your endocannabinoid system.

Switching consumption methods is another great way to do a modified tolerance break. If you are someone who regularly takes dabs that are high in THC, switch to vaping flower or smoking, or a method that involves nothing going into the lungs like edibles at low levels. This way the tolerance break can double as a smoke break to give your lung tissue some time to breathe–pun intended. I typically take smoke breaks when I come back from celebrations, conferences, or events where I'm smoking more than usual.

As you taper off of THC, it is good to add in other things into your routine that can supplement your ECS naturally, such as exercise. Exercise is one of the best ways to stimulate your ECS and is also a great way to keep your brain busy. Runner's high is the euphoric feeling you get after exercising. It was originally thought that runner's high was due to your body releasing naturally occurring opioids called endorphin's (endogenous morphines), but it was later discovered this is due to endocannabinoid release.

How to know if you need a tolerance break

There are a variety of ways your body or brain may be telling you to take a tolerance break. If you are tired of feeling like you want to consume all the time or are feeling like you don't really feel any effects anymore and are just consuming out of habit, then it may be a good time for a tolerance break.

Make sure you take the time to listen to your body and take the signals seriously when your body is telling you to change your routines, diet, or even relationships. One of the top reasons why people stop using cannabis, especially after years of use, is because cannabis suddenly makes them feel incredibly anxious, paranoid, or overwhelmed.

Although we don't have the exact scientific reason as to why that's happening, I believe it's the body's way of saying that it doesn't need THC anymore. The hormones and signaling molecules in the body fluctuate as we age, and as we are growing and maturing, our bodies are going through a lot of change. As we age and become more stable, I believe for many people there is less of a need to supplement the ECS with high levels of THC, but more of a need to supplement with the anti-inflammatory help of CBD.

SIDE EFFECTS

Despite it being very stressful to the brain, some people still prefer to do the cold turkey method of tolerance breaks because it is easier for them to follow through, and I fully respect that. If this is the case, you should be aware of some very common effects from suddenly abstaining from cannabis.

First, sleep is the most reported difficulty during a tolerance break. And I can attest to this: during my only full tolerance break in the past decade during a trip to France I ended up reading six books over a week while the rest of the world slept because my body simply would not get tired. Many people use cannabis right before bed to initiate sleep. As such, using cannabis is essentially acting as the signal that flushes through the body to tell the brain to start getting tired. When they suddenly take that signal away during a tolerance break, they don't feel sleepy and do not get any rest the first few days of a tolerance break.

If you are taking it slow and tapering into a tolerance break, one of the first things I would recommend right as you're starting is to stop consuming right before bed. Rather, start consuming a nighttime tea, or initiate a different new signal like reading a book to start to train your body away from THC as the sleep signal.

How long to take a tolerance break

Tolerance breaks can be as short or as long as you like, and research indicates that a tolerance break can be effective even for just a couple of days[2]. In general, two to four weeks of lowered use or abstinence is the most common amount of time for a tolerance break. However, because everyone has different endocannabinoid tone, medical needs, and hormonal fluctuations, I encourage you to listen to your body and journal your experience to gauge the time you need and understand the effects you're experiencing.

When and if you decide to start consuming cannabis again after your tolerance break, I highly recommend taking it slow to keep your low tolerance as long as possible and not go immediately back to where your brain was at pre-break. When I'm trying to maintain a low tolerance, I love to use my small one-hitter (vape or smoke device), which only holds a small pinch of flower and is a great way to dose low and slow throughout the day.

REGULATING OURSELVES

As cannabis consumers we have a great power with autonomy over our bodies and medicine. We most often don't have a physician or pharmacist telling us exactly what dose to take at what time of the day. Rather, we have a deep connection with our medicine that allows us to feel our bodies at a deeper level and explore our minds to new degrees.

With this power comes a lot of responsibility and honesty. Tolerance breaks are a great way to reflect on your relationship with the plant and make sure that you are still benefiting from it in the ways you intended, or determine if you need to start shifting your consumption patterns and intentions. It can be difficult, especially if you are in a group of friends who are heavy consumers, but if your relationship with cannabis is rocky, it is often a reflection of other issues that may also benefit from some unclouded attention.

Developing a tolerance or a dependence on cannabis is not shameful and does not need to be a negative thing unless it is causing negativity in your life. I recently received a message on social media from a woman who said that she was using cannabis for her GI issues and mental health issues and feels she can't live without it. It made her life significantly better; she was able to afford it, use cannabis safely, and it was benefitting her life. She felt ashamed for no reason. It's a positive thing that she has found a medicine that works for her needs, and despite it coming in a mylar bag rather than an orange pill bottle, it is still valuable medicine.

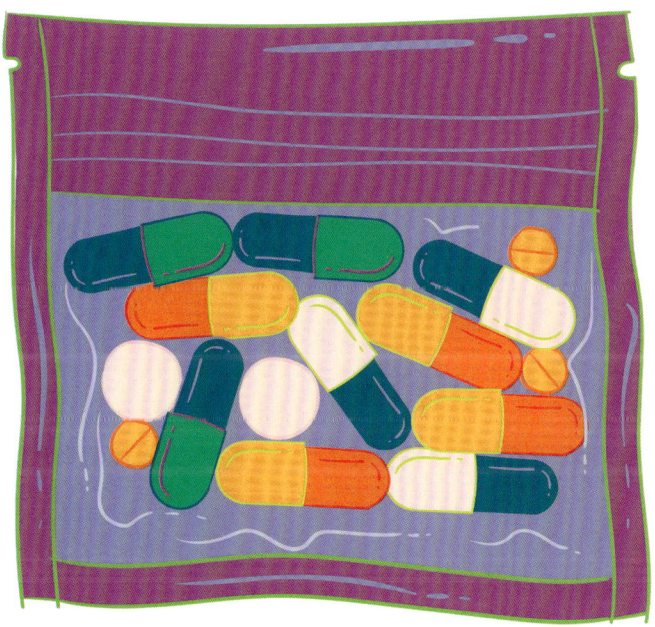

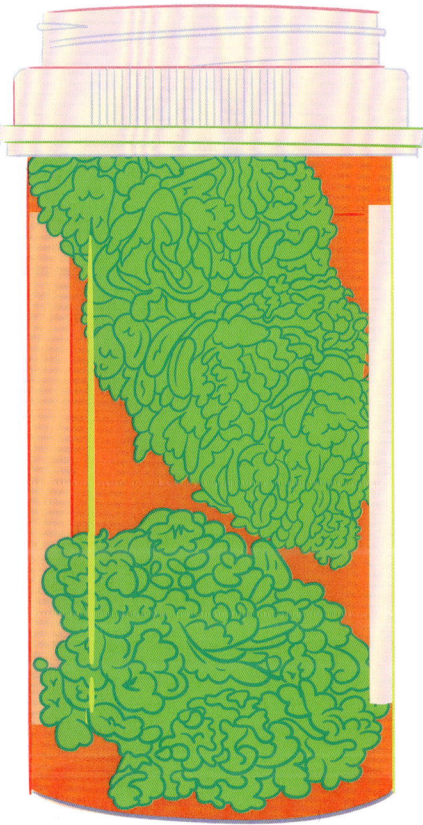

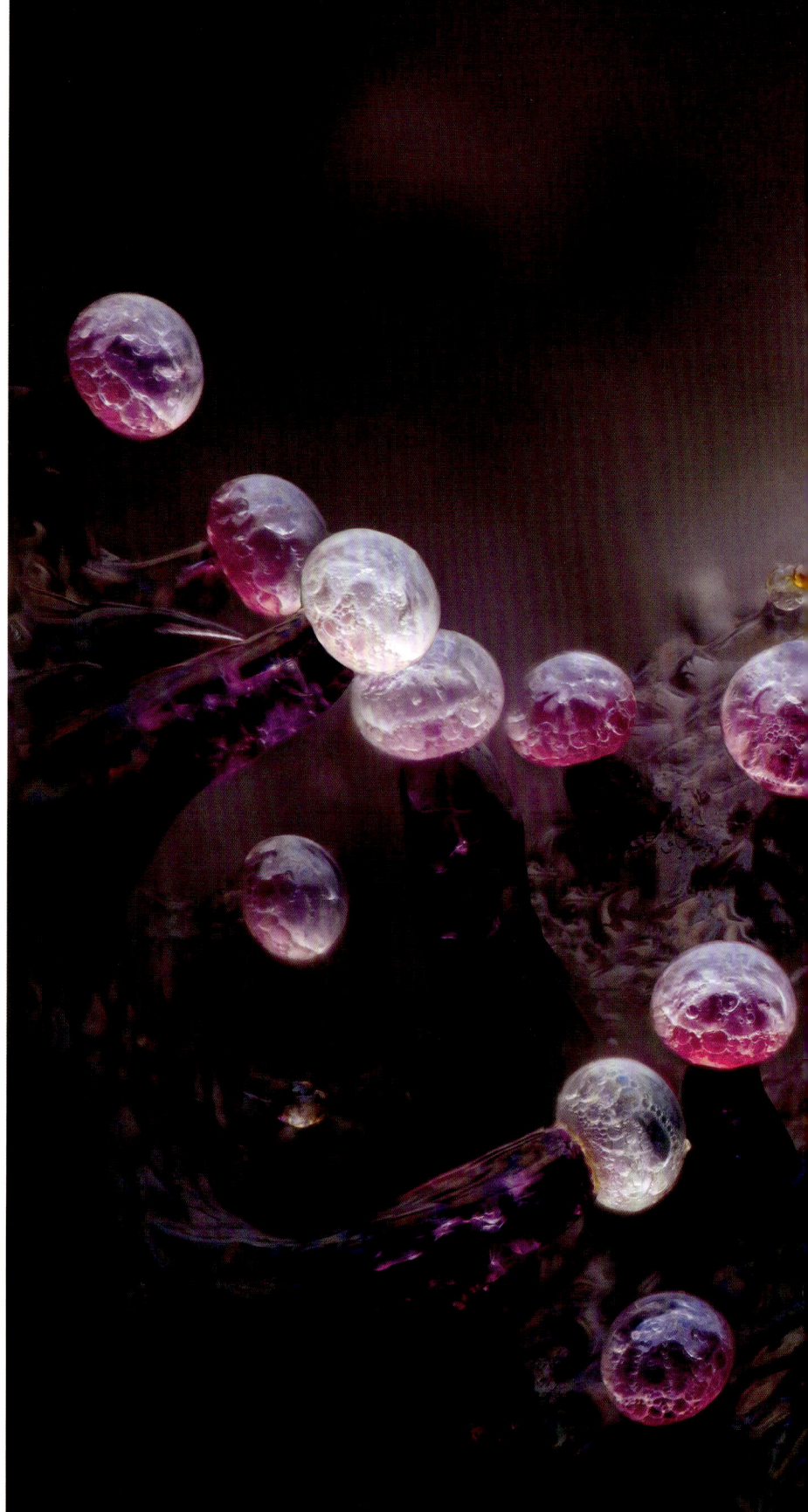

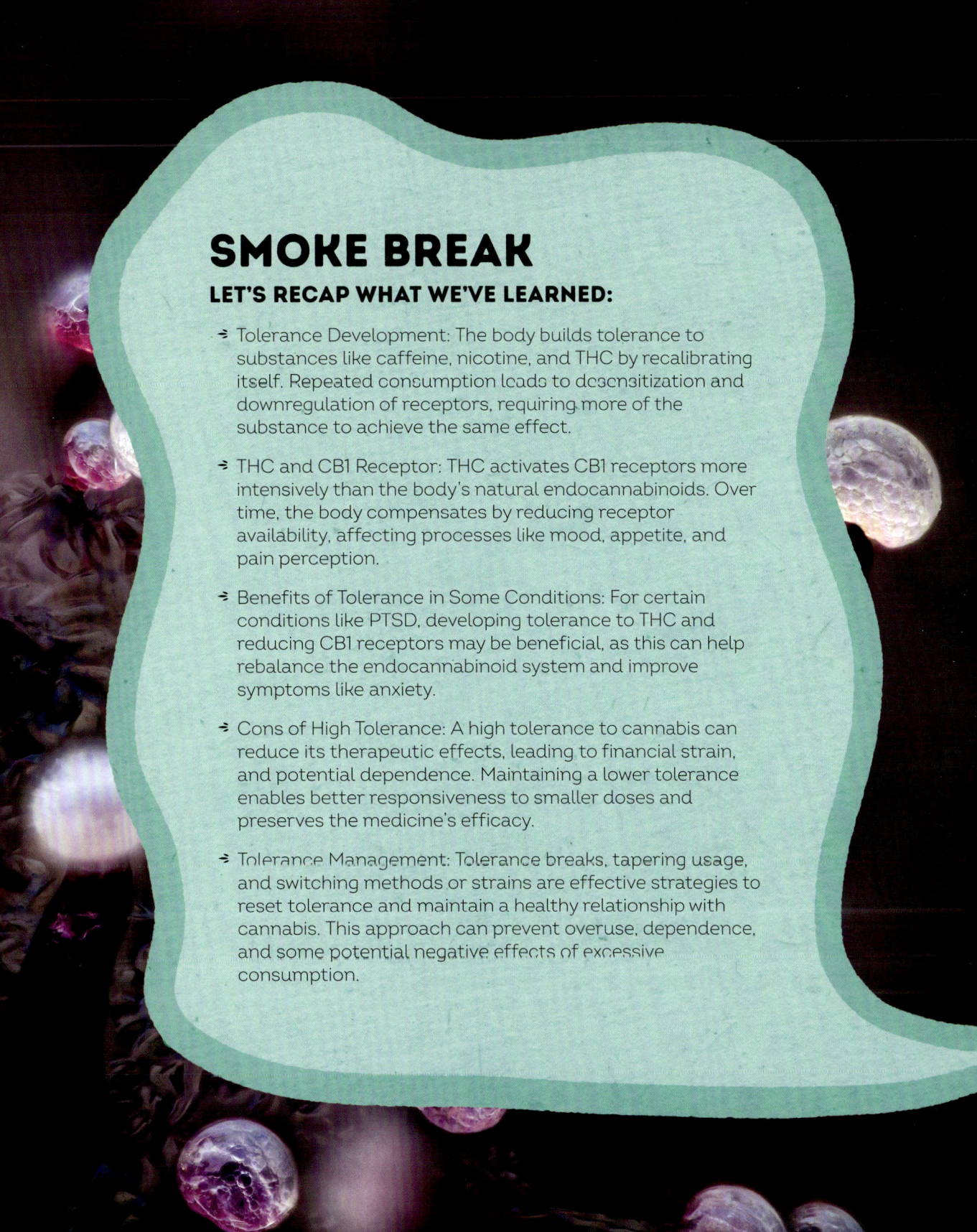

SMOKE BREAK

LET'S RECAP WHAT WE'VE LEARNED:

⇻ Tolerance Development: The body builds tolerance to substances like caffeine, nicotine, and THC by recalibrating itself. Repeated consumption leads to desensitization and downregulation of receptors, requiring more of the substance to achieve the same effect.

⇻ THC and CB1 Receptor: THC activates CB1 receptors more intensively than the body's natural endocannabinoids. Over time, the body compensates by reducing receptor availability, affecting processes like mood, appetite, and pain perception.

⇻ Benefits of Tolerance in Some Conditions: For certain conditions like PTSD, developing tolerance to THC and reducing CB1 receptors may be beneficial, as this can help rebalance the endocannabinoid system and improve symptoms like anxiety.

⇻ Cons of High Tolerance: A high tolerance to cannabis can reduce its therapeutic effects, leading to financial strain, and potential dependence. Maintaining a lower tolerance enables better responsiveness to smaller doses and preserves the medicine's efficacy.

⇻ Tolerance Management: Tolerance breaks, tapering usage, and switching methods or strains are effective strategies to reset tolerance and maintain a healthy relationship with cannabis. This approach can prevent overuse, dependence, and some potential negative effects of excessive consumption.

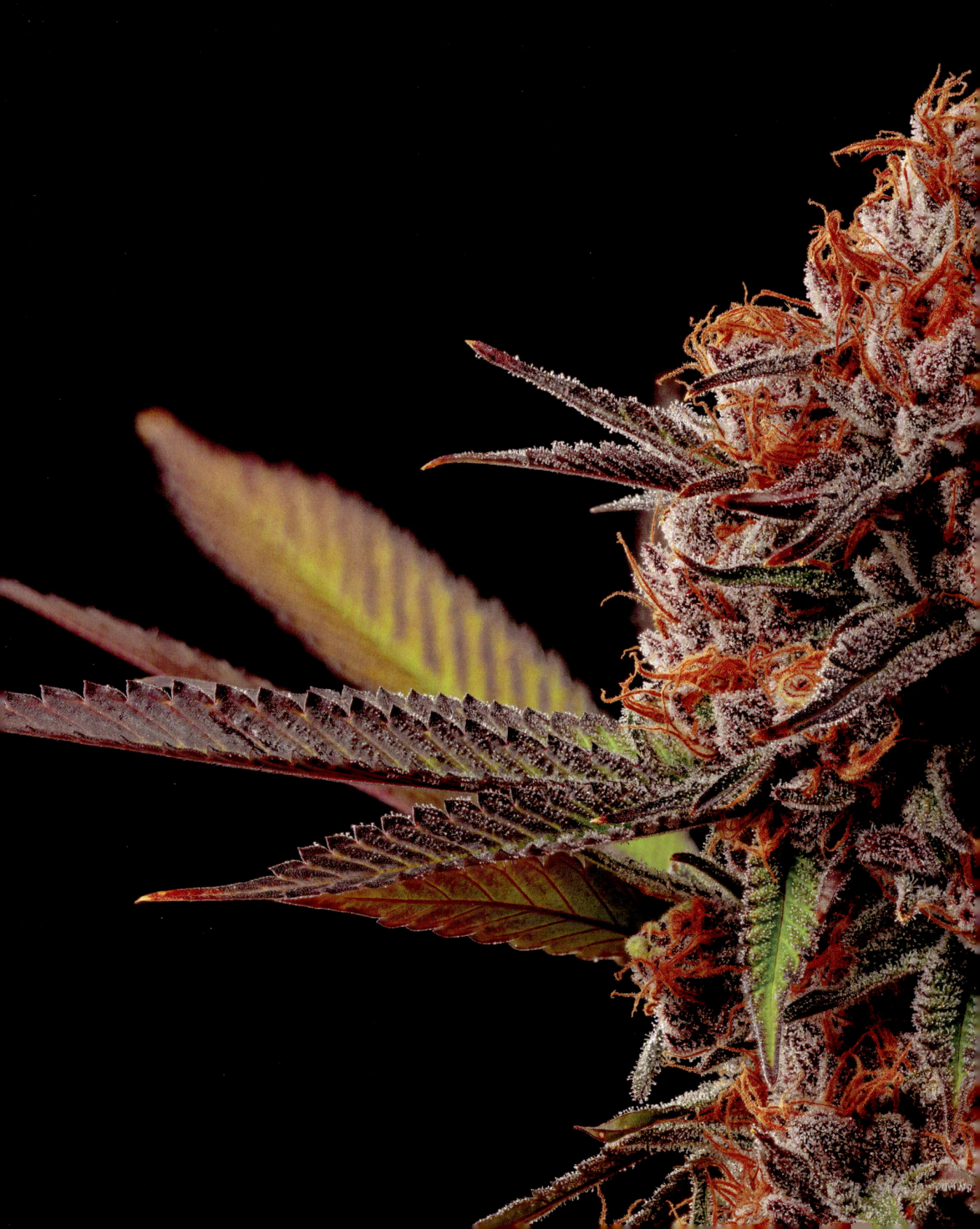

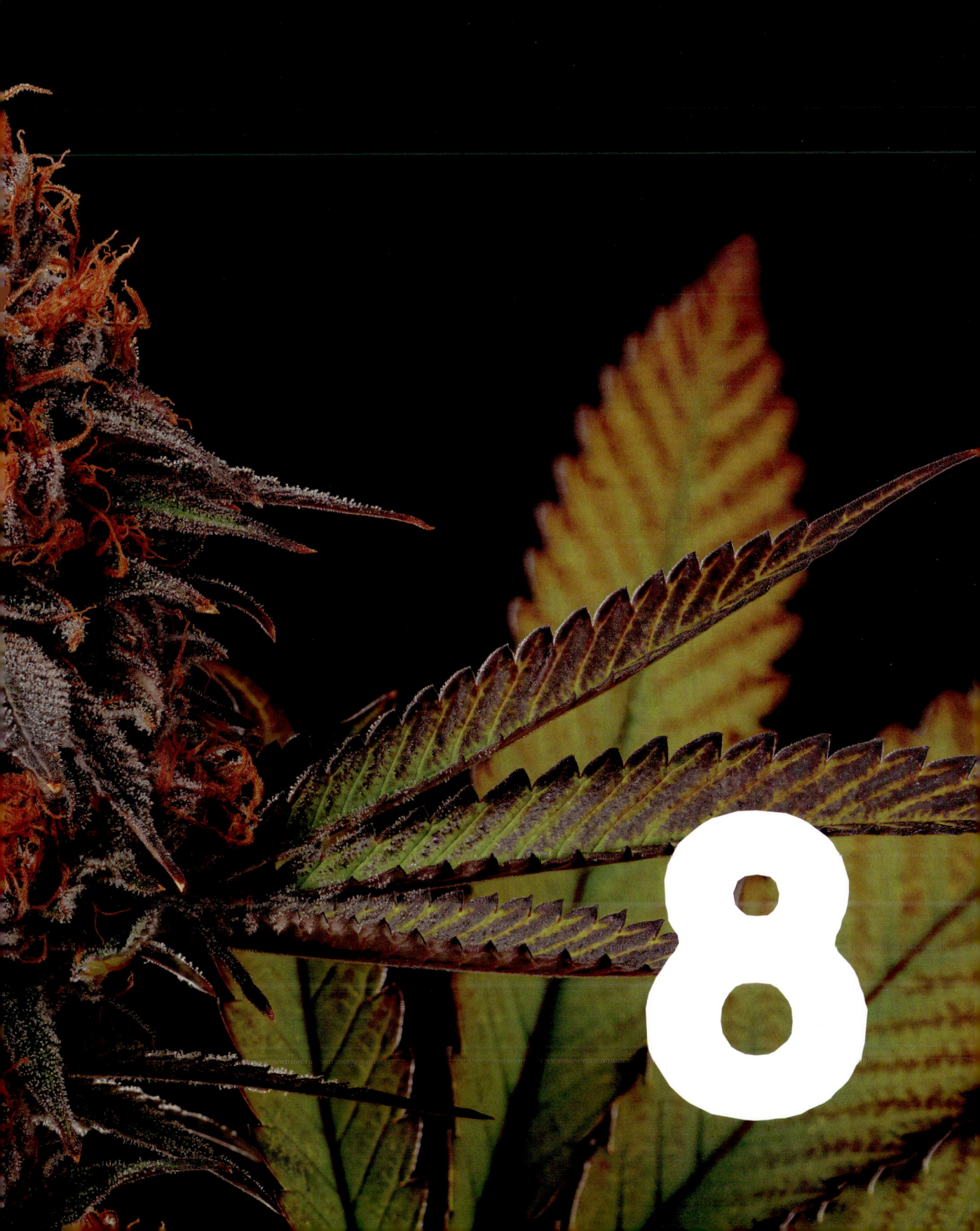

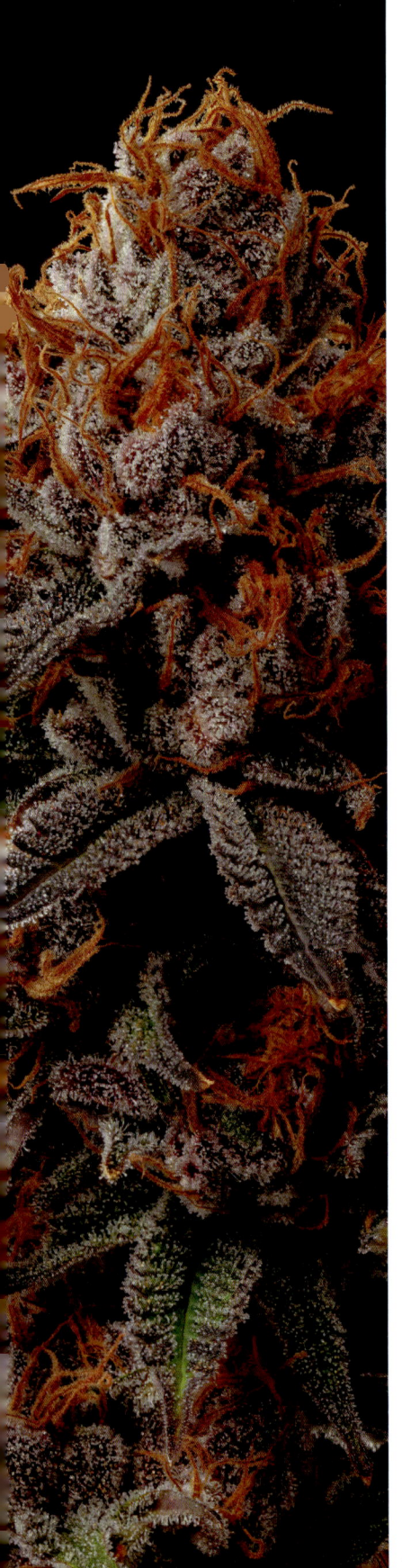

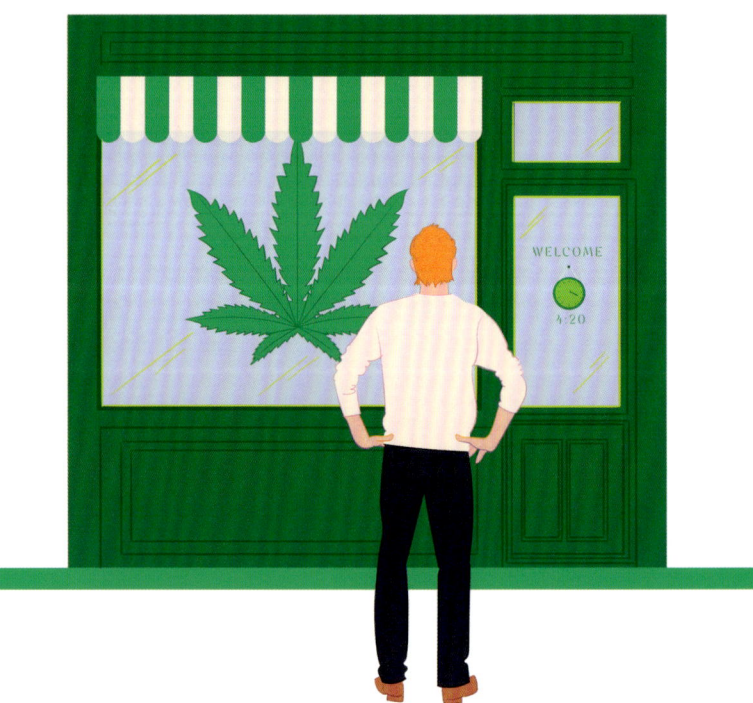

INTENTIONAL CONSUMPTION AND NAVIGATING A DISPENSARY

When you drive through some areas in the U.S., it's clear that cannabis laws vary widely from state to state. For example, in New England, you can travel from Maine where there is a dispensary on every corner, turn the corner into New Hampshire where you can get prosecuted for possessing it, and then drive another thirty minutes to Massachusetts where it again is fully legal. It does feel a bit silly.

As cannabis is still considered a schedule 1 drug, each state has developed their own rules and regulations. Some states limit consumption to medical use only, while others either permit adult use (aka recreational) or have fully prohibited cannabis.

It is important to check local cannabis laws, including purchasing, possession, public consumption, transportation, etc., when traveling from one state or country to another. Some states have medical reciprocity, allowing medical card holders to purchase cannabis at medical dispensaries, or at the very least possess cannabis, when they travel out of state. Again, this varies greatly from region to region, so check the regs before you arrive to have the safest experience. One of the best resources for staying up to date on legislative changes or legal restrictions is on the website NORML.org,; NORML is a nationwide advocacy group.

Now that you are an educated consumer and understand the plant and your body better, you are ready to enter a dispensary and begin your cannabis journey.

Instead of using the word "recreational" to describe cannabis usage, often the preferred term is "adult-use" cannabis. "Recreational" seems to imply that people only want to get high. Yet, in reality, many adults use cannabis to de-stress, socialize, initiate arousal, be creative, increase their patience, abstain from alcohol, or connect with themselves spiritually.

MEDICAL CANNABIS USE

How can you get a medical card?

In medical-only states, you must possess a medical card in order to purchase any cannabis. Medical cards are typically administered through medical professionals like your physician. However, online services can help get you a medical card if you are unable to see your physician or haven't developed that line of trust yet.

The qualifying conditions for obtaining medical cards vary in different areas. In some states, physicians can provide medical cards for any condition, as the endocannabinoid system is involved in every inflammatory and chronic condition of the human body. In other states, you may need a diagnosis of one of the qualifying conditions to get a medical card. In my opinion it is egregious that not every medical patient has the right to legally grow cannabis.

CONSULTING A SPECIALIST

While some medical professionals are educated on cannabis and how it works in the body, most are not. Medical professionals are not taught or required to learn about the ECS or cannabis medicine in medical school. If you need a medical professional who can help you learn about potential treatments using cannabinoids, consumption methods, dosing, etc., it may be worth seeking a physician, pharmacist, or nurse who specializes in cannabis medicine. The

American Nurses Association (ANA) recently recognized cannabis nursing as a specialty field, reflecting the growing expertise and need for professionals in this area.

BENEFITS

There are benefits to having a medical card, even if you live in a state with adult-use cannabis. Medical card holders have access to higher potency products, higher possession limits, the ability to grow (in some states), consultation with medical professionals, tax exemptions, higher quality products, higher testing standards, lower costs and relaxed age restrictions when needed. Cost alone is a huge factor because cannabis is currently not covered by insurance like other medicines are and can get very expensive over time. Even if you do not purchase your cannabis from a dispensary, it is much safer to travel and medicate with a medical card. Lastly, it is helpful as an industry to know how many people identify their use as medical vs. adult use for advocacy purposes.

GUN OWNERSHIP

Because cannabis prohibition is a federal issue, laws get extra sticky when the topic of gun ownership and medical cards are presented. The Gun Control Act of 1968 says that anyone who is an "unlawful user of or addicted to any controlled substance" can't own a firearm. Since cannabis is federally prohibited, technically gun ownership by cannabis medical card holders is also prohibited. This has been debated in court many times, and likely will continue to be as gun ownership and cannabis are both very polarizing topics.

In August 2024, the 5th U.S. Circuit Court of Appeals ruled that disarming cannabis users solely based on past marijuana use is unconstitutional, citing Second Amendment rights. The case involved Paola Connelly, a Texas woman who occasionally used cannabis and was charged with illegal gun possession, but the court found no historical basis for disarming sober, nonviolent citizens. This ruling challenges federal laws restricting gun ownership for cannabis users, especially in states where cannabis use is legal

Substances known to increase anger and reactive actions like alcohol remain openly available and de-scheduled and continue to contribute to gun violence. However, it is difficult to be hopeful of change when the department in charge of making these decisions in the U.S. is called The Federal Bureau of Alcohol, Tobacco, Firearms, and Explosives (ATF). Once again, it's imperative that we deconstruct the intimate association with politics and money from the alcohol, tobacco, and pharmaceutical industries to get fair and just laws for cannabis consumers.

PICKING A DISPENSARY

When you visit dispensaries, you'll notice each one has their own character and flair. Some dispensaries are designed with the Gen Z stoner crowd in mind, some are more medical focused and pharmacy-like, and I've even seen others that are gothic or underwater themed. Regardless, the first dispensary you go to may not be the right fit for what you're looking for. I encourage you to keep looking in your local area for a place that makes you feel comfortable and welcomed, and of course, that carries the medicine you are looking for.

MULTI-STATE OPERATORS

The biggest divide you will find in the types of dispensaries is craft dispensaries versus MSOs (multi-state operators). MSOs are often referred to as the Walmart of cannabis; they are the largest brands available in many different states with the most amount of money—essentially corporate cannabis.

One benefit to MSOs is that they are operating at scale, so they can often provide more affordable products. However, many people who want to support their local economy and prefer small-batch cannabis like to support local growers and craft cannabis shops. The dedication to the craft, roots to the local lands, community engagement, and quality medicine of craft cannabis are all huge advantages to supporting your local cannabis businesses. If you are not sure if the dispensary you go to is an MSO or not, head to their website. If their website says something like "available in MA, CO, CA, MI, OH, etc.," it is probably an MSO. If they have one or two shops in one area and have an "About Us" page on their website with their story, they're likely a craft operator. Some states have even set up their legal cannabis infrastructure to encourage craft growers and discourage large MSOs (I'm looking at you, Vermont).

CRAFT CANNABIS

Craft cannabis usually refers to local cannabis farms that produce small batches of flower, prioritizing quality over quantity. This often includes a more hands on approach when it comes to watering, trimming, packaging, etc. Most craft growers only focus on a few different strains to optimize their flavor profile and effects. Some craft cannabis includes local sungrown cannabis that demonstrates the local environment like the soil, air and water quality.

THE DISPENSARY EXPERIENCE

When you enter a dispensary, make sure to have your ID ready, and your medical card if applicable. Dispensaries typically will check your ID when you walk in and again when you are about to purchase products. Dispensaries that offer online/curbside pickup will check your ID when you pull up. Some medical dispensaries may ask you to fill out an intake form and see if you want to talk with a pharmacist.

THE BUDTENDER

Budtenders are employees at a dispensary who can help you find the right product—like bartenders but for weed! Budtenders are usually cannabis consumers and very well informed about cannabis products.

They are often encouraged to sample most of the dispensary's products so they can provide informed opinions based on personal experience. However, while some budtenders are educated on how cannabis works on our bodies, **budtenders are not medical professionals.**

If you want to know what product or strain is best for your fibromyalgia, IBS, plantar fasciitis, or other specific medical issue, they likely will not have the answers for you. Instead, you should consult a cannabis pharmacist, cannabis nurse, or other medical specialist in the field. Some medical dispensaries will have a cannabis pharmacist on staff that you can set a time to speak with.

When talking with your budtender, feel free to ask for more information on how a product is made, where it is made, and its effects. Other questions you can ask are things like: "Do you have any product recommendations for a cannabis topical with THC?" or, "Do you have any flower that has both THC:CBD in it?" or, "Is this flower grown at a local farm?" or,

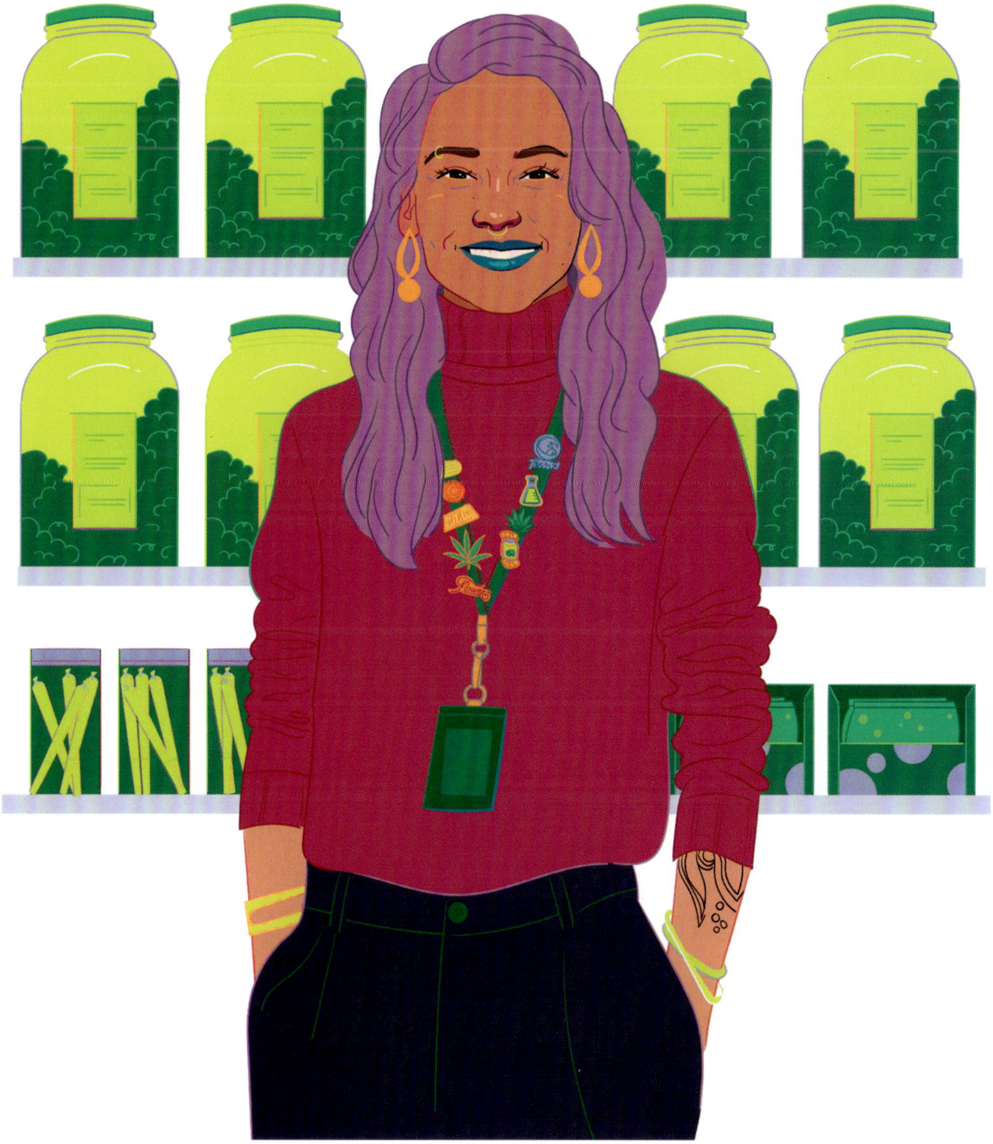

"What flower was harvested most recently?" Asking specific questions about the products, rather than their medical applications, is the best way to utilize a budtender's expertise.

Use the terpene spectrum here as well as the information in Chapter 3 to figure out what types of effects and medicinal value you're looking for to communicate with your budtender. For example, if you're seeking an uplifting daytime cannabis flower you can say, "I tried super Lemon Haze here last time, and I really like the effects. Do you have something similar to that?"

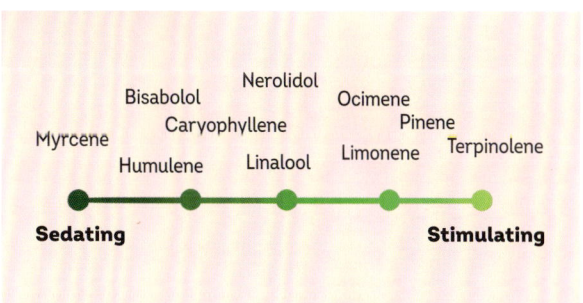

Myrcene

Bisabolol   Nerolidol
Caryophyllene   Ocimene
Humulene   Linalool   Limonene   Pinene
Terpinolene

Sedating   **Stimulating**

UNDERSTANDING DISPENSARY PRODUCTS

THE MENU

Dispensary menus can be overwhelming—there are a bunch of words you've never seen paired with numbers displaying product THC percentage and price. **If you're someone who typically looks at restaurant menus in advance, I highly recommend doing the same for dispensaries too.** Almost all dispensaries will have an online menu. I typically narrow down my choices to two to three options, then when I go in, I will ask for additional details about the products or ask if the budtenders recommend any other products.

When you enter a dispensary, it is helpful to know what type of product and effect you are looking for. For instance, if you know you want to purchase some edibles, do you want them for daytime (uplifting) or nighttime (sedating)? High dose or low dose? Fast-acting or slow release? Are you looking for a THC-only product or a balanced THC/CBD product? Do you prefer gummy or chocolate?

CANNABIS FLOWER

Cannabis flower from the dispensary is usually prepackaged into small containers or bags that are either 1 gram, ⅛ ounce, ¼ ounce, ½ ounce, or 1 ounce. It is typically much cheaper to purchase larger amounts of cannabis flower (like most things we buy). However, if you have never purchased flower from a specific farm before and you have no idea if you like a specific strain or cultivar, it is best to avoid whole ounces until you know how your body reacts to it.

Weight (ounces)	Weight (grams)
0.035 ounce	1
⅛ ounce	3.5
¼ ounce	7
½ ounce	14
1 ounce	28 (technically 28.3)

If I were going to a dispensary for the first time, I'd investigate getting a few products with very different chemical profiles (think indica, sativa, and hybrid types). Some brands even sell variety packs that let you try a few different types without breaking the bank.

PRE-ROLLS

If you want to purchase flower but don't know how to roll a joint, you can purchase pre-rolls. Pre-rolls are cannabis joints that have already been rolled up for you. Most of them come as a 1 gram joint, which is a lot for a new consumer. You don't need to finish the entire joint. You can take a couple of puffs and put it out, maybe store it back in the tube it came in and come back to it later. Some pre-rolls come in half gram or even quarter gram "dog-walker" size joints which can be a great dose for when you're starting out.

Unfortunately, many pre-rolls are cheap and smoke really harsh because they are not filled with premium cannabis flower—rather, they are filled with trim or the non-premium parts of the plant that have lower amounts of active compounds. Some pre-rolls have also been sitting on a dispensary shelf for a year or so after harvest. This can cause the flavor to diminish over time.

If I do purchase pre-rolls at a dispensary, I ask two questions: "Is this made with trim or premium bud?" and "Can I get the most recently harvested product?"

CERTIFICATE OF ANALYSIS

All products purchased from a legal dispensary must come with a certificate of analysis (COA). COAs allow you to know that your product was tested in a laboratory as well as which and how much of the active compounds are present in that product. COAs often resemble the nutritional labels on the back of food packages. Many products will link their COAs through a QR code on their packaging. Legal hemp products online also have COAs. If COAs are not available, don't buy your products there.

The COA will have different sections, one should have the different safety tests and the results from those tests, such as microbials, heavy metals, pesticides, and moisture content. All safety tests should be reported as passing. There will also be a section on cannabinoids and terpenes. The list of all the cannabinoids and terpenes that the lab tests for should be available with numbers next to each. Note that each lab doesn't test for all 150 cannabinoids that could be in the plant. Instead, labs typically test for the 12 to 20 cannabinoids that are most abundant in the plant.

Many of the compounds on the list are going to have ND, which means not detected, or <LOQ, which means that the amount present is essentially 0 because it is lower than what a lab can comfortably report. Present active compounds will typically be reported in weight (mg/g) as well as the percentage of total cannabinoids or terpenes.

There will also be a section with the sum of total cannabinoids and subsections for the sum of total THC, total CBD, and possibly some other numbers. You might notice a bit of a math equation for the "sum of total X cannabinoid." For example, for the cannabinoid CBC, the COA might read, total CBC (CBC+0.877*CBCA). In this equation, the 0.877 represents the weight of the molecule without the carboxylic acid group that is lost when cannabinoids are heated or decarboxylated.

Terpenes, or the smelly molecules in cannabis, are also reported on the COA. These will be reported in mg/g as well as percentage typically. Note that terpene concentrations are much lower than cannabinoid concentrations—on average, cannabis flower may have around 2 to 4% total terpenes. Pay special attention to the top terpenes or the ones that are most abundant in the plant because those will likely have the most effect on your experience.

CONSUMPTION METHODS AND PRODUCT PURCHASING

Before you purchase something from a dispensary, knowing how you plan on consuming cannabis can help you purchase the correct product. Chapter 4 goes into more detail about the different consumption methods, how to use them, and what to expect.

Keeping Track of Consumption

Cannabis consumers notoriously have bad memory, as impaired short-term memory is a side effect of chronic THC consumption. Do not trust your brain to remember important things; **write it down.** If you purchase a new cultivar or strain of cannabis with a unique chemical profile that reacts really well with

your body, don't do the classic "Oh there's no way I would forget about this." **Write it down.**

It is also important to write down products or varieties that don't mesh well with your body so you know what to avoid in the future. Other things to note would be if a product made you hungry, if it improved your mood, if you were on your period, what your mental state was like that day, etc.

You don't need to do this forever, although some people do, but when you're first getting started with cannabis it can be overwhelming and difficult to remember some strain names like Glitter Titties, Floss Sugar, or Mulanje Gold.

Tracking consumption is also incredibly important if you are a medical patient who visits a physician or pharmacist. Recording this information can help them understand what products react well with your body and how that relates to your medication and needs.

There are apps that you can download to keep track of the products that you try, what doses you take, etc. You can also purchase a cannabis tracking journal if you have the funds, or you can use a regular notebook to make your own cannabis journal.

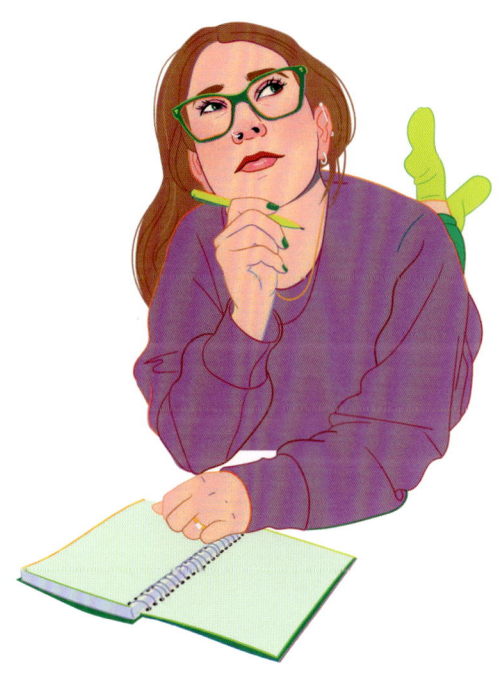

HERE ARE SOME THINGS YOU MAY WANT TO RECORD IN YOUR CANNABIS JOURNAL:

- **Date:**

  Time (circle one):   Morning   Afternoon   Evening

- **Product:** Strain name or product name (may be helpful to write where you purchased it as well)

- **Consumption method:** Smoke, Vape, Edible, Other

  THC: % or mg

  CBD: % or mg

- **Other cannabinoids:** List and concentration.

  Main terpenes: I like to write top 3

- **Dose (amount):** 3 puffs, 1 small dab, 5 mg edible, etc.

  Effects (circle):
  Sleepy 1 2 3 4 5 6 7 8 9 10 Stimulating

- **Overall desirability:**
  Ew 1   2   3   4   5   6   7   8   9   10 Amazing

- **Notes:**

Tracking your consumption doesn't have to be sterile and boring. If you have fun with it, you will be much more consistent. If you already journal, you can add a small section into your journal to note your cannabis use. You could also use colored pencils and pens to express how you feel with color and shapes. If you have a group of friends who also use cannabis, start a group chat to discuss what products you're trying and how you react to them.

- **Date:** April 20, 2025
- **Time:** (Morning)   Afternoon   Evening
- **Product:** Headbanger from Riley's Dispo in Maine
- **Consumption method:** Smoking a ½g J
- **THC:** 22%
- **CBD:** 1%
- **Other cannabinoids:** CBG 1%
- **Main terpenes:** Caryophyllene, Limonene, Linalool
- **Dose (amount):** ½ g Joint
- **Effects (circle):**
  Sleepy 1 2 3 4 5 6 7 8 (9) 10 Stimulating
- **Overall desirability:**
  Ew 1 2 3 4 5 6 (7) 8 9 10 Amazing
- **Notes:** Loved the stimulating effects of the flower, would purchase again for daytime use but it did make me a little anxious and it was very dry and difficult to roll. Effects lasted 1.5 hours and the pain in my stomach was alleviated for most of that time. Would add some CBD flower next time to help with the anxiety.

NUGS OF KNOWLEDGE

Pro tip, if the COA that your product comes with is on a sticker, you can put the entire sticker directly into your weed journal.

RELIEF WITHOUT THE HIGH

For many people, using cannabis is associated with getting high. While some desire this elevated feeling, others consider it an adverse effect they want to avoid. Whether it's anxiety, work, sobriety, or just not liking the feeling of THC, there are ways to use cannabis without feeling high.

Most of the compounds in the cannabis plant don't get you high but have other benefits to the body and mind like reducing inflammation, reducing oxidative damage, promoting bone health, enhancing mood, etc. THC is the main compound to avoid when you don't want to feel high. However, if you are seeking a "little bit of a high" effect, CBN may be worth trying. CBN is naturally produced during the smoking process but is not present in any appreciable amounts in the cannabis flower because it is a breakdown product of THC. CBN is often formulated into sleep products in gummy, tincture, or capsule form. It is about one third to one fourth the intensity of THC but still has the benefits of activation of the CB1 receptor for pain relief, anxiety, sleep, etc.

The best researched and most used nonintoxicating compound is CBD. CBD products can be found in literally almost every form imaginable from CBD bath bombs to CBD gummies, tinctures, pillows, suppositories and lotions. You won't feel the effects from CBD products, so it can be difficult to know if they're working. If you are new to taking CBD, make sure to use it consistently for at least a week or two before gauging the effects.

Although CBD products legally have to have less than or equal to 0.3% THC in them, smoking CBD-flower or hemp may cause more of a high feeling as CBD partially converts to THC during the smoking process. So, if you are very sensitive to THC or don't want to feel any mental state change, I would recommend topicals, tinctures (with <0.3%), capsules, or suppositories, but not smoking or high temperature vaping. If you're looking for a low dose of THC that you can feel a little bit, smoking or high temperature dry herb vaping is a nice medium ground.

CANNABIS AS A SPIRITUAL GUIDE

The science of cannabis can only take you so far. There is a lot we still don't know about the exact molecules and mechanisms that the plant works. Cannabis is incredibly complex and so is the human body, and we currently don't have the ability to map that level of complexity. However, we do know that cannabis allows you to be more in touch with your body, mind, and spirit.

Cannabis can help with expressing yourself in your truest form. It allows many people, me included, to feel a deeper connection with others and communicate our thoughts into words.

Yet, this effect can sometimes also be negative. This expansion of consciousness, thought, and perception can be difficult to handle, especially if you're already at a vulnerable place in life. These are other things that may be worth putting in your cannabis journal OR, if your counselor is accepting of plant medicine, incorporating cannabis into your treatment plan to allow you to heal in the way that is most comfortable to you.

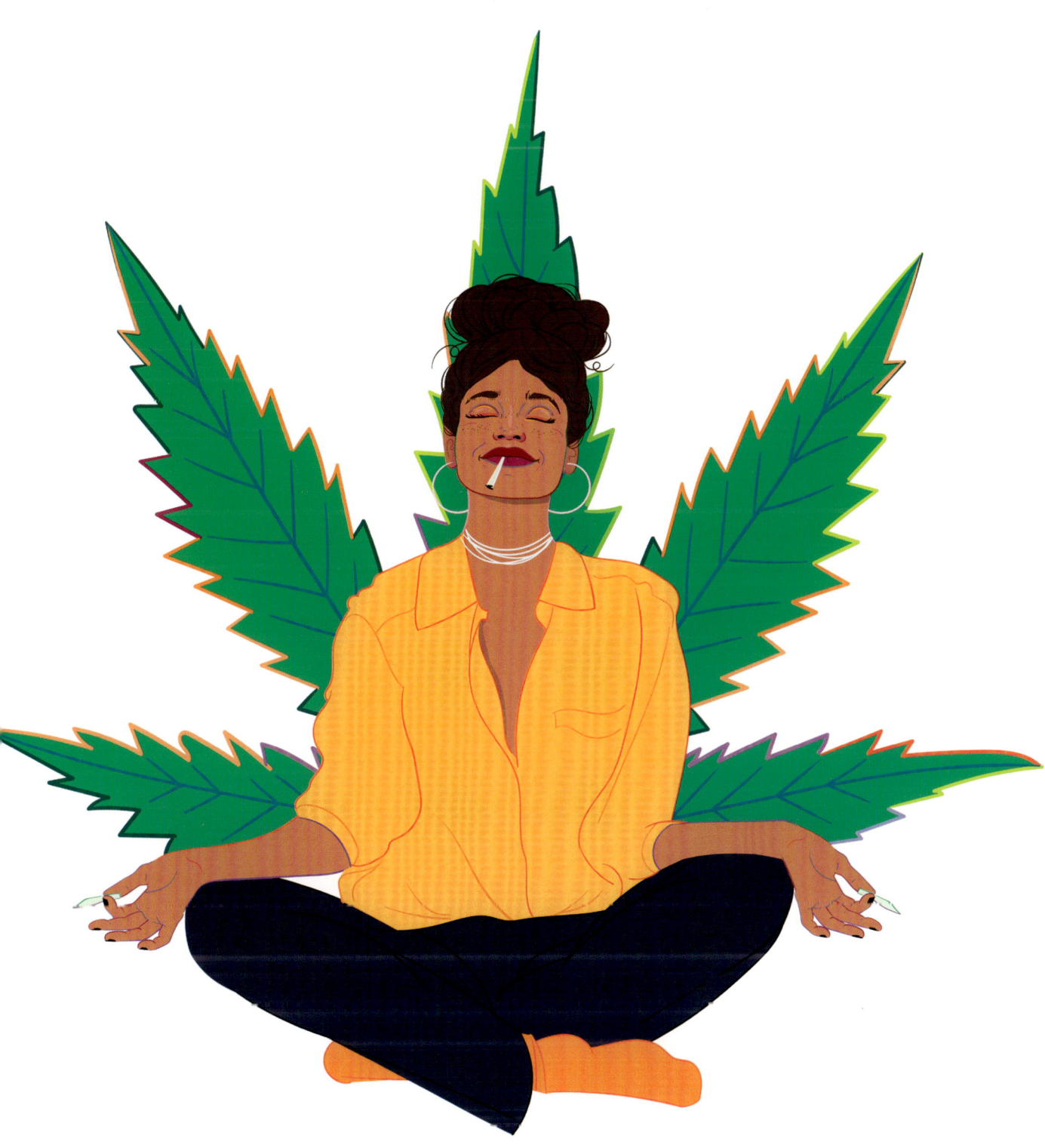

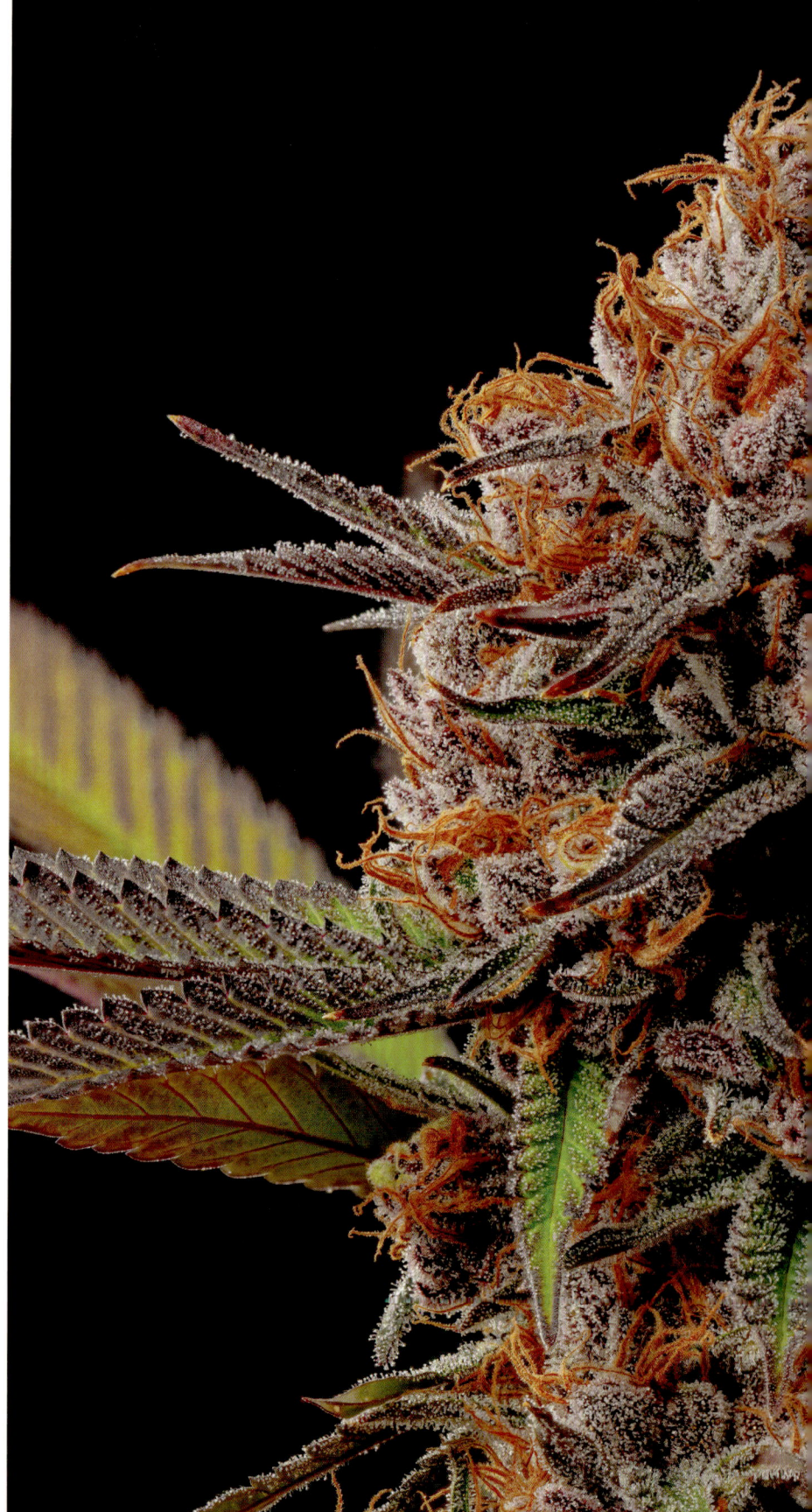

SMOKE BREAK

LET'S RECAP WHAT WE'VE LEARNED:

⇉ Cannabis Laws and Variability: Cannabis laws vary significantly between states, with some allowing medical or adult-use cannabis and others strictly prohibiting it. It's essential to research local laws before traveling, and NORML.org is a valuable resource for staying updated on regulations.

⇉ Medical Cannabis Benefits: Having a medical card provides access to higher-potency products, tax exemptions, and the ability to grow cannabis in some states. Medical cardholders may also benefit from consultations with cannabis specialists, which is especially helpful as many medical professionals lack training in cannabis medicine.

⇉ Choosing a Dispensary: Dispensaries vary widely in character, from corporate-run MSOs (multi-state operators) to local, craft cannabis shops. Craft dispensaries often provide higher-quality, locally grown products, while MSOs can offer more affordable pricing due to larger operations.

⇉ Budtenders and Product Selection: Budtenders, while knowledgeable about products, are not medical professionals. It's important to consult specialists for medical issues. Asking budtenders specific questions about product content (like cannabinoids and terpenes) can help you make informed choices about cannabis strains or products.

⇉ Tracking and Managing Cannabis Use: Keeping a cannabis journal helps track strains, effects, and doses, making it easier to understand what works best for your body. It's especially useful for medical patients, and tools like apps or simple notebooks can help in organizing this information.

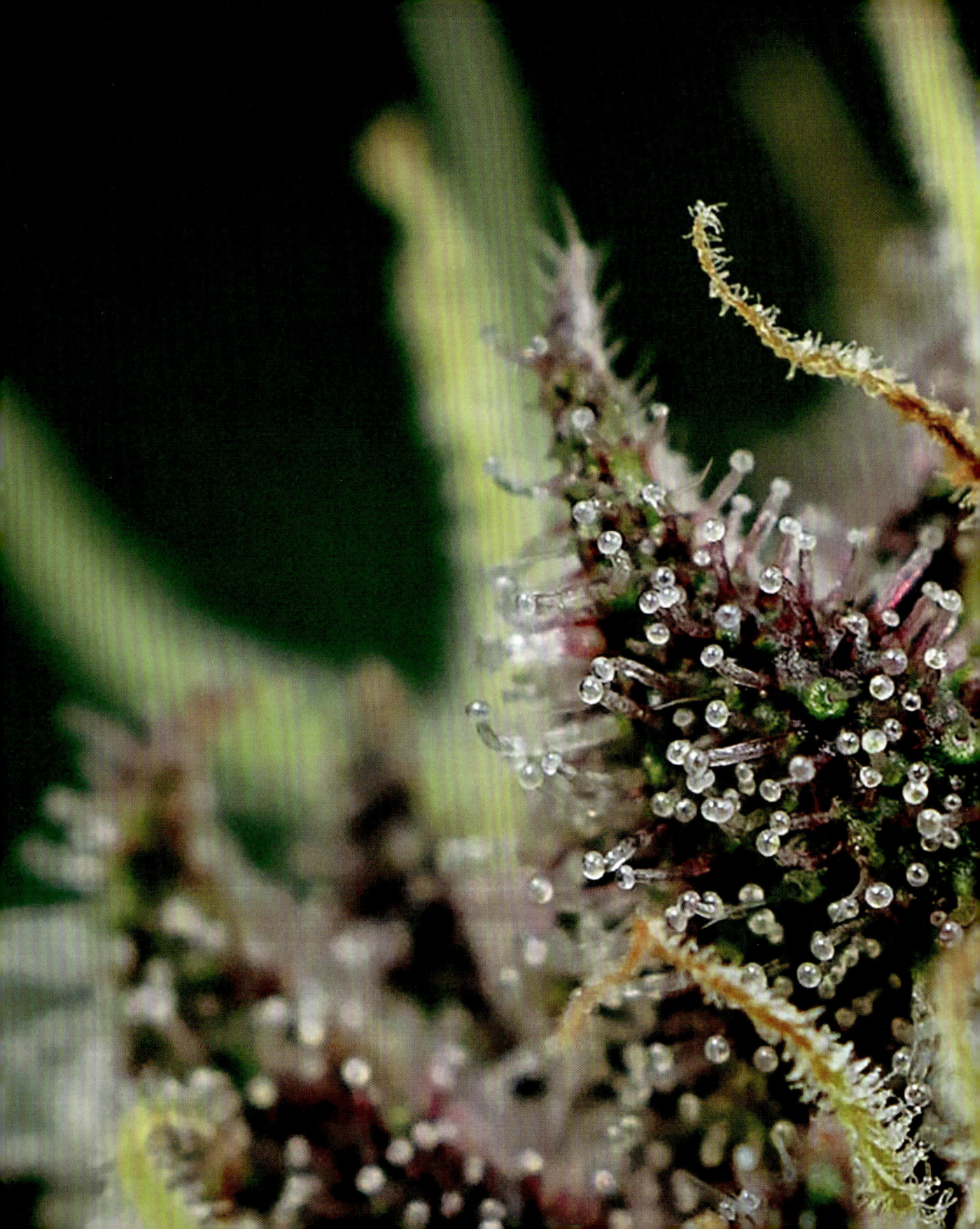

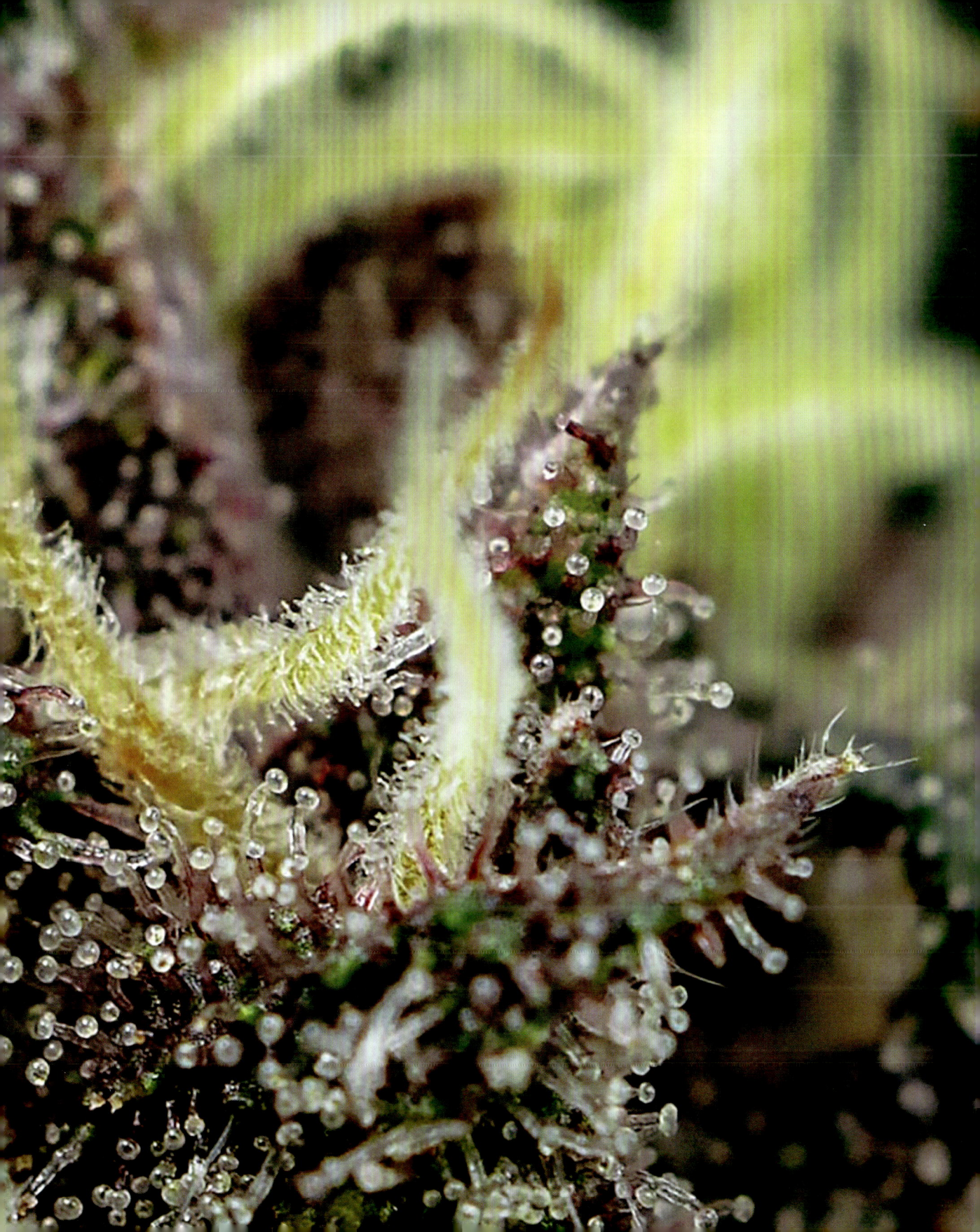

WORKS CITED

CHAPTER 1: NATURE AND DRUGS

1 Newman, DJ., and Cragg, G.M. "Natural Products as Sources of New Drugs over the Nearly Four Decades from 01/1981 to 09/2019." *J Nat Prod.* 2020 Mar 27;83(3):770-803. doi: 10.1021/acs.jnatprod.9b01285. Epub 2020 Mar 12. PMID: 32162523.

2 Clarke, T.L., et al. "The Endocannabinoid System and Invertebrate Neurodevelopment and Regeneration." *Int J Mol Sci.* 2021 Feb 20;22(4):2103. doi: 10.3390/ijms22042103. PMID: 33672634; PMCID: PMC7924210.

3 Miyabe Shields, C., and Kirk, R.D., (2022). "Pharmaceutical Applications of Hemp." In: Belwal, T., Belwal, N.C. (eds) *Revolutionizing the Potential of Hemp and Its Products in Changing the Global Economy.* Springer, Cham. https://doi.org/10.1007/978-3-031-05144-9_5

CHAPTER 2: A BRIEF HISTORY OF CANNABIS

1 Columbia History of the World, Harper & Row, New York, 1981. The emperor wears no clothes, Jack Herer

2 Godlaski, T. M. (2012). "Shiva, Lord of Bhang". *Substance Use & Misuse,* 47(10), 1067–1072. https://doi.org/10.3109/10826084.2012.684308

3 Columbia History of the World, Harper & Row, New York, 1981. The emperor wears no clothes, Jack Herer.

4 Crocq, Marc-Antoine. "History of Cannabis and the Endocannabinoid System." *Dialogues in Clinical Neuroscience,* vol. 22, no. 3, Sept. 2020, pp. 223–228. https://doi.org/10.31887/DCNS.2020.22.3/mcrocq.

Godlaski, T. M. (2012). "Shiva, Lord of Bhang". *Substance Use & Misuse,* 47(10), 1067–1072. https://doi.org/10.3109/1

Zuardi, A. W. "History of Cannabis as a Medicine: A Review." *Brazilian Journal of Psychiatry,* vol. 28, no. 2, June 2006, pp. 153–157, https://doi.org/10.1590/s1516-44462006000200015. PMID: 16810401.

Hussain, T., G. Jeena, T. Pitakbut, N. Vasilev, and O. Kayser. "Cannabis Sativa Research Trends, Challenges, and New-Age Perspectives." *iScience,* vol. 24, no. 12, 1 Nov. 2021, p. 103391, https://doi.org/10.1016/j.isci.2021.103391. PMID: 34841230; PMCID: PMC8605354.

CHAPTER 3: MOLECULES, RECEPTORS, AND THE ENDOCANNABINOID SYSTEM

1 Laprairie, R.B., et al. "Cannabidiol is a negative allosteric modulator of the cannabinoid CB1 receptor". *Br J Pharmacol.* 2015 Oct;172(20):4790-805. doi: 10.1111/bph.13250. Epub 2015 Oct 13. PMID: 26218440; PMCID: PMC4621983.

2 Lu, D., et al. "Translational potential of allosteric modulators targeting the cannabinoid CB1 receptor". *Acta Pharmacol Sin* 40, 324–335 (2019). https://doi.org/10.1038/s41401-018-0164-x

3 Fuerte-Hortigón, A., et al. "Distribution of the Cannabinoid Receptor Type 1 in the Brain of the Genetically Audiogenic Seizure-Prone Hamster GASH/Sal." *Front Behav Neurosci.* 2021 Mar 24;15:613798. doi: 10.3389/fnbeh.2021.613798. PMID: 33841106; PMCID: PMC8024637.

4 Komorowska-Müller, J.A. and Schmöle, A.C. "CB2 Receptor in Microglia: The Guardian of Self-Control." *Int. J. Mol. Sci.* 2021, 22, 19. https://doi.org/10.3390/ijms22010019

5 Elmes, M.W., et al. "Fatty acid-binding proteins (FABPs) are intracellular carriers for Δ9-tetrahydrocannabinol (THC) and cannabidiol (CBD)." *J Biol Chem.* 2015 Apr 3;290(14):8711-21. doi: 10.1074/jbc.M114.618447. Epub 2015 Feb 9. PMID: 25666611; PMCID: PMC4423662.

6 Silver, R., et al. "The Endocannabinoid System and Endocannabinoidome." In: Cital, S., Kramer, K., Hughston, L., Gaynor, J.S. (eds) *Cannabis Therapy in Veterinary Medicine.* Springer, Cham. https://doi.org/10.1007/978-3-030-68317-7_1

7 Pete, D.D. and Narouze, S.N. "Endocannabinoids: Anandamide and 2-Arachidonoylglycerol (2-AG)." *Narouze, S.N. (eds) Cannabinoids and Pain.* Springer, Cham. 2021 https://doi.org/10.1007/978-3-030-69186-8_9

8 Pete, D.D. and Narouze, S.N. "Endocannabinoids: Anandamide and 2-Arachidonoylglycerol (2-AG)." *Narouze, S.N. (eds) Cannabinoids and Pain.* Springer, Cham 2021 https://doi.org/10.1007/978-3-030-69186-8_9

9 Front. Pharmacol. 14 December 2020 Sec. Neuropharmacology Volume 11 - 2020 https://doi.org/10.3389/fphar.2020.595635

10 Gertsch, J., et al. "Phytocannabinoids beyond the Cannabis plant - do they exist?" *Br J Pharmacol.* 2010 Jun;160(3):523-9. doi: 10.1111/j.1476-5381.2010.00745.x. PMID: 20590562; PMCID: PMC2931553.

11 Rock, E.M., et al. "Tetrahydrocannabinolic acid reduces nausea-induced conditioned gaping in rats and vomiting in Suncus murinus." *Br J Pharmacol.* 2013 Oct;170(3):641-8. doi: 10.1111/bph.12316. PMID: 23889598; PMCID: PMC3792001.

12 Verhoeckx, K.C., et al. "Unheated Cannabis sativa extracts and its major compound THC-acid have potential immuno-modulating properties not mediated by CB1 and CB2 receptor coupled pathways." *Int Immunopharmacol.* 2006; 6:656–665.

13 Editors: David Kendall, Stephen P.H. Alexander. "Cannabis Pharmacology: The Usual Suspects and a Few Promising Leads." *Advances in Pharmacology*, Academic Press, Volume 80, 2017, Pages 67-134,

14 Blebea, N.M., et al. "Phytocannabinoids: Exploring Pharmacological Profiles and Their Impact on Therapeutical Use." *Int J Mol Sci.* 2024 Apr 10;25(8):4204. doi: 10.3390/ijms25084204. PMID: 38673788; PMCID: PMC11050509.

15 Abioye, A., et al. "Δ9-Tetrahydrocannabivarin (THCV): a commentary on potential therapeutic benefit for the management of obesity and diabetes." *J Cannabis Res* 2, 6 (2020). https://doi.org/10.1186/s42238-020-0016-7

16 Jadoon, K.A., et al. "Efficacy and Safety of Cannabidiol and Tetrahydrocannabivarin on Glycemic and Lipid Parameters in Patients With Type 2 Diabetes: A Randomized, Double-Blind, Placebo-Controlled, Parallel Group Pilot Study." *Diabetes Care* 1 October 2016; 39 (10): 1777–1786. https://doi.org/10.2337/dc16-0650

17 Iannotti, F.A., et al. "Nonpsychotropic plant cannabinoids, cannabidivarin (CBDV) and cannabidiol (CBD), activate and desensitize transient receptor potential vanilloid 1 (TRPV1) channels in vitro: potential for the treatment of neuronal hyperexcitability." *ACS Chem Neurosci.* 2014; 5(11):1131-1141. DOI: 10.1021/cn5000524.

18 Blebea, N.M., et al. "Phytocannabinoids: Exploring Pharmacological Profiles and Their Impact on Therapeutic Use." *Int J Mol Sci.* 2024 Apr 10;25(8):4204. doi: 10.3390/ijms25084204. PMID: 38673788; PMCID: PMC11050509.

19 Bonn-Miller, M.O., et al. "A Double-Blind, Randomized, Placebo-Controlled Study of the Safety and Effects of CBN with and without CBD on Sleep Quality." *Experimental and Clinical Psychopharmacology,* vol. 32, no. 3, June 2024, pp. 277–284. APA PsycNet, https://doi.org/10.1037/pha0000682.

20 McCartney, L.I., et al. "Cannabinol (CBN; 30 and 300 mg) effects on sleep and next-day function in insomnia disorder ('CUPID' study): protocol for a randomised, double-blind, placebo-controlled, cross-over, three-arm, proof-of-concept trial." *BMJ Open.* 2023 Aug 23;13(8):e071148. doi: 10.1136/bmjopen-2022-071148. PMID: 37612115; PMCID: PMC10450062.

21 Gojani, E.G., et al. "Anti-Inflammatory Effects of Minor Cannabinoids CBC, THCV, and CBN in Human Macrophages." *Molecules.* 2023; 28(18):6487. https://doi.org/10.3390/molecules28186487

22 Zavala-Tecuapetla, C., et al. "Advances and Challenges of Cannabidiol as an Anti-Seizure Strategy: Preclinical Evidence." *Int J Mol Sci.* 2022 Dec 19;23(24):16181. doi: 10.3390/ijms232416181. PMID: 36555823; PMCID: PMC9783044.

23 Peltner, L.K., et al. "Cannabidiol acts as molecular switch in innate immune cells to promote the biosynthesis of inflammation-resolving lipid mediators". *Cell Chemical Biology*, Volume 30, Issue 12, 1508 - 1524. e7

24 Mlost, J., et al. "Cannabidiol for Pain Treatment: Focus on Pharmacology and Mechanism of Action." *Int J Mol Sci.* 2020 Nov 23;21(22):8870. doi: 10.3390/ijms21228870. PMID: 33238607; PMCID: PMC7700528.

25 Chagas, M.H., et al. "Effects of acute systemic administration of cannabidiol on sleep-wake cycle in rats." *J Psychopharmacol.* 2013;27(3):312–6.

26 Arnold, J.C., et al. "The safety and efficacy of low oral doses of cannabidiol: An evaluation of the evidence." *Clin Transl Sci.* 2023 Jan;16(1):10-30. doi: 10.1111/cts.13425. Epub 2022 Oct 19. PMID: 36259271; PMCID: PMC9841308.

27 Arnold, J.C., et al. "The safety and efficacy of low oral doses of cannabidiol: An evaluation of the evidence." *Clin Transl Sci.* 2023 Jan;16(1):10-30. doi: 10.1111/cts.13425. Epub 2022 Oct 19. PMID: 36259271; PMCID: PMC9841308.

28 Martins, A.M., et al. "Cannabis-Based Products for the Treatment of Skin Inflammatory Diseases: A Timely Review." *Pharmaceuticals (Basel).* 2022 Feb 9;15(2):210. doi: 10.3390/ph15020210. Erratum in: Pharmaceuticals (Basel). 2022 Jul 11;15(7):849. doi: 10.3390/ph15070849. PMID: 35215320; PMCID: PMC8878527.

29 Pérez-Segura, I., et al. "PPARs and Their Neuroprotective Effects in Parkinson's Disease: A Novel Therapeutic Approach in α-Synucleinopathy?" *Int J Mol Sci.* 2023 Feb 7;24(4):3264. doi: 10.3390/ijms24043264. PMID: 36834679; PMCID: PMC9963164.

30 Calapai, F., et al. "Pharmacological Aspects and Biological Effects of Cannabigerol and Its Synthetic Derivatives." *Evid Based Complement Alternat Med.* 2022 Nov 8;2022:3336516. doi: 10.1155/2022/3336516. PMID: 36397993; PMCID: PMC9666035.

31 Luz-Veiga, M., et al. "Cannabidiol and Cannabigerol Exert Antimicrobial Activity without Compromising Skin Microbiota." *Int J Mol Sci.* 2023 Jan 25;24(3):2389. doi: 10.3390/ijms24032389. PMID: 36768709; PMCID: PMC9917174.

32 Udoh, M., et al. "Cannabichromene is a cannabinoid CB2 receptor agonist." *Br J Pharmacol.* 2019 Dec;176(23):4537-4547. doi: 10.1111/bph.14815. Epub 2019 Nov 21. PMID: 31368508; PMCID: PMC6932936.

33 Shinjyo, N. and Di Marzo, V. "The effect of cannabichromene on adult neural stem/progenitor cells." *Neurochem Int.* 2013 Nov;63(5):432-7. doi: 10.1016/j.neuint.2013.08.002. Epub 2013 Aug 11. PMID: 23941747.

34 Vučković, S., et al. "Cannabinoids and Pain: New Insights From Old Molecules." *Front Pharmacol.* 2018 Nov 13;9:1259. doi: 10.3389/fphar.2018.01259. PMID: 30542280; PMCID: PMC6277878.

35 Vučković, S., et al. "Cannabinoids and Pain: New Insights From Old Molecules." *Front Pharmacol.* 2018 Nov 13;9:1259. doi: 10.3389/fphar.2018.01259. PMID: 30542280; PMCID: PMC6277878.

36 Sukul, P., et al. "Origin of breath isoprene in humans is revealed via multi-omic investigations." *Commun Biol.* 2023 Sep 30;6(1):999. doi: 10.1038/s42003-023-05384-y. PMID: 37777700; PMCID: PMC10542801.

37 Smith, C.J., et al. "The phytochemical diversity of commercial Cannabis in the United States." *PLoS One.* 2022 May 19;17(5):e0267498. doi: 10.1371/journal.pone.0267498. PMID: 35588111; PMCID: PMC9119530.

38 Kim, K.Y. "Anti-inflammatory and ECM gene expression modulations of β-eudesmol via NF-κB signaling pathway in normal human dermal fibroblasts." *Biomed Dermatol.* 2, 3 (2018). https://doi.org/10.1186/s41702-017-0014-3

39 Surendran, S., et al. "Myrcene-What Are the Potential Health Benefits of This Flavouring and Aroma Agent?" *Front Nutr.* 2021 Jul 19;8:699666. doi: 10.3389/fnut.2021.699666. PMID: 34350208; PMCID: PMC8326332.

40 Hartley, N and McLachlan, C.S. "Aromas Influencing the GABAergic System." *Molecules.* 2022 Apr 8;27(8):2414. doi: 10.3390/molecules27082414. PMID: 35458615; PMCID: PMC9026314.

41 Abdoul-Latif, M., et al "Exploring the Potent Anticancer Activity of Essential Oils and Their Bioactive Compounds: Mechanisms and Prospects for Future Cancer Therapy." *Pharmaceuticals (Basel).* 2023 Jul 31;16(8):1086. doi: 10.3390/ph16081086. PMID: 37631000; PMCID: PMC10458506.

42 Bie, B. Wu., et al "An overview of the cannabinoid type 2 receptor system and its therapeutic potential." *Curr Opin Anaesthesiol.* 2018 Aug;31(4):407-414. doi: 10.1097/ACO.0000000000000616. PMID: 29794855; PMCID: PMC6035094.

43 Yeo, D., et al. "Humulene Inhibits Acute Gastric Mucosal Injury by Enhancing Mucosal Integrity." *Antioxidants (Basel).* 2021 May 11;10(5):761. doi: 10.3390/antiox10050761. PMID: 34064830; PMCID: PMC8150829.

44 Eddin, L.B., et al. "Neuroprotective Potential of Limonene and Limonene Containing Natural Products." *Molecules.* 2021 Jul 27;26(15):4535. doi: 10.3390/molecules26154535. PMID: 34361686; PMCID: PMC8348102.

45 Yu, X., et al. "D-limonene exhibits antitumor activity by inducing autophagy and apoptosis in lung cancer." *Onco Targets Ther.* 2018 Apr 4;11:1833-1847. doi: 10.2147/OTT.S155716. PMID: 29670359; PMCID: PMC5894671.

46 Harada, H., et al. "Linalool Odor-Induced Anxiolytic Effects in Mice." *Front Behav Neurosci.* 2018 Oct 23;12:241. doi: 10.3389/fnbeh.2018.00241. PMID: 30405369; PMCID: PMC6206409.

47 Weston-Green, K., et al. "A Review of the Potential Use of Pinene and Linalool as Terpene-Based Medicines for Brain Health: Discovering Novel Therapeutics in the Flavours and Fragrances of Cannabis." *Front Psychiatry*. 2021 Aug 26;12:583211. doi: 10.3389/fpsyt.2021.583211. PMID: 34512404; PMCID: PMC8426550.

48 Masyita, A., et al, "Terpenes and terpenoids as main bioactive compounds of essential oils, their roles in human health and potential application as natural food preservatives." *Food Chem X*. 2022 Jan 19;13:100217. doi: 10.1016/j.fochx.2022.100217. PMID: 35498985; PMCID: PMC9039924.

49 Salehi, B., et al. "Therapeutic Potential of α- and β-Pinene: A Miracle Gift of Nature." *Biomolecules*. 2019 Nov 14;9(11):738. doi: 10.3390/biom9110738. PMID: 31739596; PMCID: PMC6920849.

50 Ito, K. and Ito, M. "The sedative effect of inhaled terpinolene in mice and its structure-activity relationships." *J Nat Med*. 2013 Oct;67(4):833-7. doi: 10.1007/s11418-012-0732-1. Epub 2013 Jan 22. PMID: 23339024.

51 Oswald, I.W.H., et al. "Nonterpenoid Volatile Compounds Drive the Aroma Differences of Exotic Cannabis." *ACS Omega*. 2023 Oct 12;8(42):39203-39216. doi: 10.1021/acsomega.3c04496. PMID: 37901519; PMCID: PMC10601067.

52 Bautista, J.L. "Flavonoids in Cannabis sativa: Biosynthesis, Bioactivities, and Biotechnology." *ACS Omega*. 2021 Feb 18;6(8):5119-5123. doi: 10.1021/acsomega.1c00318. PMID: 33681553; PMCID: PMC7931196.

53 Al-Khazaleh, A.K., et al. "The Neurotherapeutic Arsenal in Cannabis sativa: Insights into Anti-Neuroinflammatory and Neuroprotective Activity and Potential Entourage Effects." *Molecules*. 2024 Jan 15;29(2):410. doi: 10.3390/molecules29020410. PMID: 38257323; PMCID: PMC10821245.

54 Abdel-Kader, Maged S., et al. "Chemistry and Biological Activities of Cannflavins of the Cannabis Plant." *Cannabis and Cannabinoid Research*, vol. 8, no. 6, 2023, pp. 974–985. https://doi.org/10.1089/can.2023.0052.

CHAPTER 4: HOW TO CONSUME CANNABIS

1 Meier, E., et al. "Cigarette Smokers Versus Cousers of Cannabis and Cigarettes: Exposure to Toxicants." *Nicotine Tob Res*. 2020 Jul 16;22(8):1383-1389. doi: 10.1093/ntr/ntz199. PMID: 31616939; PMCID: PMC7366295.

2 Kaplan, A.G. "Cannabis and Lung Health: Does the Bad Outweigh the Good?." *Pulm Ther*. 7, 395–408 (2021). https://doi.org/10.1007/s41030-021-00171-8

3 Moir, D., et al. "A comparison of mainstream and sidestream marijuana and tobacco cigarette smoke produced under two machine smoking conditions." *Chem Res Toxicol*. 2008;21(2):494–502.

4 Patel, S., et al. "Physiology, Oxygen Transport And Carbon Dioxide Dissociation Curve." [Updated 2023 Mar 27]. In: *StatPearls* [Internet]. Treasure Island (FL): StatPearls Publishing; 2024 Jan-. Available from: https://www.ncbi.nlm.nih.gov/books/NBK539815/

5 Eran, Nizri., et al. "Activation of the Cholinergic Anti-Inflammatory System by Nicotine Attenuates Neuroinflammation via Suppression of Th1 and Th17 Responses." *J Immunol* 15 November 2009; 183 (10): 6681–6688. https://doi.org/10.4049/jimmunol.0902212

Mahmoudzadeh, L., et al. "Effect of Nicotine on Immune System Function." *Adv Pharm Bull*. 2023 Jan;13(1):69-78. doi: 10.34172/apb.2023.008. Epub 2022 Jan 4. PMID: 36721811; PMCID: PMC9871277.

6 Van der Kooy, F., et al. "Cannabis smoke condensate II: influence of tobacco on tetrahydrocannabinol levels." *Inhalation toxicology.* vol. 21,2 (2009): 87-90. doi:10.1080/08958370802187296

7 https://www.who.int/news-room/fact-sheets/detail/tobacco

8 Centers for Disease Control and Prevention (US); National Center for Chronic Disease Prevention and Health Promotion (US); Office on Smoking and Health (US). How Tobacco Smoke Causes Disease: The Biology and Behavioral Basis for Smoking-Attributable Disease: A Report of the Surgeon General. Atlanta (GA): Centers for Disease Control and Prevention (US); 2010. 3, Chemistry and Toxicology of Cigarette Smoke and Biomarkers of Exposure and Harm. https://www.ncbi.nlm.nih.gov/books/NBK53014/

9 Jiries, M.A., et al. "Toxicant Formation in Dabbing" *ACS Omega* 2017, 2, 9, 6112–6117 Publication Date:September 22, 2017. https://doi.org/10.1021/acsomega.7b01130

10 McDaniel, C., et al. "Metals in Cannabis Vaporizer Aerosols: Sources, Possible Mechanisms, and Exposure Profiles." *Chemical research in toxicology* vol. 34,11 (2021): 2331-2342. doi:10.1021/acs.chemrestox.1c00230

11 Kirk, R.D., et al. "Evaluations of Skin Permeability of Cannabidiol and Its Topical Formulations by Skin Membrane-Based Parallel Artificial Membrane Permeability Assay and Franz Cell Diffusion Assay." *Med Cannabis Cannabinoids.* 2022 Oct 10;5(1):129-137. doi: 10.1159/000526769. PMID: 36467778; PMCID: PMC9710319.

12 Casiraghi, A., et al. "Topical Administration of Cannabidiol: Influence of Vehicle-Related Aspects on Skin Permeation Process." *Pharmaceuticals (Basel).* 2020 Oct 23;13(11):337. doi: 10.3390/ph13110337. PMID: 33114270; PMCID: PMC7690861.

13 Luz-Veiga, M., et al. "Cannabidiol and Cannabigerol Exert Antimicrobial Activity without Compromising Skin Microbiota." *Int. J. Mol. Sci.* 2023;24:2389. doi: 10.3390/ijms24032389.

CHAPTER 5: SAFETY, ADVERSE EFFECTS, AND OTHER CONSIDERATIONS

1 Schwabe A.L., et al. "Uncomfortably high: Testing reveals inflated THC potency on retail Cannabis labels." *PLOS One.* 2023 Apr 12;18(4):e0282396. doi: 10.1371/journal.pone.0282396. PMID: 37043421; PMCID: PMC10096267.

2 Zandkarimi, F., et al. "Comparison of the Cannabinoid and Terpene Profiles in Commercial Cannabis from Natural and Artificial Cultivation." *Molecules.* 2023 Jan 13;28(2):833. doi: 10.3390/molecules28020833. PMID: 36677891; PMCID: PMC9861703.

3 Alengebawy, A., et al. "Heavy Metals and Pesticides Toxicity in Agricultural Soil and Plants: Ecological Risks and Human Health Implications." *Toxics.* 2021 Feb 25;9(3):42. doi: 10.3390/toxics9030042. PMID: 33668829; PMCID: PMC7996329.

4 McDaniel, C., et al. "Metals in Cannabis Vaporizer Aerosols: Sources, Possible Mechanisms, and Exposure Profiles." *Chem Res Toxicol.* 2021 Nov 15;34(11):2331-2342. doi: 10.1021/acs.chemrestox.1c00230. Epub 2021 Oct 27. PMID: 34705462.

5 Seltenrich, N. "Into the Weeds: Regulating Pesticides in Cannabis." *Environ Health Perspect.* 2019 Apr;127(4):42001. doi: 10.1289/EHP5265. PMID: 31021196; PMCID: PMC6785225.

6 Curran, H. Valerie, et al. "Keep off the Grass? Cannabis, Cognition and Addiction." *Nature Reviews Neuroscience*, vol. 17, 2016, pp. 293–306. Nature, https://doi.org/10.1038/nrn.2016.28.

7 Bonnet, U., et al. "Abstinence phenomena of chronic cannabis-addicts prospectively monitored during controlled inpatient detoxification: cannabis withdrawal syndrome and its correlation with delta-9-tetrahydrocannabinol and -metabolites in serum." *Drug Alcohol Depend*. 2014.

8 Russo, E.B. et al. *"Cannabinoid Hyperemesis Syndrome Survey and Genomic Investigation." Cannabis Cannabinoid Res*. 2022 Jun;7(3):336-344. doi: 10.1089/can.2021.0046. Epub 2021 Jul 5. PMID: 34227878; PMCID: PMC9225400.

9 Kocis, P.T. and Vrana, K. "Delta-9-tetrahydrocannabinol and cannabidiol drug-drug interactions." *Med Cannabis* Cannabinoids. (2020) 3:61–73. doi: 10.1159/000507998

10 Pasha, Ahmed K.., et al. "Cardiovascular Effects of Medical Marijuana: A Systematic Review." *The American Journal of Medicine*, vol. 134, no. 2, 2021, pp. 182–193. Elsevier, https://doi.org/10.1016/j.amjmed.2020.07.012.

11 Radhakrishnan, R., et al. "Acute Effects of Cannabis on Psychosis-Related Outcomes: A Systematic Review." Frontiers in Psychiatry, vol. 5, 2014, *Addictive Disorders Section*, 21 May 2014, https://doi.org/10.3389/fpsyt.2014.00054.

12 Manseau, M. W., and D. C. Goff. "Cannabinoids and Schizophrenia: Risks and Therapeutic Potential." *Neurotherapeutics*, vol. 12, 2015, pp. 816–824, https://doi.org/10.1007/s13311-015-0382-6.

13 Koethe, D., et al. "Anandamide Elevation in Cerebrospinal Fluid in Initial Prodromal States of Psychosis." *The British Journal of Psychiatry*, vol. 194, no. 4, 2009, pp. 371–372, https://doi.org/10.1192/bjp.bp.108.053843.

14 Zuardi, A. W., et al. "Cannabidiol for the treatment of psychosis in Parkinson's disease." *Journal of Psychopharmacology* 23 (8), 979–983. 2009. doi: 10.1177/ 0269881108096519

15 Russo, E. "Cannabis Treatments in Obstetrics and Gynecology: A Historical Review." *Journal of Cannabis Therapeutics*. vol. 2, no. 3-4, 2002, pp. 5–35. https://doi.org/10.1300/J175v02n03_02.

16 Pollan, Michael. *The Botany of Desire : A Plant's Eye View of the World*. New York, Random House, 2002.

17 Grywacheski, V., et al, "Opioid and cannabis use during pregnancy and breastfeeding in relation to sociodemographics and mental health status: A descriptive study." *Journal of Obstetrics and Gynaecology Canada*, 43(3), 329–336. 2021. https://doi.org/10.1016/j.jogc.2020.09.017.

18 Gabrys, R. and Porath, A. Clearing the Smoke on Cannabis: Regular Use and Cognitive Functioning. *Canadian Centre on Substance Use and Addiction*, 2019.

19 Linn, S., et al. "The Association of Marijuana Use with Outcome of Pregnancy." *American Journal of Public Health*, vol. 73, no. 10, Oct. 1983, pp. 1161–1164, https://doi.org/10.2105/ajph.73.10.1161. PMID: 6604464; PMCID: PMC1651077.

20 National Academies of Sciences, Engineering, and Medicine; Health and Medicine Division; Board on Population Health and Public Health Practice; Committee on the Health Effects of Marijuana: An Evidence Review and Research Agenda. The Health Effects of Cannabis and Cannabinoids: The Current State of Evidence and Recommendations for Research. Washington (DC): National Academies Press (US); 2017 Jan 12. 10, Prenatal, Perinatal, and Neonatal Exposure to Cannabis. Available from: https://www.ncbi.nlm.nih.gov/books/NBK425751/

21 Wang, G.S. "Pediatric Concerns Due to Expanded Cannabis Use: Unintended Consequences of Legalization." *J Med Toxicol.* 2017 Mar;13(1):99-105. doi: 10.1007/s13181-016-0552-x. Epub 2016 May 2. PMID: 27139708; PMCID: PMC5330955.

22 Gaitán, A.V., et al., "Endocannabinoid Metabolome Characterization of Transitional and Mature Human Milk." *Nutrients.* 2018 Sep 12;10(9):1294. doi: 10.3390/nu10091294. PMID: 30213124; PMCID: PMC6165354.

23 US Department of Transportation. National Highway Traffic Safety Administration. State of Knowledge of Drugged Driving: FINAL REPORT. op. cit. Other summaries include: Ramaekers et al. 2006. Cognition and motor control as a function of Delta-9-THC concentration in serum and oral fluid: Limits of impairment. Drug and Alcohol Dependence 85: 114-122; David Hadorn. "A Review of Cannabis and Driving Skills," In: The Medicinal Uses of Cannabis and Cannabinoids. (eds: Guy et al). Pharmaceutical Press, 2004; Canadian Senate Special Committee on Illegal Drugs, Cannabis: Summary Report: Our Position for a Canadian Public Policy. 2002. (See specifically: Chapter 8: "Driving Under the Influence of Cannabis"); Alison Smiley. "Marijuana: On-Road and Driving-Simulator Studies," In: The Health Effects of Cannabis. (eds. Kalant et al) Canadian Centre for Addiction and Mental Health, 1999.

24 Ménétrey, A., et al. "Assessment of driving capability through the use of clinical and psychomotor tests in relation to blood cannabinoids levels following oral administration of 20 mg dronabinol or of a cannabis decoction made with 20 or 60 mg Delta9-THC." *Journal of analytical toxicology* vol. 29,5 (2005): 327-38. doi:10.1093/jat/29.5.327

25 Skopp, G., et al. "Cannabinoidbefunde im Serum 24 bis 48 Stunden nach Rauchkonsum" [Serum cannabinoid levels 24 to 48 hours after cannabis smoking]. *Archiv fur Kriminologie* vol. 212,3-4 (2003): 83-95.

Toennes, S.W., et al. "Comparison of cannabinoid pharmacokinetic properties in occasional and heavy users smoking a marijuana or placebo joint." *Journal of analytical toxicology* vol. 32,7 (2008): 470-7. doi:10.1093/jat/32.7.470

Karschner, E. L., et al. "Do Delta9-tetrahydrocannabinol concentrations indicate recent use in chronic cannabis users?." *Addiction* (Abingdon, England) vol. 104,12 (2009): 2041-8. doi:10.1111/j.1360-0443.2009.02705.x

26 National Highway Traffic Safety Administration, Fatalities and Fatality Rates By State, 1994-2009. Online document access September 6, 2011.

27 Zhao, S., et al. "The effect of cannabis edibles on driving and blood THC." *J Cannabis Res.* 2024 May 31;6(1):26. doi: 10.1186/s42238-024-00234-y. PMID: 38822413; PMCID: PMC11140993.

28 Ramaekers, J.G., et al. "Tolerance and cross-tolerance to neurocognitive effects of THC and alcohol in heavy cannabis users." *Psychopharmacology* 214: 391-401. 2010.

29 Ramaekers, J.G., et al. "Dose related risk of motor vehicle crashes after cannabis use." *Drug and Alcohol Dependence* 73: 109-119. 2004.

30 Herkenham, M., et al. "Cannabinoid receptor localization in brain." *Proc Natl Acad Sci U S A.* 1990 Mar;87(5):1932-6. doi: 10.1073/pnas.87.5.1932. PMID: 2308954; PMCID: PMC53598.

CHAPTER 6: THE MANY MEDICINAL USES OF CANNABIS

1 Stromsnes, K., et al. "Anti-Inflammatory Properties of Diet: Role in Healthy Aging." *Biomedicines*, 9(8), Jul 30 2021:922. doi: 10.3390/biomedicines9080922. PMID: 34440125; PMCID: PMC8389628.

2 Chiurchiù, V., et al. "The Differential Characterization of GPR55 Receptor in Human Peripheral Blood Reveals a Distinctive Expression in Monocytes and NK Cells and a Proinflammatory Role in These Innate Cells." *Int. Immunol* 27 (3), 2015, 153–160. 10.1093/intimm/dxu097.

3 Anil, SM., et al. "Medical Cannabis Activity Against Inflammation: Active Compounds and Modes of Action." *Front Pharmacol* 13:908198, May 9 2022. doi: 10.3389/fphar.2022.908198. PMID: 35614947; PMCID: PMC9124761.

4 Correa, F., et al. "A Role for CB2 Receptors in Anandamide Signalling Pathways Involved in the Regulation of IL-12 and IL-23 in Microglial Cells." *Biochem Pharmacol* 77 (1), 2009, 86–100. 10.1016/j.bcp.2008.09.014

5 Capozzi, A., et al. "Anti-inflammatory Activity of a CB2 Selective Cannabinoid Receptor Agonist: Signaling and Cytokines Release in Blood Mononuclear Cells." *Molecules,* 27 (1), 2021, 64. 10.3390/molecules27010064.

6 Sangiovanni, E., et al. "Cannabis Sativa L. Extract and Cannabidiol Inhibit In Vitro Mediators of Skin Inflammation and Wound Injury." *Phytother.* Res. 33 (8), 2019, 2083–2093. 10.1002/ptr.6400.

7 Gaffal, E., et al. "Anti-inflammatory Activity of Topical THC in DNFB-Mediated Mouse Allergic Contact Dermatitis Independent of CB1 and CB2 Receptors." *Allergy* 68 (8), 2013, 994–1000. 10.1111/all.12183.

8 Gugliandolo, A., et al. "In Vitro model of Neuroinflammation: Efficacy of Cannabigerol, a Non-psychoactive Cannabinoid." *Int. J. Mol. Sci.* 19 (7), 2018, 1992. 10.3390/ijms19071992.

Cuttler, C., et al. "A Naturalistic Examination of the Perceived Effects of Cannabis on Negative Affect." *Journal of Affective Disorders*, vol. 235, 1 Aug. 2018, pp. 198–205, https://doi.org/10.1016/j.jad.2018.04.054. PMID: 29656267.

9 Childs, E., et al. "Dose-related effects of delta-9-THC on emotional responses to acute psychosocial stress." *Drug Alcohol Depend* 177, 2017, 136-144. doi:10.1016/j.drugalcdep.2017.03.030.

10 Somaini, L., et al. "Psychobiological responses to unpleasant emotions in cannabis users." *Eur Arch Psychiatry Clin Neurosci* 262(1), 2012, 47–57. doi:10.1007/s00406-011-0223-5.

11 Le, K., et al. "The Role of Medicinal Cannabis as an Emerging Therapy for Opioid Use Disorder." *Pain Ther* 13, 2024, 435–455. https://doi.org/10.1007/s40122-024-00599-1.

12 Raman, S. and Bradford, A.C. "Recreational cannabis legalizations associated with reductions in prescription drug utilization among Medicaid enrollees." *Health economics* 31(7) 2022, 1513-1521. doi:10.1002/hec.4519.

13 Reiman, A. "Cannabis as a substitute for alcohol and other drugs." *Harm Reduct J* 6, 2009 35. https://doi.org/10.1186/1477-7517-6-35.

14 Bachhuber, M.A., et al. "Medical Cannabis Laws and Opioid Analgesic Overdose Mortality in the United States, 1999-2010." *JAMA Intern Med.* 2014,174(10).1668 1673. doi:10.1001/jamainternmed.2014.4005.

15 Naef M., et al. "The analgesic effect of oral delta-9-tetrahydrocannabinol (THC), morphine, and a THC-morphine combination in healthy subjects under experimental pain conditions." *Pain*, 105 (1–2), 2003, pp. 79-88. doi:10.1016/s0304-3959(03)00163-5.

16 Pertwee, R.G., et al. "International Union of Basic and Clinical Pharmacology. LXXIX. Cannabinoid receptors and their ligands: beyond CB1 and CB2." *Pharmacological Reviews*, 62 (4), 2010, pp. 588-631. doi:10.1124/pr.110.003004.

17 Zhang, L.R., et al. "Cannabis and Respiratory Disease Research Group of New Zealand; Brhane Y, Liu G, Hung RJ. Cannabis smoking and lung cancer risk: Pooled analysis in the International Lung Cancer Consortium." *Int J Cancer*. 2015 Feb 15;136(4):894-903. doi: 10.1002/ijc.29036. Epub 2014 Jun 30. PMID: 24947688; PMCID: PMC4262725.

18 Khan, M.I., et al. "The therapeutic aspects of the endocannabinoid system (ECS) for cancer and their development: From nature to laboratory." *Curr. Pharm. Des*. 2016;22:1756–1766. doi:10.2174/1381612822666151211094901.

19 Melck, D., et al. "Suppression of nerve growth factor Trk receptors and prolactin receptors by endocannabinoids leads to inhibition of human breast and prostate cancer cell proliferation." *Endocrinology*. 2000;141:118–126. doi: 10.1210/endo.141.1.7239v.

20 Ramer, R. and Hinz, B. "Antitumorigenic targets of cannabinoids–Current status and implications." *Expert Opin. Ther. Targets*. 2016;20:1219–1235. doi: 10.1080/14728222.2016.1177512.

21 Huang, M., et al. Terpenoids: natural products for cancer therapy" *Expert opinion on investigational drugs* 21,12, 2012, 1801-18. doi:10.1517/13543784.2012.727395.

22 Matsuo, A.L., et al. "α-Pinene isolated from Schinus terebinthifolius Raddi (Anacardiaceae) induces apoptosis and confers antimetastatic protection in a melanoma model." *Biochem Biophys Res Commun*. 2011;411(2):449–454.

23 Yang, H., et al. "α-Pinene, a major constituent of pine tree oils, enhances non-rapid eye movement sleep in mice through GABAA-benzodiazepine receptors." *Mol Pharmacol*. 2016;90(5):530–539. doi: 10.1124/mol.116.105080.

24 Park, K.R., et al. "β-Caryophyllene oxide inhibits growth and induces apoptosis through the suppression of PI3K/AKT/mTOR/S6K1 pathways and ROS-mediated MAPKs activation." *Cancer Lett*. 2011;312(2):178–188.

25 Thomas, A.A., et al. "Association between cannabis use and the risk of bladder cancer: results from the California Men's Health Study." *Urology*. 2015 Feb;85(2):388-92. doi: 10.1016/j.urology.2014.08.060. Epub 2014 Nov 1. PMID: 25623697.

26 Tomko, A.M., et al. "Anti-cancer properties of cannflavin A and potential synergistic effects with gemcitabine, cisplatin, and cannabinoids in bladder cancer." *J Cannabis Res*. 2022 Jul 22;4(1):41. doi: 10.1186/s42238-022-00151-y. PMID: 35869542; PMCID: PMC9306207.

27 Gurney, J., et al. "Cannabis exposure and risk of testicular cancer: a systematic review and meta-analysis." *BMC Cancer*. 2015 Nov 11;15:897. doi: 10.1186/s12885-015-1905-6. PMID: 26560314; PMCID: PMC4642772.

28 Gojani, E.G., et al. "Anti-Inflammatory Effects of Minor Cannabinoids CBC, THCV, and CBN in Human Macrophages." *Molecules*. 2023, 28, 6487. https://doi.org/10.3390/molecules28186487

29 Mlost, J., et al. "Cannabidiol for Pain Treatment: Focus on Pharmacology and Mechanism of Action." *Int J Mol Sci*. 2020 Nov 23;21(22):8870. doi: 10.3390/ijms21228870. PMID: 33238607; PMCID: PMC7700528.

30 Louis-Gray, K., et al. "TRPV1: A Common Denominator Mediating Antinociceptive and Antiemetic Effects of Cannabinoids." *International journal of molecular sciences* vol. 23,17 10016. 2 Sep. 2022, doi:10.3390/ijms231710016

31 Berliocchi, L., et al. "(-)-Linalool attenuates allodynia in neuropathic pain induced by spinal nerve ligation in c57/bl6 mice." *International review of neurobiology* vol. 85 (2009): 221-35. doi:10.1016/S0074-7742(09)85017-4

32 McDougall J.J. and McKenna, M.K. "Anti-Inflammatory and Analgesic Properties of the Cannabis Terpene Myrcene in Rat Adjuvant Monoarthritis." *Int J Mol Sci.* 2022 Jul 17;23(14):7891. doi: 10.3390/ijms23147891. PMID: 35887239; PMCID: PMC9319952.

33 Lurie, J., et al. "Visualizing Global Chronic Pain." *Anesthesia & Analgesia* 138(4):p 918-919, April 2024. | DOI: 10.1213/ANE.0000000000006564

34 Woodhams, S.G., et al "The Role of the Endocannabinoid System in Pain." *Schaible, HG. (eds) Pain Control. Handbook of Experimental Pharmacology*, vol 227. 2015. Springer, Berlin, Heidelberg. https://doi.org/10.1007/978-3-662-46450-2_7

35 Hameed, M., et al. "Medical Cannabis for Chronic Nonmalignant Pain Management." *Curr Pain Headache Rep.* 2023 Apr;27(4):57-63. doi: 10.1007/s11916-023-01101-w. Epub 2023 Mar 10. PMID: 36897501; PMCID: PMC9999073.

36 Kiesel, L., M. Vogel, Q. K. Le, and S. D. Schäfer. "Pathogenesis of Endometriosis: Progesterone Resistance in Women with Endometriosis." *Endometriosis and Adenomyosis*, edited by E. Oral, Springer, Cham, 2022, https://doi.org/10.1007/978-3-030-97236-3_7

37 Andrade M.A., et al. "The Effect of Neuromodulatory Drugs on the Intensity of Chronic Pelvic Pain in Women: A Systematic Review." *Rev. Bras. Hematol. Hemoter.* 2022;44:891–898. doi: 10.1055/s-0042-1755459.

38 Walker, O.S., et al. "The role of the endocannabinoid system in female reproductive tissues." *J. Ovarian Res.* 2019;12:3. doi: 10.1186/s13048-018-0478-9.

Dmitrieva, N., et al. "Endocannabinoid Involvement in Endometriosis." *Pain*, vol. 151, no. 3, Dec. 2010, pp. 703–710. https://doi.org/10.1016/j.pain.2010.08.037. Accessed Sept. 15, 2010. PMID: 20833475; PMCID: PMC2972363.

39 Hirao, M., et al. "Plasma Levels of Endocannabinoids and Related N-Acylethanolamines in Women with Endometriosis." *Journal of Clinical Endocrinology & Metabolism.* 2012

40 Fernandes, E.S., et al. "The functions of TRPA1 and TRPV1: moving away from sensory nerves." *Br J Pharmacol.* 2012;166(2):510-521.

41 Bisogno, T., et al. "Molecular targets for cannabidiol and its synthetic analogues: effect on vanilloid VR1 receptors and on the cellular uptake and enzymatic hydrolysis of anandamide." *Br J Pharmacol.* 2001;134:845–852

42 Crowley, K., et al. "Effects of Cannabinoids on Intestinal Motility, Barrier Permeability, and Therapeutic Potential in Gastrointestinal Diseases." *Int. J. Mol. Sci.* 2024, 25, 6682. https://doi.org/10.3390/ijms25126682

43 Wright, K., et al. "Differential expression of cannabinoid receptors in the human colon: Cannabinoids promote epithelial wound healing." *Gastroenterology.* 2005;129:437–453. doi: 10.1016/j.gastro.2005.05.026.

44 Ahmed, W. and Seymour, K. "Therapeutic Use of Cannabis in Inflammatory Bowel Disease." *Gastroenterology & Hepatology*, vol. 12, no. 11, Nov. 2016, pp. 668–679. PMID: 28035196; PMCID: PMC5193087.

45 Alhamoruni, A., et al. "Cannabinoids mediate opposing effects on inflammation-induced intestinal permeability." *British journal of pharmacology* vol. 165,8 (2012): 2598-610. doi:10.1111/j.1476-5381.2011.01589.x

46 Alhamoruni, A., et al. "Cannabinoids mediate opposing effects on inflammation-induced intestinal permeability." *British journal of pharmacology* vol. 165,8 (2012): 2598-610. doi:10.1111/j.1476-5381.2011.01589.x

47 D'Argenio, G., et al. "Up-regulation of anandamide levels as an endogenous mechanism and a pharmacological strategy to limit colon inflammation." *FASEB J.* 2006;20:568–570.

48 Izzo, A.A., et al. "Cannabinoid CB1-receptor mediated regulation of gastrointestinal motility in mice in a model of intestinal inflammation." *Br J Pharmacol.* 2001;134:563–570.

49 Croci, T., et al. "Role of cannabinoid CB1 receptors and tumor necrosis factor-alpha in the gut and systemic anti-inflammatory activity of SR 141716 (rimonabant) in rodents." *Br J Pharmacol.* 2003;140:115–122.

50 Wright, K.L., et al. "Cannabinoid CB2 receptors in the gastrointestinal tract: a regulatory system in states of inflammation." *Br J Pharmacol.* 2008;153:263–270.

51 Marquéz, L., et al. "Ulcerative colitis induces changes on the expression of the endocannabinoid system in the human colonic tissue." *PLoS One.* 2009;4:e6893. doi: 10.1371/journal.pone.000

52 Duncan, M., et al. "Cannabinoid CB2 receptors in the enteric nervous system modulate gastrointestinal contractility in lipopolysaccharide-treated rats." *Am J Physiol Gastrointest Liver Physiol.* 2008;295:G78–G87. doi: 10.1152/ajpgi.90285.2008

53 Ihenetu, K., et al. "Inhibition of interleukin-8 release in the human colonic epithelial cell line HT-29 by cannabinoids. *Eur J Pharmacol.* 2003;458:207–215.

54 Mathison, R., et al. "Effects of cannabinoid receptor-2 activation on accelerated gastrointestinal transit in lipopolysaccharide-treated rats." *Br J Pharmacol.* 2004;142:1247–1254.

55 Yu, X., et al. "TRP channel functions in the gastrointestinal tract." *Semin Immunopathol* 38, 385–396 (2016). https://doi.org/10.1007/s00281-015-0528-y

56 Naftali .T., et al. "Cannabis induces a clinical response in patients with crohn's disease: a prospective placebo-controlled study." *Clin Gastroenterol Hepatol.* 2013;11(10):1276–1280.e1. doi: 10.1016/j.cgh.2013.04.034

57 Nicolodi, M., et al. "Fibromyalgia and headache. Failure of serotonergic analgesia and N-methyl-D-aspartate-mediated neuronal plasticity: their common clues." *Cephalalgia.* 1998;18(Suppl 21):41–44

58 Chang, F.Y. and Lu, C.L. "Irritable bowel syndrome and migraine: bystanders or partners?" *J Neurogastroenterol Motil.* 2013 Jul;19(3):301-11. doi: 10.5056/jnm.2013.19.3.301. Epub 2013 Jul 8. PMID: 23875096; PMCID: PMC3714407.

59 Richardson, J.D., et al. "Hypoactivity of the spinal cannabinoid system results in NMDA-dependent hyperalgesia." *J Neurosci.* 1998;18:451–457

60 Ware, M.A., et al. "The effects of nabilone on sleep in fibromyalgia: results of a randomized controlled trial. *Anesth Analg.* 2010;110:604–610

61 Fiz, J., et al. "Cannabis use in patients with fibromyalgia: effect on symptoms relief and health-related quality of life." *PLoS One.* 2011;6:e18440.

62 van de Donk, T., et al. "An experimental randomized study on the analgesic effects of pharmaceutical-grade cannabis in chronic pain patients with fibromyalgia." *Pain vol.* 160,4 (2019): 860-869. doi:10.1097/j.pain.0000000000001464

63 Del Giorno, R., et al. "Palmitoylethanolamide in Fibromyalgia: Results from Prospective and Retrospective Observational Studies." *Pain and therapy* vol. 4,2 (2015): 169-78. doi:10.1007/s40122-015-0038-6

64 Raggi, A., et al. "Hallmarks of Primary Headache: Part 1 – Migraine." *The Journal of Headache and Pain*, vol. 25, 2024, p. 189, https://doi.org/10.1186/s10194-024-01889-x.

65 Rossi, M., et al. "Sex and Gender Differences in Migraines: A Narrative Review." *Neurological Sciences*, vol. 43, 2022, pp. 5729–5734, https://doi.org/10.1007/s10072-022-06178-6.

66 Hoffmann, J., and Charles, A. "Glutamate and Its Receptors as Therapeutic Targets for Migraine." *Neurotherapeutics*, vol. 15, 2018, pp. 361–370, https://doi.org/10.1007/s13311-018-0616-5.

67 Poudel, S., et al. Medical Cannabis, Headaches, and Migraines: A Review of the Current Literature. *Cureus.* 2021 Aug 24;13(8):e17407. doi: 10.7759/cureus.17407. PMID: 34589318; PMCID: PMC8459575.

68 Ceccarelli, I., et al. "Frontiers in Neuroscience, Neuropharmacology Section." *Frontiers in Neuroscience*, vol. 14, 17 Aug. 2020, https://doi.org/10.3389/fnins.2020.00850.

69 LeBlanc, Erin S., et al. "Insomnia Is Associated with an Increased Risk of Type 2 Diabetes in the Clinical Setting." *BMJ Open Diabetes Research & Care*, vol. 6, 2018, e000604, https://doi.org/10.1136/bmjdrc-2018-000604.

70 Liu, Y., et al. "Association between perceived insufficient sleep, frequent mental distress, obesity and chronic diseases among US adults, 2009 behavioral risk factor surveillance system." *BMC Public Health* 13, 84 (2013). https://doi.org/10.1186/1471-2458-13-84

71 Hombali, A., et al. "Prevalence and Correlates of Sleep Disorder Symptoms in Psychiatric Disorders." *Psychiatry Research*, vol. 279, 2019, pp. 116–122, https://doi.org/10.1016/j.psychres.2019.02.041.

72 Edwards, D and Filbey, F.M. "Are Sweet Dreams Made of These? Understanding the Relationship Between Sleep and Cannabis Use." *Cannabis Cannabinoid Res.* 2021 Dec;6(6):462-473. doi: 10.1089/can.2020.0174. Epub 2021 Jun 18. PMID: 34143657; PMCID: PMC8713269.

73 Morena, M., et al. "Endogenous Cannabinoid Release within Prefrontal-Limbic Pathways Affects Memory Consolidation of Emotional Training." *Proc. Natl. Acad. Sci. USA.* 2014;111:18333–18338. doi: 10.1073/pnas.1420285111.

74 Kaul, M., et al. "Effects of Cannabinoids on Sleep and their Therapeutic Potential for Sleep Disorders." *Neurotherapeutics* 18, 217–227 (2021). https://doi.org/10.1007/s13311-021-01013-w

75 DeLarge A.F. and Winsauer P.J. "Effects of Δ9-THC on Memory in Ovariectomized and Intact Female Rats." *Horm. Behav.* 2021;127:104883. doi: 10.1016/j.yhbeh.2020.104883.

76 Kaul, M., et al. "Effects of Cannabinoids on Sleep and their Therapeutic Potential for Sleep Disorders." *Neurotherapeutics* 18, 217–227 (2021). https://doi.org/10.1007/s13311-021-01013-w

77 Nicholson, Anthony N., et al. "Effect of Delta-9-tetrahydrocannabinol and cannabidiol on nocturnal sleep and early-morning behavior in young adults." *Journal of clinical psychopharmacology* vol. 24,3 (2004): 305-13. doi:10.1097/01.jcp.0000125688.05091.8f

78 Carlini EA, Cunha JM. Hypnotic and antiepileptic effects of cannabidiol. J Clin Pharmacol. 1981 Aug-Sep;21(S1):417S-427S. doi: 10.1002/j.1552-4604.1981.tb02622.x. PMID: 7028792.

79 Linck V.M., et al. "Effects of inhaled Linalool in anxiety, social interaction and aggressive behavior in mice." *Phytomedicine.* 2010 Jul;17(8-9):679-83. doi: 10.1016/j.phymed.2009.10.002. Epub 2009 Dec 3. PMID: 19962290.

80 Lee, B.K., et al. "Linalool Ameliorates Memory Loss and Behavioral Impairment Induced by REM-Sleep Deprivation through the Serotonergic Pathway." *Biomolecules & therapeutics* vol. 26,4 (2018): 368-373. doi:10.4062/biomolther.2018.081

81 O'Brien, K and Blair, P. "Routes of Administration, Pharmacokinetics and Safety of Medicinal Cannabis." *Medicinal Cannabis and CBD in Mental Healthcare.* (2021) Springer, Cham. https://doi.org/10.1007/978-3-030-78559-8_11

82 Zipursky, Jonathan S., et al. "Edible cannabis." *CMAJ : Canadian Medical Association journal = journal de l'Association medicale canadienne* vol. 192,7 (2020): E162. doi:10.1503/cmaj.191305

83 Marsicano, G., et al. "The endogenous cannabinoid system controls extinction of aversive memories." *Nature.* 2002;418(6897):530–4.

84 Neumeister, A., et al. "Elevated brain cannabinoid CB receptor availability in post-traumatic stress disorder: a positron emission tomography study." *Mol Psychiatry.* 2013;18(9):6.

85 Carr, M., et al. "Reduced REM Sleep Percent in Frequent Cannabis Versus Non-Cannabis Users." *Sleep* vol. 43, suppl. 1, Apr. 2020, pp. A62–A63, https://doi.org/10.1093/sleep/zsaa056.157.

86 Fraser, G.A. "The use of a synthetic cannabinoid in the management of treatment-resistant nightmares in posttraumatic stress disorder (PTSD)." *CNS neuroscience & therapeutics* vol. 15,1 (2009): 84-8. doi:10.1111/j.1755-5949.2008.00071.x

87 Passie, T., et al. "Mitigation of post-traumatic stress symptoms by Cannabis resin: a review of the clinical and neurobiological evidence." *Drug Test Anal.* 2012;4(7–8):649–59.

88 Budney, Alan J., et al. "Review of the validity and significance of cannabis withdrawal syndrome." *The American journal of psychiatry* vol. 161,11 (2004): 1967-77. doi:10.1176/appi.ajp.161.11.1967

89 Kaul, M., et al. "Effects of Cannabinoids on Sleep and their Therapeutic Potential for Sleep Disorders." *Neurotherapeutics 18*, 217–227 (2021). https://doi.org/10.1007/s13311-021-01013-w

90 Salari, N., et al. "Global prevalence of sleep disorders during menopause: a meta-analysis." *Sleep & breathing = Schlaf & Atmung* vol. 27,5 (2023): 1883-1897. doi:10.1007/s11325-023-02793-5

91 Slavin, M.N., et al. "Expectancy mediated effects of marijuana on menopause symptoms." *Addict Res Theory* 2016;24:322–329. doi: 10.3109/16066359.2016.1139701

92 Stanley, C., et al. "O'Sullivan SE. Vascular targets for cannabinoids: animal and human studies. "*Br J Pharmacol* 2014;171:1361–1378. doi: 10.1111/bph.12560

93 Childs, E., et al. "Dose-related effects of delta-9-THC on emotional responses to acute psychosocial stress." *Drug Alcohol Depend.* 2017 Aug 1;177:136-144. doi: 10.1016/j.drugalcdep.2017.03.030. Epub 2017 May 30. PMID: 28599212; PMCID: PMC6349031.

94 Linares, I.M., et al. "Cannabidiol presents an inverted U-shaped dose-response curve in a simulated public speaking test." *Braz J Psychiatry.* 2019 Jan-Feb;41(1):9-14. doi: 10.1590/1516-4446-2017-0015. Epub 2018 Oct 11. PMID: 30328956; PMCID: PMC6781714.

95 Langlois, C., et al. "Down and High: Reflections Regarding Depression and Cannabis." *Front Psychiatry.* 2021 May 14;12:625158. doi: 10.3389/fpsyt.2021.625158. PMID: 34054594; PMCID: PMC8160288.

96 Yoshida, K., et al. "Inhalation of a racemic mixture (R, S)-linalool by rats experiencing restraint stress alters neuropeptide and MHC class I gene expression in the hypothalamus" *Neurosci. Lett.*, 653 (2017), pp. 314-3

97 Piccinelli, A.C., et al. "Antihyperalgesic and antidepressive actions of (R)-( )-limonene, α-phellandrene, and essential oil from Schinus terebinthifolius fruits in a neuropathic pain model." *Nutr. Neurosci.*, 18 (2015), pp. 217-22

98 Su, T., et al. "Endocannabinoid System Unlocks the Puzzle of Autism Treatment via Microglia." *Front Psychiatry.* 2021 Oct 22;12:734837. doi: 10.3389/fpsyt.2021.734837. PMID: 34744824; PMCID: PMC8568770.

99 Silva, E.A.D. Junior, et al. "Cannabis and cannabinoid use in autism spectrum disorder: a systematic review." *Trends in psychiatry and psychotherapy* vol. 44 e20200149. 13 Jun. 2022, doi:10.47626/2237-6089-2020-0149

100 Aran, A., et al. "Lower circulating endocannabinoid levels in children with autism spectrum disorder." *Mol. Autism.* 2019;10:1–11. doi: 10.1186/s13229-019-0256-6.

Aran, A., Eylon M., et al "Lower circulating endocannabinoid levels in children with autism spectrum disorder." *Mol. Autism.* 2019;10:1–11. doi: 10.1186/s13229-019-0256-6.

101 Thomas, R., et al. "Prevalence of attention-deficit/hyperactivity disorder: a systematic review and meta-analysis." *Pediatrics.* 2015;135:e994–1001.

102 Cooper, R.E., et al. "Cannabinoids inattention-deficit/hyperactivity disorder: a randomised-controlled trial." *Eur Neuropsychopharmacol.* 2017;27:795–808.

103 Cooper, R.E., et al. "Cannabinoids inattention-deficit/hyperactivity disorder: a randomised-controlled trial." *Eur Neuropsychopharmacol.* 2017;27:795–808.

104 Greer G.R., et al. " PTSD symptom reports of patients evaluated for the New Mexico Medical Cannabis Program." *J Psychoact Drugs.* 2014;46(1):73–7.

105 Parker, L. *Cannabinoids and the Brain.* Cambridge, Massachusetts, The Mit Press, 2018.

106 Sylantyev, S., et al. "Cannabinoid- and lysophosphatidylinositol-sensitive receptor GPR55 boosts neurotransmitter release at central synapses." *Proceedings of the National Academy of Sciences of the United States of America* vol. 110,13 (2013): 5193-8. doi:10.1073/pnas.1211204110

107 Kaczor, E.E., et al. "The Potential Proconvulsant Effects of Cannabis: a Scoping Review." *J. Med. Toxicol.* 18, 223–234 (2022). https://doi.org/10.1007/s13181-022-00886-3

108 de Oliveira, Cleide Correia., et al. "Anticonvulsant activity of β-caryophyllene against pentylenetetrazol-induced seizures." *Epilepsy & behavior : E&B* vol. 56 (2016): 26-31. doi:10.1016/j.yebeh.2015.12.040

109 de Oliveira, Cleide Correia., et al. "Anticonvulsant activity of β-caryophyllene against pentylenetetrazol-induced seizures." *Epilepsy & behavior : E&B* vol. 56 (2016): 26-31. doi:10.1016/j.yebeh.2015.12.040

110 de Oliveira, Cleide Correia., et al. "Anticonvulsant activity of β-caryophyllene against pentylenetetrazol-induced seizures." *Epilepsy & behavior : E&B* vol. 56 (2016): 26-31. doi:10.1016/j.yebeh.2015.12.040

111 Limebeer, C. L., et al. "Inverse agonism of cannabinoid CB1 receptors potentiates LiCl-induced nausea in the conditioned gaping model in rats." *British journal of pharmacology* vol. 161,2 (2010): 336-49. doi:10.1111/j.1476-5381.2010.00885.x

112 Maresz, K., et al. "Direct suppression of CNS autoimmune inflammation via the cannabinoid receptor CB1 on neurons and CB2 on autoreactive T cells." *Nat Med.* 2007;13:492–497. doi: 10.1038/nm1561

113 Kishimoto, S., et al. "2-Arachidonoylglycerol, an endogenous cannabinoid receptor ligand, induces accelerated production of chemokines in HL-60 cells." *J Biochem.* 2004;135:517–524. doi: 10.1093/jb/mvh063

114 Kishimoto, S., et al. "2-Arachidonoylglycerol, an endogenous cannabinoid receptor ligand, induces accelerated production of chemokines in HL-60 cells." *J Biochem.* 2004;135:517–524. doi: 10.1093/jb/mvh063

115 Giorgi, V., et al. "Cannabis and Autoimmunity: Possible Mechanisms of Action." *Immunotargets Ther.* 2021 Jul 21;10:261-271. doi: 10.2147/ITT.S267905. PMID: 34322454; PMCID: PMC8313508.

Nuutinen, T. "Medicinal properties of terpenes found in Cannabis sativa and Humulus lupulus." European journal of medicinal chemistry vol. 157 (2018): 198-228. doi:10.1016/j.ejmech.2018.07.076

116 Paolicelli, D., et al. "Long-term data of efficacy, safety, and tolerability in a real-life setting of THC/CBD oromucosal spray-treated multiple sclerosis patients." *J Clin Pharmacol.* 2016;56:845–851. doi:

117 Zettl U.K., et al. "Evidence for the efficacy and effectiveness of THC-CBD oromucosal spray in symptom management of patients with spasticity due to multiple sclerosis." *Ther Adv Neurol Disord.* 2016;9:9–30. doi: 10.1177/1756285615612659

Klein, T.W., et al. "Delta 9-tetrahydrocannabinol treatment suppresses immunity and early IFN-gamma, IL-12, and IL-12 receptor beta 2 responses to Legionella pneumophila infection." *J Immunol.* 2000 Jun 15;164(12):6461-6. doi: 10.4049/jimmunol.164.12.6461. PMID: 10843702.

118 Webb, M., et al. "Genetic deletion of Fatty Acid Amide Hydrolase results in improved long-term outcome in chronic autoimmune encephalitis." *Neurosci Lett.* 2008;439:106–110. doi: 10.1016/j.neulet.2008.04.090

119 Vrechi, T.A., et al. "Cannabinoid Receptor Type 1 Agonist ACEA Protects Neurons from Death and Attenuates Endoplasmic Reticulum Stress-Related Apoptotic Pathway Signaling." *Neurotox Res.* 2018 May;33(4):846-855. doi: 10.1007/s12640-017-9839-1. Epub 2017 Nov 13. PMID: 29134561.

120 Sarne Y., et al. "Reversal of age-related cognitive impairments in mice by an extremely low dose of tetrahydrocannabinol." *Neurobiol Aging.* 2018 Jan;61:177-186. doi: 10.1016/j.neurobiolaging.2017.09.025. Epub 2017 Oct 6. PMID: 29107185.

121 Aghazadeh, M., et al. "Medicinal chemistry, pharmacology, and potential therapeutic benefits of cannabinoid CB2 receptor agonists" *Chem. Rev.*, 116 (2016), pp. 519-560

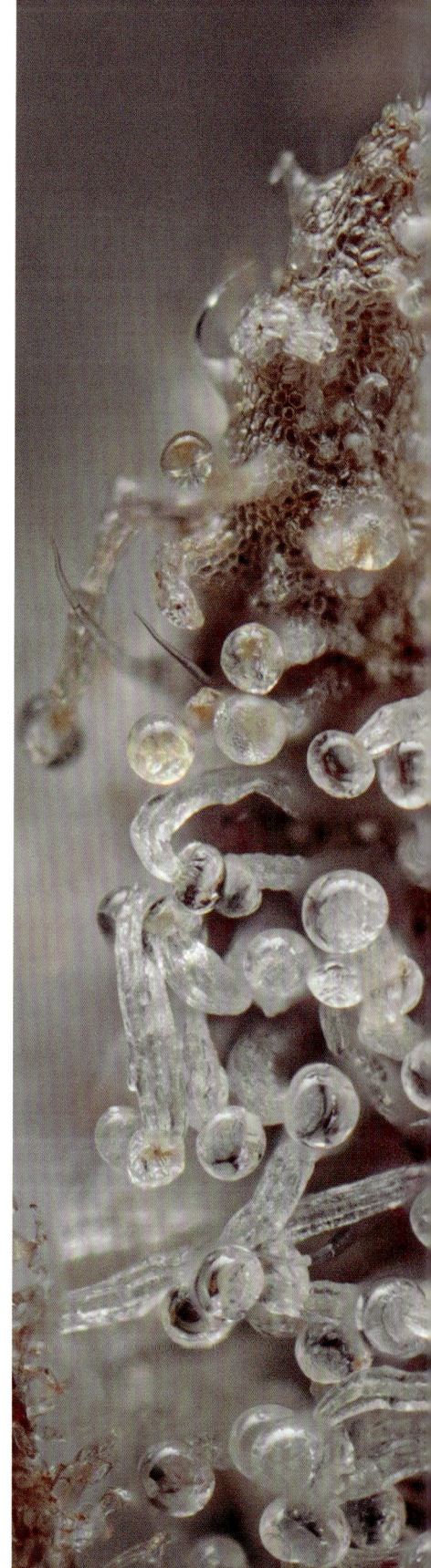

122 Viveros-Paredes, Juan M., et al. "Neuroprotective Effects of β-Caryophyllene against Dopaminergic Neuron Injury in a Murine Model of Parkinson's Disease Induced by MPTP." *Pharmaceuticals* (Basel, Switzerland) vol. 10,3 60. 6 Jul. 2017, doi:10.3390/ph10030060

CHAPTER 7: TOLERANCE

1 Neumeister, A., et al. "Elevated brain cannabinoid CB1 receptor availability in post-traumatic stress disorder: a positron emission tomography study." *Molecular Psychiatry*, 2013; DOI: 10.1038/mp.2013.61.

2 Neumeister, A., et al. "Elevated brain cannabinoid CB1 receptor availability in post-traumatic stress disorder: a positron emission tomography study." *Molecular Psychiatry*, 2013; DOI: 10.1038/mp.2013.61.

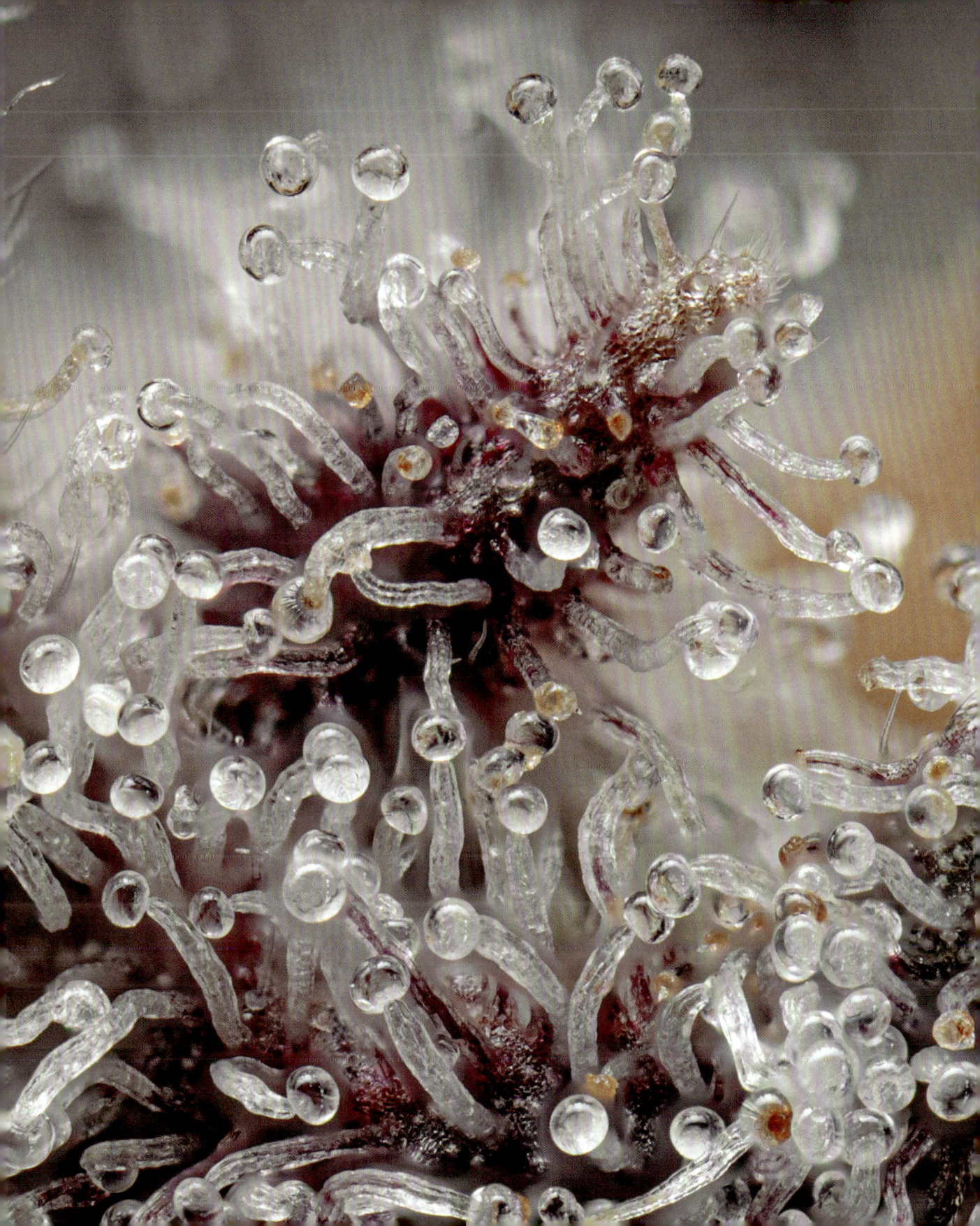

ACKNOWLEDGMENTS

My perspective on cannabis is shaped not only by my personal experiences and knowledge but also by the countless unique stories and emotional connections people share with this plant every day. These narratives have profoundly influenced my understanding of cannabis's impact on human lives. I am deeply grateful to the hundreds of thousands of individuals on social media who have shared their personal journeys, offering a glimpse into their worlds of healing. Your voices have transformed the way I teach about cannabis and approach its use as a personalized medicine.

This book was born from this vibrant online community. I owe a heartfelt thanks to Jane Kinney Denning, who reached out, encouraged me to write the proposal, and helped make this vision a reality. For years, we dreamed of this book before it was even a possibility. Thank you as well to the other amazing team members that contributed to the art and vision of this book—from the various editors, reviewers, and illustrators that turned some high thoughts into a work of art. This non-inclusive list includes Molly Ahuja, Lindsay Dobbs, and Mallory Heyer.

I am immensely grateful to Dr. Matthew Bertin, my mentor and advisor, whose resources, guidance, and encouragement allowed me to delve deeply into the complexities of natural product chemistry. Your challenges to think outside the box and explore innovative approaches to education and communication have been invaluable. Thank you to Dr. Miyabe Shields for embracing curiosity, provoking divergent thinking, and highlighting the incredible diversity of minds in this industry and beyond. Together, our research will continue to push boundaries in the cannabis field, while always prioritizing community and quality of life.

A special thanks to my parents, Linda and John Kirk, who were the first to shape my understanding of cannabis and its consumers while providing a sanctuary of support growing up. To my brothers, Bill and Dan, for being the best stoner role models, keeping me grounded and always finding something to laugh about.

I am especially grateful to my biggest supporter, no matter how crazy life gets, my husband Jake, for his love and encouragement, always reminding me to be bold, proud, and to trust in nature as the ultimate teacher. Thank you for consistently making me get outside even if I have a million things to do on my computer. To my furry sidekicks Joey, Ric and Hazel for kicking around at all hours of the night and the best anti-anxiety snuggles.

Lastly, this book's value hinges on the policies that govern cannabis. Thank you to the trailblazers in this industry—past and present—who tirelessly advocate for equitable access to quality plant medicine. Your efforts pave the way for progress and empowerment and your efforts do not go unnoticed.

PHOTOGRAPHY CREDITS

INTRODUCTION
Robert Beutelspacher

CHAPTER 1
Sarah Capparuccini

CHAPTER 2
Joanna "JoJoSnaps" Valente

CHAPTER 3
Colton Bridge

CHAPTER 4
Robert Beutelspacher

CHAPTER 5
Zoom Gardens

CHAPTER 6
Sean Scott

CHAPTER 7
Kandi Kush

CHAPTER 8
Chris Romaine · Kandid Kush

WORKS CITED
Sarah Capparuccini (pg. 174)
Sean Scott (pg. 192)

ENDPAPERS (FRONT & BACK)
Merlin B "Billy Bob"

INDEX

2-AG (2-Arachidonoylglycerol)
    about, 50, 53
    CB1/CB2 receptors and, 50, 54, 152
    changing levels of, 154
    endometriosis and, 134
    gut permeability and, 137
    newborn suckling response and, 120
    pain relief and, 132
5-HT1A receptor, 57, 63, 64, 133
5HTXX receptor, 47
5-hydroxytryptamine (5-HT), 47
8-chlorocannabiorcichromenic acid, 54
11-hydroxy-THC, 97
11-OH-THC, 97
60/60 method, 28

A

α-2 adrenoceptor, 65
Abstrax Tech, 39
acetaminophen, 115–116
acidic cannabinoids, 57
action potential, 47–48
activated cannabinoids, 58–59
acute psychosis, 116
addiction, 33, 48, 101, 111, 131, 143
ADHD, 65, 111, 142, 143–144
adrenocorticotropic hormone, 130
adult-use (recreational) programs, 37
AEA (anandamide), 50, 53, 54
    childbirth and, 118
    colitis/colon biopsies and, 137
    endometriosis and, 134
Afghan ash, 92
Afghan hash, 92
aging, 112, 114, 156
agonist receptors, 47
AIDS patients, THC for weight loss in, 58, 145
AIDS wasting syndrome, 145
AKT1 gene, 116
alcohol (use), 33
    driving and, 120, 121–122
    infused drinks as an alternative to, 131

submerging cannabis flower in, 57
    THC interactions with using, 116
alcoholic gastritis, 71
alcohol industry, 33
alkylamides, 54
allergic inflammation, 71
allosteric binding sites, 46, 144
alpha caryophylene. See humulene
alpha-linolenic acid (ALA), 49
alpha phellandrene, 72, 143, 146
Alzheimer's disease, 48, 70, 142
American Civil Liberties Union (ACLU), 35
American Nurses Association (ANA), 163
Amnesia Haze, 155
amorfrutins, 54
Amorpha fruticosa, 54
anandamide (AEA), 50, 53, 54
    anesthesia and, 129
    autism and, 143
    CB2 receptor and, 66
    changing levels of, 154
    colitis research and, 137
    eating disorders and, 145
    inflammatory gut conditions and, 137
    obesity and, 146
    pain relief and, 132
    PTSD and, 153
    schizophrenia and, 116–117
anesthesia, 129
animals, 123
anorexia, 145, 146
Anslinger, Henry, 37
antagonist receptors, 47
anticancer activity, 70, 132. See also cancer
anticancer effects, 70, 71, 132
antihypertensive agents, 65
anti-inflammatory effects. See inflammation
antimicrobial activity, 65, 71, 99
anti-nausea activity, 57, 58
antipsychotic effects of CBD, 117
anti-seizure activity, 70, 71, 144
anxiety
    aging and, 112, 114
    CB1 receptor for, 153, 170
    CBDA and, 57
    CBD and, 63, 64, 131, 142

combining CBD with THC and, 46
    dabbing and, 94
    limonene and, 71
    linalool and, 71
    PTSD and, 144
    THC and, 59, 60, 142
appearance (sight), identifying quality of cannabis flower by, 27
appetite, 22, 58, 60, 145, 153
apps, 167
arthritis, 66, 70–71, 134, 146
Aspergillus, 109
atropine, 32
autism, 142, 143, 153
autoimmune diseases, 63, 92, 137, 146

B

bacteria, lab testing of products for, 109
balanced strains, 107
Banana OG strain, 134
Bantus, 33
Barbados, 35
basal signaling, 50
BCP. See beta caryophyllene (BCP)
BDNF (brain derived neurotrophic factor), 116
Beckstead, H.D., 25
beta caryophyllene (BCP), 81
    about, 69, 70–71
    cancer and, 132
    endometriosis and, 134
    epilepsy and, 144
    inflammation and, 129
    melanoma and, 132
    migraines and, 138
    neuroprotective effects, 147
    pain reducing benefits, 133
    sleep and, 140
beta-caryophyllene oxide, 69, 71
BIA 10-2474 (drug), 49
binge-eating disorder, 145
bioaccumulation, heavy metals and, 109
bioactive compounds, 20, 106, 107
Biochanin A, 49
bisabolol
    about, 70
    anxiety and, 142

against cannabis community, 33, 37
related to use of marijuana, 34

dispensaries
budtenders at, 164–165
cannabis flower from, 166
cannabis pharmacists at, 164
certificate of analysis on products from, 166–167
choosing a, 164
entering, 164
MSOs (multi-state operators) vs., 164
pre-rolls from, 27

dispensary menus, 166

dispensary products
beginning with a low dose of, 82
lab testing of products from, 108
pre-rolls, 27, 167
safety of, 82
understanding, 166–167

distillate, 95

District of Columbia, 14

dizziness, 59, 81, 116, 139

D-limonene, 146

dogs
cannabinoid receptors in, 123
drug-sniffing, 71
THC consumed by, 123

dopamine, 22, 47, 52, 111, 116, 145

dorsal horn, 132

dose layering, 133

doses/dosing
acute symptoms of psychosis and, 116
for autism, 143
breastfeeding and, 120
CBD, 63–64
dabbing and, 94
edibles, 96
homemade products and, 82
for migraines, 138–139
during pregnancy, 119
for sleep, 139–140
taking too much cannabis, 81
THC and, 59
of THC for anxiety, 142
of THC for sleep, 140
titrating, 81

Do-Si-Dos, 71

dreams/dreaming, 140–141, 144

driving, cannabis use during, 120–122

drugs. See also pharmaceutical drugs/industry

defined, 20
before industrialization, 20

drug-sniffing dogs, 71

drug targets, 49

dry herb vaping, 72, 90, 93–94, 101

drying cannabis plant, 28

Durban Poison, 60, 72, 145

E

Early Jewish People, 33

eating disorders, 145

E coli, 109

ECS. See endocannabinoid system (ECS)

edibles/edible consumption. See also gummies
about, 96
activating cannabinoids for, 58
acute psychosis and, 116
CBC products and, 66
differences in consumption method effects and, 81
dose layering and, 133
dosing, 59, 81
driving and, 122
for endometriosis pain management, 135
homemade, 97–98
micro-dosing, 135
not feeling, 97
for pain relief, 133
palliative care and, 132
pets/animals consuming, 123
for sleep, 140
taking too much THC using, 114
waiting period when using, 96–97

electronic devices, 94

Emerald Cup, 25

endocannabinoids. See also 2AG (2-Arachidonoylglycerol); anandamide (AEA)
about, 22, 51
anticancer effects of, 132
autism and, 143
cancer cells and, 132
as combinations of neurotransmitters, 52
endocannabinoid tone, 52, 153
endometriosis and, 134
enzymes and, 49, 50
exercise and, 112

fibromyalgia and, 138
inflammatory gut conditions and, 137
migraines and, 138
molecular structure of, 52
multiple sclerosis and, 146
not producing enough, 128
obesity and, 146
pain relief and, 132, 133
related to endometriosis, 134
schizophrenia and, 116
structure of, 52
trauma and, 144

endocannabinoid system (ECS), 13–14. See also cannabinoid receptors; endocannabinoids; receptors
about, 22
in animals, 123
autism and, 143
bringing balance/homeostasis, 22
CB1 activation and, 152
dopamine system and, 111
enzymes, 45, 49–50
estrogen levels and, 141
exercise and, 156
food intake and, 145
gut conditions and, 137
"high" feeling after exercise and, 112
insomnia and, 139
neuroprotective properties of, 147
pain relief and, 132–133
PTSD and, 140
as retrograde signaling system, 22, 48
roles of, 22, 39, 111, 118, 128
therapeutic effect of cannabis and, 128
trauma and, 144
without cannabis, 22

endocannabinoid tone, 52, 153

endogenous morphine compounds, 38, 156. See also endorphins

endometriosis, 100, 133, 134–135

endometriosis-related chronic pelvic pain (CPP), 134

endorphins, 38, 112, 145

The Entourage Effect, 22–23, 70, 81

entourage of edibles, 97

enzymes, 45, 49–50, 129

epidermolysis bullosa, 62

Epidiolex, 33, 62, 64, 144

epilepsy, 49, 142, 144

escapism, 101, 112

estrogen, 134, 141

humulene, 67, 69, 71, 72
    sleep and, 140
hunger hormones, 145
Huntingtons disease, 64
hybrids, 24
hyperalgesia, 138
hyperemesis gravidarum, 118

I

IBD. *See* irritable bowel disease (IBD)
IBS. *See* irritable bowel syndrome (IBS)
Ice Cream Cake strain, 135
ice hash rosin, 94–95
IFN-gamma pro-inflammatory compound, 146
IFN-y pro-inflammatory cytokine, 146
IL-1 pro-inflammatory compound, 146
IL-6 inflammatory cytokine, 146
IL-10 anti-inflammatory compound, 146
immune cells, 129
India, 33, 35, 37
Indian charas, 37
indica(s), 24, 26, 140, 166
indole molecule, 40, 72, 73
inflammation
    beta caryophyllene, 70–71
    CB2 receptor and, 48, 66, 129–130, 133
    CBDA and, 57
    CBD and, 57, 62, 63, 64, 130, 146
    CBG and, 64, 65
    CBN and, 61
    flavonoids and, 73–74
    herbal teas and, 90
    humulene and, 71
    limonene and, 71
    neuroinflammation, 14, 64, 147
    receptors and, 21, 22
    rheumatoid arthritis and, 146
    THCA and, 57
    THC and, 58
    topicals and, 99
    TRPV1 receptor and, 63
inflammatory bowel syndrome. *See* irritable bowel disease (IBD)
inflammatory gut conditions, 64, 137
infused butter, 114

infused coconut oil, 100
infused drinks, 131
infused products, 98, 101
inhalation methods. *See* smoking (consumption method); vaping
insects, relationship between plants and, 18
insomnia, 63, 112, 139
intoxication, driving and evaluating, 120–121
irritable bowel disease (IBD), 52, 128, 134, 137
irritable bowel syndrome (IBS), 128, 133, 134, 137, 143

J

Jack Herer, 72, 144, 155
Jacks and Hazes, 25
Jamaica, 35
joints
    lighting a, 89
    rolling, 84–88
    smoking, 89, 90
    trying out the flavor of, before smoking, 89
journaling, 81, 156, 167–169, 170

K

kaempferol, 49
kanap'is, 34
κάναβις, 34
kendir, 34
kief, 25, 83–84
konoplija, 34

L

lab testing/test results, 108–110, 166–167
lavender, 66, 70, 71, 140, 142
leaky gut conditions, 137
leaves, cannabis plant, 25–26
legislation, cannabis
    differences in state, 162–163
    first state to legalize medical cannabis, 37
    history of, 35, 37

lobbying slowing progress toward, 33
    synthetic cannabinoids and, 111
    synthetic cannabis and, 111
legumes, 54
Lemon Skunk, 71
lightheadness, 59, 116
limonene, 67
    about, 68, 69, 71
    ADHD and, 144
    anticancer potential of, 132
    linalool and, 66
    rheumatoid arthritis and, 146
    as a topical, 99
linalool, 66, 67, 70
    about, 69, 71
    analgesic effects, 133
    for anxiety, 142
    anxiety and, 142
    memory consolidation and, 140, 154–155
    rheumatoid arthritis and, 146
    sleep and, 140
liquid diamonds, 95
liquid shatter, 95
live extracts, 94
liver cancer, 132
liver, drug-drug interactions and the, 115–116
liver enzymes, 97, 115, 116
live resin, 94, 95, 107
live rosin, 94, 95
lotions, 45, 98, 99, 170
lozenges, 97, 100
lung cancer, 132

M

MAGL 9 (monoacylglycerol lipase), 50
marijuana plant. *See* cannabis plant
marijuana, use of word, 34
Marinol, 33, 58
maternal health, 118–119
MCT oil, 57, 98
Mechoulam, Raphael, 38
medical cannabis. *See* therapeutic uses and benefits of cannabis
medical cards
    benefits to having, 163
    gun ownership and, 163
    how to obtain, 163

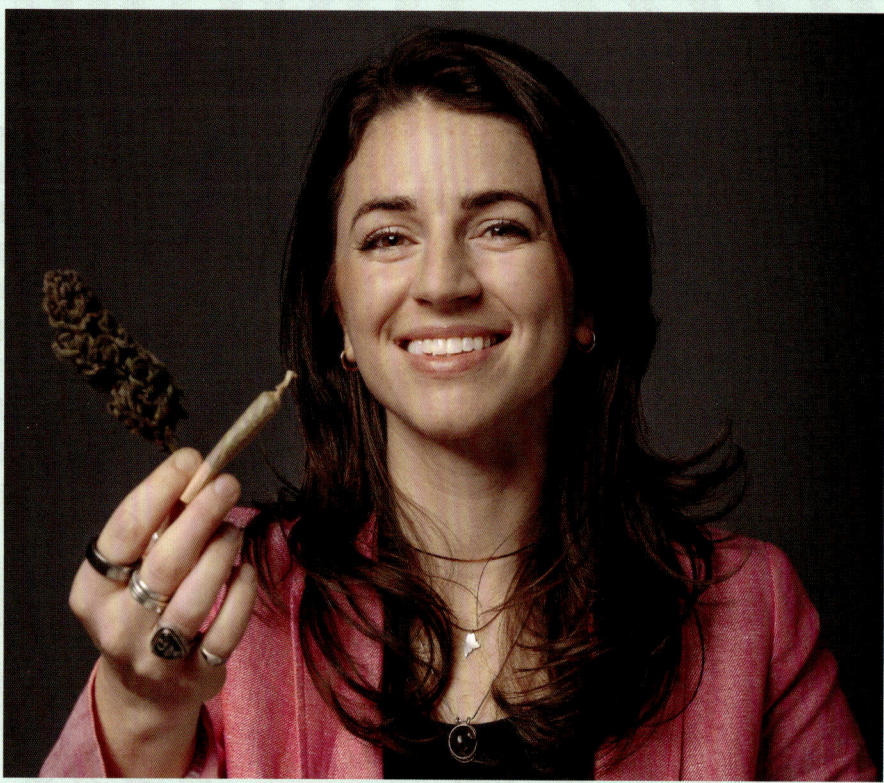

DR. RILEY KIRK is a cannabis research scientist, science communicator, and daily cannabis consumer. She earned her Ph.D. in Pharmaceutical Sciences from the University of Rhode Island where her research spans a broad spectrum of natural products, including many traditionally used medicinal plants and fungi.

Dr. Kirk is the co-founder of the Network of Applied Pharmacognosy (NAP), a research nonprofit organization dedicated to exploring the intersection of biochemistry and real-world data to develop a deeper understanding of how natural medicines like cannabis can benefit people. She is a skilled communicator, creating social media content that is both educational and approachable with the username @Cannabichem, bridging the gap between complex science and everyday understanding.

Beyond her work in cannabis science, Dr. Kirk is an avid outdoorswoman with a commitment to sustainability, often harvesting and growing much of her own food. Her unique blend of expertise, creativity, and connection to nature informs her holistic approach to research, education, and advocacy.